Cardiovascular Biomaterials

Garth W. Hastings (Ed.)

Cardiovascular Biomaterials

With 77 Figures

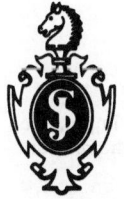

Springer-Verlag
London Berlin Heidelberg New York
Paris Tokyo Hong Kong
Barcelona Budapest

Garth W. Hastings, PhD, DSc, FRSC, CChem, FPRI
Department of Biomedical Engineering, North Staffordshire
Polytechnic, College Road, Stoke-on-Trent ST4 2DE, UK

ISBN-13:978-1-4471-1849-7   e-ISBN-13:978-1-4471-1847-3
DOI: 10.1007/978-1-4471-1847-3

Cover illustration: Ch. 3, Fig. 19. Hancock aortic porcine heart valve prosthesis

British Library Cataloguing in Publication Data
Hastings, Garth W.
    Cardiovascular biomaterials.
    I. Title
    617.95

Library of Congress Cataloging-in-Publication Data
Cardiovascular biomaterials/[edited by] Hastings Garth W.
        p.   cm.
    Includes index.
    ISBN-13:978-1-4471-1849-7
    1. Heart valve prosthesis.   2. Blood vessel prosthesis.
    3. Biocompatibility.   I. Hastings, Garth W.
    [DNLM: 1. Bioprosthesis.   2. Blood Vessel Prosthesis.   3. Heart
    Valve Prosthesis.   WG 169 C2679]
    RD598.35.H42C37   1991
    617.4'120592—dc20
    DNLM/DLC
    for Library of Congress   91-4854
                                                            CIP

Typeset by Best-set Typesetter Ltd. Hong Kong

69/3830-543210 Printed on acid-free paper

Preface

The study and development of materials for use in the cardiovascular system addresses requirements that are more demanding than those for materials to be used in other parts of the human body. There is of course the overall requirement for biocompatibility, or biological performance, which is directly relevant to the intended use. In addition, though, to the usual requirements for the absence of toxic, immunological or carcinogenic reactions and for mechanical properties suited to use in a dynamic situation (i.e. fatigue life, wear resistance, controlled porosity and kink resistance) there is the fact of blood contact. It is this last factor which imposes its own constraints on the materials used.

Since the first attempts to produce thrombo-resistant materials by attachment of heparin to polymer surfaces via graphite intermediates, the science and technology of haemocompatible materials has advanced considerably. Heparin analogue materials, as well as better heparin binding, have been studied in detail and new polymers, for example various types of polyurethanes for vascular prostheses and heart assist devices, have been evaluated. The whole train of events in the blood clotting sequence is now better understood and thus the possibility of minimal interference with blood chemistry and physiology is improved.

Arterial disease is one of the major problems of the developed world. It is one of the main causes of death. Narrowing of the vessel lumen (atherosclerosis) in the abdominal aorta, the iliac artery and in the arteries of the lower limb can eventually lead to gangrene. Occlusion of the arteries of the head leads to angina, myocardial infarcts, strokes and other neurological episodes. Surgical reconstruction of the arteries solves the problems but does not deal with the disease process, which is not understood fully.

The materials for vascular replacement used in bypass surgery often illustrate textile technology rather than polymer science as regards their porosity and weave or knit structures. New materials have been investigated clinically, because there is a continuing need for small vessel replacement (i.e. less than 4 mm diameter). Polyurethanes appeared at one stage to be likely candidates for small vessel replacements, but long-term stability was not satisfactory. The majority of prosthetic vessels are made from polyethylene terephthalate (Dacron) or polytetrafluorethylene (PTFE, Gore-Tex). Patency rates are good in general. The invasion of the graft structure by fibrous tissue and the deposition of endothelial cells on the inner wall is observed in animal studies but not in humans, where the deposition of compacted fibrin is observed. Long-term problems are now being observed. Mechanical and possibly chemical degradation of the materials is leading to rupture or aneurysm formation. Fatigue failure or creep in the polymeric fibre is a factor to be considered and may be addressed by changes in the construction of prostheses.

In replacement of the abdominal aorta and the iliac arteries knitted Dacron is the common choice, whilst for the femoropopliteal and femorotibial bypass, expanded PTFE is used as well as knitted Dacron. In the lower limb autologous vein grafts give better results than do synthetic materials and have compliance similar to that of the normal artery.

Prevention of occlusion, long-term stability and degradation resistance of the synthetic polymers are the current issues under consideration. It is thus hoped to avoid the late failure now being observed. It is the reactions of and on the surface in direct contact with blood that are critical for the acceptance of the prosthesis and control of tissue proliferation is a main research topic. How do the characteristics of the material affect protein deposition, cell adsorption and activation, and cell proliferation? Some of the proposals include cell seeding on the synthetic surface, the use of biodegradable components to promote ingrowth of tissue and the use of growth factors. The porosity of knitted Dacron grafts is still an area for study and initial patency has been achieved by pre-clotting with the patient's blood. More recently sealing with protein has been proposed and cross-linked gelatin is being investigated. Degradation is controlled by the extent of cross-linking given.

For heart (ventricular) assist devices, polyurethanes do seem to be suitable and there have been studies in many centres on ventricular assist devices as well as on the total artificial heart. There is a whole range of devices and techniques ranging from extracorporeal systems to totally implantable devices. The various aspects of these systems were reviewed in the Fourth European Symposium on Biomaterials which was a part of the European Community Concerted Action on Replacement of Body Parts and Functions: Eurobiomat. It was organised at the University of Siena by CRISMA in April 1991.

This Concerted Action has had several symposia and instructional courses dealing with blood-contacting materials. The group has faced the fact that materials currently available do not satisfy all the demands for safe clinical use. Controversial hypotheses and ill-defined approaches are seen as reasons for the stagnation in biomaterials development. Eurobiomat has therefore started to collect information on all biocompatibility test methods and the fully documented series is to be published. To assist in standardisation six reference materials have been given to participating laboratories and test results will thus be obtained from identical surfaces. These will be available as a European Standard. It is hoped to enhance the evolution of better haemocompatible surfaces as a result of this initiative.

This present book has a similar aim. It does not seek to be fully comprehensive, because such a treatise could become unwieldy. It is selective, but draws attention to some of the main areas from which developments have come or are likely to follow. The issues referred to above have been addressed by the contributing authors. In addition to synthetic materials the natural materials themselves are discussed. A better knowledge of these should help in the search for improved replacements. The authors are all leading experts in their fields and have written from their own experience of the problems in developing materials for blood contact. It is hoped that the book will be of value to research workers and to clinical practitioners who are engaged in this challenging area of biomaterials science.

July 1991   Garth W. Hastings

Contents

Contributors

J.A. Awad
Professor of Surgery, Laboratory of Experimental Surgery, Laval University, Quebec City, QC, Canada

M.M. Black
Department of Medical Physics and Clinical Engineering, Royal Hallamshire Hospital, Sheffield S10 2JF, UK

J.M. Courtney
Bioengineering Unit, University of Strathclyde, Glasgow G4 0NW, UK

C.D. Forbes
University of Dundee, Department of Medicine, Ninewells Hospital & Medical School, Dundee DD1 9SY

J.D.S. Gaylor
Bioengineering Unit, University of Strathclyde, Glasgow G4 0NW, UK

D.F. Gibbons
Biosciences Laboratory, 3M Company, St Paul, MN 55144, USA

R. Guidoin
Professor of Surgery, Laboratory of Experimental Surgery, Laval University, Quebec City, QC, Canada

T.V. Ilow
Institute of Medical and Dental Engineering, University of Liverpool, Liverpool L69 3BX, UK

L. Irvine
Bioengineering Unit, University of Strathclyde, Glasgow G4 0NW, UK

M.W. King
Associate Professor of Clothing and Textiles, University of Manitoba, Winnipeg, Manitoba, Canada

M.E. Nimni
Professor of Biochemistry, Medicine and Orthopaedics, University
of California School of Medicine and Orthopaedic Hospital in Los
Angeles, Los Angeles, CA 90007-2697, USA

H. Reul
Helmholtz Institute for Biomedical Engineering, 5100 Aachen,
Germany

R.W. Snyder
Lecor Inc., League City, Texas, USA

K.M. Taylor
British Heart Foundation Chair of Cardiac Surgery, Cardiothoracic
Surgical Unit, Royal Postgraduate Medical School, Hammersmith
Hospital, Du Cane Road, London W12 0HS

A.P. Yoganathan
Professor, School of Chemical Engineering, Georgia Institute of
Technology, Atlanta, GA 30332, USA

Chapter 1

Mechanical Properties of Arteries and Arterial Grafts

T.V. How

Introduction

Arterial prostheses made from synthetic textile fibres have been used in man for nearly 40 years. During the early period a variety of synthetic polymers were evaluated, but most were later abandoned when it became apparent that some polymers can lose mechanical strength as a result of degradation following implantation. Polyethlene terephthalate (PET) (trade name: Dacron) and polytetrafluoroethylene (PTFE) (trade name: Teflon) are the two polymers currently used for the fabrication of large and medium-size arterial prostheses. Although these prostheses have more than adequate strength to withstand the loads encountered in vivo, complications due to aneurysmal dilatation, fibre breakdown and rupture occur in a small percentage of patients. It is therefore important to study the effect of degradation and to characterize the creep and fatigue properties of arterial prostheses in order that the long-term mechanical performance may be predicted.

The arteries of the body behave as distensible cylindrical conduits whilst the commercially available textile prostheses have essentially rigid walls. The insertion of a rigid prosthesis in a compliant pulsatile flow system may have significant effects on blood pulse wave propagation and local flow velocity field. Theoretical studies [1] of pulse wave reflection show that a rigid tube inserted in a compliant arterial system acts as a "low pass filter", damping out the higher harmonics and introducing phase distortion. Attenuation of the pulse wave increases with the rigid tube length. The change in elasticity at the union between a rigid prosthesis and the compliant artery leads to an abrupt change in diameter which in turn produces a distortion of the local flow field [2,3]. The effect is similar to flow through constrictions or expansions, where undesirable flow patterns such as flow separation, vortex formation and turbulence may be present [4]. These effects may be more severe if there is a large initial discrepancy between the internal diameter of the prosthesis and the artery.

Although PET and PTFE prostheses perform satisfactorily in the replacement of large and medium-size arteries they normally fail when used to replace small diameter arteries. The high failure rate of small diameter fabric prostheses has been ascribed by many authors to their low distensibility compared with the normal artery [5,6]. Consequently, it is argued that small bore prostheses should have distensibility or compliance matched closely to that of the artery.

In this chapter the mechanical properties of natural arteries and various types of currently used arterial grafts, both of synthetic and biological origin, are outlined. In addition, the properties of elastomeric prostheses which have similar compliance to that of natural arteries are also described.

Mechanical Properties of Arteries

Structure of the Arterial Wall

The blood vessel wall has a complex structure which varies from site to site. Its architecture and composition is thought to be determined by the mechanical stresses to which it is subjected [7]. The walls of arteries are made up of three concentric layers: the tunica intima, the tunica media and the tunica adventitia. The intima consists of a single layer of endothelial cells which are in contact with blood and a thin subendothelial layer containing collagen fibres. Between the intima and the media is the internal elastic lamina, a layer of cross-linked elastin fibres.

The media is usually the thickest layer in the wall and has different structure in different parts of the vascular system. In the large arteries near the heart, the media is composed of a number of fenestrated elastic laminae with alternate layers made up of connective tissues, collagen fibres and smooth muscle fibres. These large arteries are known as elastic arteries, because of their relatively large amount of elastic fibres in the media. In the smaller arteries (muscular arteries), the media consists mostly of smooth muscle cells and small amounts of connective tissue, collagen and elastic fibres. The smooth muscle cells are arranged in a spiral of small variable pitch and are organized in multiple layers.

The adventitia, which may be as thick as the media, is composed of densely-packed bundles of collagen fibres in a predominantly longitudinal direction. Elastic fibres are relatively sparse in this region.

In arteries with diameter greater than 1 mm the innermost layer of the wall is nourished from blood flowing in the lumen while the outer layers (the adventitia and part of the media) are supplied from small blood vessels called vasa vasorum.

Wall Distensibility In Vivo

Arteries are firmly attached or tethered to the surrounding tissue. With each heartbeat the artery wall moves both radially and longitudinally. In the longitudinal direction, movement is restrained because of the tethering and is roughly 1% [8] compared with radial distensibility of up to 14% [9]. Wall distensibility is usually defined as the ratio of diameter change during a heartbeat to the diastolic diameter and expressed as a percentage value.

In general, arterial distensibility decreases with distance from the heart [10]. Actual values, however, vary widely. In the thoracic aorta, for example, these range from 2.5% to 8.5% [8,11–13]. This large variation is due partly to uncontrolled factors such as pulse pressure, diastolic pressure, heart rate and age. Various methods have been used to measure diameter changes. Those employing electrical calipers which require mechanical contact with the exposed artery have been found to yield much smaller values of distensibility than non-invasive methods. For example, human carotid artery distensibility measured with electrical calipers was 0.93% [14] compared with 14.3% [9] using an ultrasonic phase-locked pulsed echo technique. This large difference raises the possibility that the distensibility of exposed arteries freed from the surrounding tissue may be lower than that of intact vessels. However, in a subsequent study by Mozersky et al. [15] using the ultrasonic technique, it was shown that any pressure exerted by the transducer over the skin surface could result in an over-estimate of the compliance. Consequently, the distensibility of the human femoral artery measured by these authors compared well with those determined by invasive methods. Some of the observed differences, however, may arise from geometric consideration. When an elastic cylinder is pressurized it undergoes a larger change in internal than external diameter. Therefore, distensibility determined from internal diameter measurements (for example, the radiographic method of Luchsinger et al. [12] and Arndt et al. [16]) would yield higher values than external diameter measurements using electrical calipers. With the ultrasonic method it is assumed that the instrument records the internal diameter plus one wall thickness [15].

Elastic Properties

The mechanical properties of the arterial tissue depend on the properties of each component of the wall and the way they are arranged within the wall. Elastin and collagen have widely different physical properties. The former is a rubber-like material and has a non-linear stress–strain relationship. Its Young's modulus is approximately 3×10^5 Pa at strain levels of about 40% [17]. Collagen, on the other hand, is much stiffer, with a Young's modulus in the order of 10^8 Pa [18]. Its elongation at break is only about 3–4% compared with about 130% for elastin fibres. At low strains the collagen fibres in arterial tissue are slack and most of the load is borne by elastin fibres. At higher strains however, the collagen fibres straighten out causing the artery wall to become inextensible [19] (collagen fibres provide strength to the blood vessel and prevent excessive deformation under high loads). Thus at low pressure the artery is highly distensible but as pressure is increased it becomes stiffer.

This non-linear behaviour of blood vessels had been described since 1880 [20] but it was only after the 1960s that significant improvements have been made on measurement techniques and the development of more realistic mathematical models. A variety of experimental methods has been developed for the study of arterial elasticity. These include the use of isolated strips or rings cut from the blood vessels, excised cylindrical segments normally maintained at their in vivo lengths and in vivo measurements on the intact blood vessel under normal physiological loads.

Uniaxial tensile measurements on strips or rings have been carried out to determine the stress–strain relationship of various types of blood vessels and their directional properties [21,22]. Although this technique has the advantage that it requires relatively simple measuring equipment and data analysis it has not been widely used because of the difficulty in describing cylindrical properties from studies on strips. Cox [23] has compared the properties of dog carotid arteries determined from ring samples and cylindrical segments and showed that significant differences exist. This was attributed to the interaction between the strains present when an intact vessel is loaded which cannot be reproduced with strips.

To overcome this problem, a long segment of the artery in its original cylindrical geometry can be used. Since the artery may shorten by up to 40% when it is excised, it is necessary to maintain it at its in vivo length during measurement [24]. Changes in the vessel dimensions (external diameter, length and wall thickness) in response to changes in internal pressure can be measured. Wall thickness is more difficult to measure but it can be estimated from external diameter provided the wall volume can be assumed to remain constant during pressurization (i.e. the arterial tissue is incompressible). Carew et al. [25] have demonstrated that arteries subjected to physiological loads can be considered as incompressible.

When static or quasi-static properties are of interest, pressure is usually applied in a step-wise [26] fashion or continuously [27]. Because of its non-linear stress–strain relationship, there is no unique elastic modulus which characterizes arterial elasticity. An incremental Young's modulus E_{inc} can be defined on the assumption that the wall is incompressible, homogeneous and isotropic [26]:

$$E_{inc} = \frac{\Delta P R_o R_i^2 2(1 - \sigma^2)}{\Delta R_o (R_o^2 - R_i^2)} \tag{1.1}$$

where R_i is the inner and R_o the outer radius, ΔR_o, the change in outer radius in response to an increment of pressure, ΔP, and σ, the Poisson's ratio, has a value of 0.5 for an incompressible material subjected to small strains.

Equation (1.1) adequately describes the elasticity of the arterial segment around the mean pressure and length at which the measurements are made. The mean pressure must be specified in order that comparison with other data can be made. Incremental Young's modulus is difficult to determine in vivo since internal diameter or wall thickness cannot be easily measured. Peterson et al. [28] proposed a "pressure–strain elastic modulus", E_p given by:

$$E_p = \frac{\Delta P R_o}{\Delta R_o}. \tag{1.2}$$

E_p is a measure of the overall stiffness of arterial wall and does not involve the wall thickness in its calculation. The relationship between E_{inc} and E_p can be shown to be:

$$E_{inc} = 1.5 E_p (1 - \gamma)^2 / [1 - (1 - \gamma)^2] \tag{1.3}$$

where $\gamma = h/R_o$; h being the wall thickness of the vessel. The Poisson's ratio is assumed to be 0.5. Because of its simplicity, E_p has been widely used to compare the results of various investigators including both in vivo and in vitro experiments [24]. This can be misleading since E_p would, in general, be greater under dynamic loads in vivo than under static pressures in vitro.

A major limitation in the use of equation (1.1) is the assumption of isotropy. It is well known that the arterial wall is anisotropic, i.e. the mechanical properties vary in different directions. Moreover it has been shown that there exists an elastic symmetry about the planes perpendicular to the principal axes indicating that blood vessels may be considered as cylindrically orthotropic [29]. This finding greatly simplifies the analysis since an orthotropic blood vessel subjected to an axial elongation and an internal pressure undergoes negligible shearing strains. A detailed analysis of incremental deformations has been presented by Vaishnav and Vossoughi [30].

The anisotropic incremental moduli have been determined for the canine aorta [31,32], carotid artery [27,33–35] and coronary artery [34,35] and rat carotid artery [36]. In the aorta it was reported that $E_z > E_\theta > E_r$, where E is the incremental elastic modulus, in the axial (z) circumferential (θ) and radial (r) directions. All these moduli were found to increase with axial stretch as well as pressure. In the carotid arteries, however, E_θ was found to be much greater than E_z [27,35].

A different approach to the study of arterial elasticity, based on the continuum mechanical theory of finite deformation of rubber-like materials, was first presented by Tickner and Sacks [37]. The theory assumes the existence of a strain energy density function which may be expressed in terms of the principal strains. The stresses may then be obtained by taking derivatives of the strain energy function with respect to the strains. Since arterial tissue is not elastic but viscoelastic, Fung et al. [38] introduced the term pseudo-elasticity to preconditioned arteries. When an artery is subjected to cyclic deformations at constant strain rates its response reaches a steady state and becomes stable and reproducible. Arteries thus preconditioned can be treated as being pseudo-elastic and their response during either loading or unloading can be described by a unique strain energy density function. Several forms of strain energy functions, in terms of the principal strains, have been proposed. Patel and Vaishnav [39] and Vaishnav et al. [32] made use of a polynomial function in terms of the circumferential and longitudinal strains to fit experimental data from the aorta which was assumed to be incompressible and orthotropic. They demonstrated that a polynomial containing terms up to the third order, resulting in seven material constants, gave a good fit.

Fung et al. [38] employed an exponential form of the strain energy density function to study the properties of rabbit arteries with reasonably good fit with experimental data. When compared with the polynomial strain energy density function these authors found that their model was more suitable, especially for the study of mechanical properties at various sites or to assess the effects of drugs and hypertension. The exponential constants showed significantly smaller variations than polynomial constants for arteries of the same type. Both the methods of Vaishnav et al. and Fung et al. are essentially two-dimensional since the vessel walls are assumed to be thin (i.e. the radial stresses are uniform) and the stresses in the circumferential and longitudinal directions are much greater than in the radial direction.

Viscoelastic Properties

Arteries are subjected to constantly changing loads as a result of the pulsatile pressure accompanying each heartbeat. Their response to these dynamic loads is therefore dependent on the viscoelastic properties. In common with other viscoelastic materials, arterial tissue exhibits hysteresis, stress relaxation and creep. Hysteresis loops can be observed on a stress–strain plot when an artery undergoes cyclic deformation. Stress relaxation and creep are transient responses in the time domain; stress relaxation being the change in stress, with time, in response to a step change in strain while creep is the change in strain in response to a step change in stress. Stress relaxation and creep measurements have been carried out on isolated arterial strips or rings [21,22,40,41] and intact cylindrical segments [42,43]. When stress is plotted against logarithm of time, a linear relationship exists but this is restricted to about two decades of time [22,24]. The degree of stress relaxation depends on the stress level, orientation of the specimen and anatomical site. It is generally greater in the circumferential than in the longitudinal direction and there is also a progressive increase in relaxation with distance towards the peripheral arteries. This is to be expected since there is a correlation between the proportion of smooth muscle and stress relaxation [44,45].

A more widely used alternative to creep or stress relaxation tests is to study the response of arterial tissue to small sinusoidal strains (dynamic mechanical tests). These tests can be carried out on isolated strips of rings [44–48] or on intact cylindrical segments in vitro [49–51] or in vivo [52–54]. When the applied sinusoidal force is small, the resulting deformation will vary sinusoidally but it will be out of phase. A complex incremental modulus, E_c can be defined for an isotropic, incompressible viscoelastic cylinder as $|E_c| \exp (j\phi)$ where $|E_c|$ is given by equation (1.1), ϕ is the phase difference and $j = \sqrt{-1}$. E_c can also be expressed as:

$$E_c = |E_c| \cos \phi + j|E_c| \sin \phi \qquad (1.4)$$

where $|E_c| \cos \phi = E_{dyn}$ is known as the dynamic elastic modulus and $|E_c| \sin \phi = \eta\omega$, the viscous modulus [49].

To study the dynamic behaviour of arteries in vivo, it is necessary first to determine the frequency components of the pressure and diameter waveforms by Fourier analysis. Since Fourier analysis is applicable only to linear systems the applied strains should be sufficiently small to minimize errors due to non-linearity [52]. The dynamic properties exhibit a strong dependence on anatomical site and there appears to be a correlation between E_{dyn} and the amount of smooth muscle and the degree of activation in the arterial wall. Bergel [49] showed that the ratio E_{dyn} to E_{stat} (the static incremental Young's modulus) in excised canine arteries dog ranged from about 1.10 in the thoracic aorta to 1.65 in the femoral artery. At low frequencies E_{dyn} increased sharply with frequency but remained relatively constant above 2 Hz whilst $\eta\omega$ increased slightly with frequency. In vivo, however, Cox [50] observed a monotonic increase in E_{dyn} but a decrease in $\eta\omega$ with frequency.

Patel et al. [54] have extended their treatment of static anisotropic incremental elastic properties of canine aorta to include viscoelastic behaviour.

They also noted that after an initial increase, the dynamic elastic moduli remained relatively constant above 2 Hz. The moduli were a function of the circumferential and longitudinal strains because of the non-linear behaviour of the arterial wall.

Although non-linear anisotropic viscoelastic models based on continuum mechanical theory have been presented by several authors (see review by Barbenel [55]) they have not found much practical application. This is due mainly to the considerable difficulties associated with experimental measurement and interpretation of the results.

Effect of Age and Disease on Arterial Elasticity

The alteration in the mechanical properties of arteries with age and disease has long been recognized [20]. Ageing is accompanied by a progressive increase in systemic arterial pressure and changes in connective tissue composition and arterial morphology [56]. Its effect on viscoelastic properties appears to be dependent upon species and anatomical site. No significant changes have been found in the dynamic elastic properties with age in rabbit and rat aortas [57,58], but in the human aorta and iliac artery, a loss of distensibility with age has been reported [59–63], an observation also made in the dog aorta [28,48]. In peripheral arteries in humans, Learoyd and Taylor [60] reported a reduction in elastic modulus with age. Using a transcutaneous technique, Mozersky et al. [15] found that the average E_p in the femoral artery increased with age. Both arterial diameter and wall thickness change [59–61] and since the ratio of wall thickness to diameter may increase [61], the elastic modulus will be lower even though E_p is increased.

Since pulse wave transmission is governed to a large extent by the mechanical properties of the blood vessel, the measurement of pulse wave velocity can provide an indirect method of determining the changes in viscoelasticity associated with ageing. This has been carried out in the human aorta by Hallcock [64] and O'Rourke et al. [65] and in dogs by Miller et al. [66], who clearly demonstrated a correlation between pulse wave velocity with age.

In atherosclerosis most of the changes in the arterial wall occur in the intima as a result of lipid deposits which develop into atherosclerotic plaques. As the disease progresses other layers of the artery may be affected by fibrosis. Calcium may also be deposited in the plaques or in the media. The effects of dietary-induced atherosclerosis on arterial wall properties have been studied in various animal models [67–69]. Experimental atherosclerosis in rabbits is associated with an increase in dynamic elastic modulus whilst no change has been observed in rats [68]. Cockerels fed on an atherogenic diet have an increased aortic distensibility, but with more severe atherosclerosis distensibility decreased progressively to below normal values due to increasing calcification and fibrosis [67].

Because atherosclerosis is such a widespread disease in man, and increases in severity with age, difficulties arise as to whether arterial wall properties due to ageing and atherosclerosis can be separated. By comparing the distensibility of aortas obtained from individuals of the same age but with varying degrees of atherosclerosis, Butcher and Newton [70] and Nakashima and Tanikawa [62] demonstrated that atherosclerosis per se had little effect unless extensive medial calcification was present. In such cases, the distensibility is significantly reduced.

PET and PTFE Prostheses

PET and PTFE Fabric Prostheses

Most fabric vascular prostheses in current use are constructed from either PET or PTFE fibres. The mechanical properties of PET and PTFE fibres are given in Table 1.1. PET and PTFE prostheses are manufactured in two basic constructions; woven or knitted. The woven prosthesis is made up of yarns of filaments running both longitudinally and circumferentially, as shown in Fig. 1.1. In order to avoid fraying of the prosthesis at the cut edges the yarns are usually closely packed together, resulting in a tube of relatively low porosity. Knitted prostheses are produced by looping the yarns around the needles. The number and size of needles and the yarn size determine the spacing between the yarns. The yarns in the knitted prosthesis, shown in Fig. 1.2, run predominantly in the longitudinal direction. This is known as a warp knit. In prostheses where the yarns run in the circumferential direction, the term used is weft knitting (see Maarek et al. [73] and Guidoin et al. [74] for details of

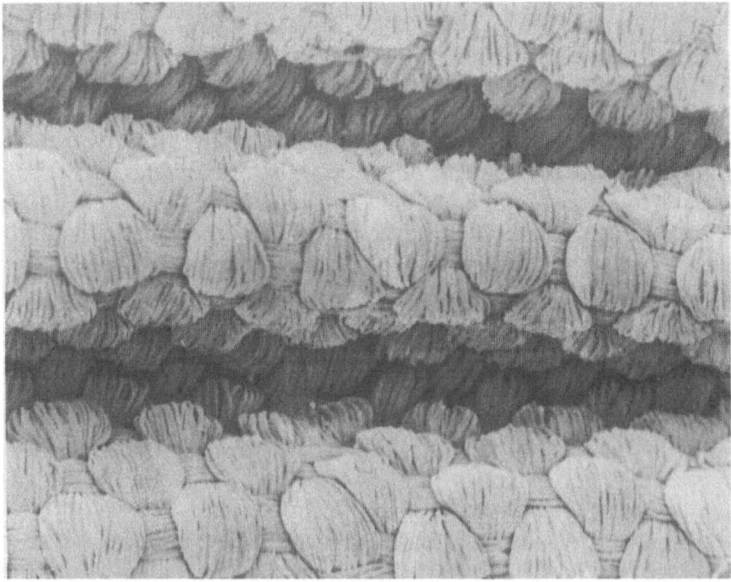

Fig. 1.1. Scanning electron micrograph of the internal surface of a woven prosthesis (Vascutek Extra Soft Woven). Scale bar = 200 μm.

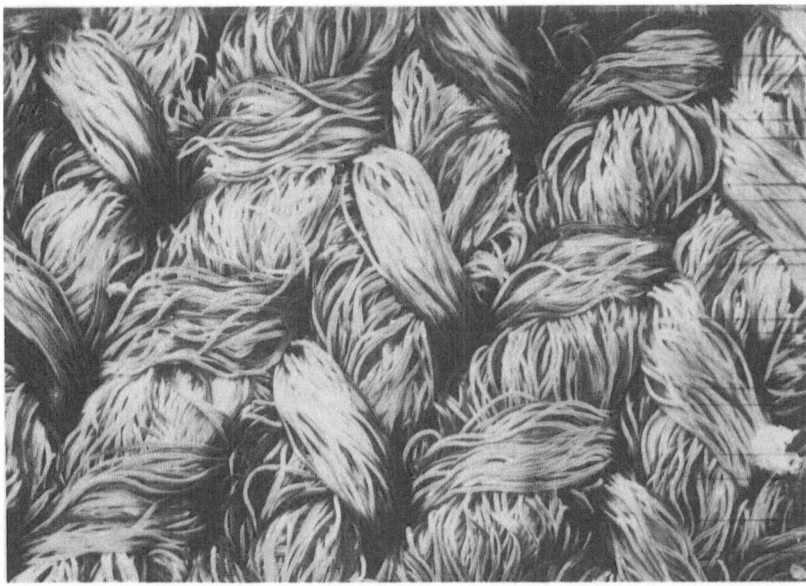

Fig. 1.2. Scanning electron micrograph of the internal surface of a knitted prosthesis (Vascutek Triaxial). Scale bar = 200 μm.

construction of currently available prostheses). Knitted prostheses are more conformable and are easier to handle and suture than woven prostheses. They are less susceptible to fraying and are therefore better at retaining sutures. However, being more porous, knitted prostheses must be preclotted with the patient's blood prior to implantation.

Knitted velour prostheses were introduced in the 1970s in order to promote better healing and incorporation of the prosthesis into the surrounding tissue. They are constructed in such a way that loops of yarn extend into the lumen and the outside wall.

The majority of fabric prostheses, woven or knitted, have crimps which can be either circular or helical. Crimping was introduced to prevent buckling of the prosthesis when the prosthesis is bent. Although lateral flexibility and axial compressibility is improved this is achieved at the expense of circumferential

Table 1.1. Mechanical properties of PET and PTFE fibres [71,72]

Property	PET	PTFE
Specific gravity	1.39	2.1–2.3
Tenacity (g/denier)[a]	4.5–5.5	1.5
Tensile strength (MPa)	550–675	290
Elongation at break (%)	15–25	13

[a] The tensile strength of a fibre is usually expressed in terms of tenacity which is the breaking strength per fibre. The denier is a measure of the size of fibres expressed as the weight, in g, of 9000 m of fibre.

distensibility. Crimping does not impart sufficient radial stiffness to the prosthesis to prevent flattening of the cross-section and buckling when crossing the knee joint [75]. Because of the damage caused by crimping [76] and the adverse blood flow behaviour (e.g. secondary flow and vortex formation) along the corrugated surface of crimped prostheses, their usefulness is now being questioned. These effects become more pronounced in smaller diameter prostheses as the size of the corrugations represents a greater proportion of the conduit diameter. More recently, a non-crimped graft, supported externally by means of a polypropylene coil fused to the graft's outer surface, had been developed [77]. Angiographic examination of these grafts placed in below-knee femoropopliteal bypasses has demonstrated that the external support prevents kinking and compression of the graft during knee flexion [78]. Although their compliance is very much reduced by the rigid polypropylene coil, externally supported Dacron grafts appear to perform better, presumably because of the improved flow surface, than crimped non-supported grafts in the femoropopliteal position [77].

Expanded PTFE Prostheses

Small diameter arterial prostheses made of microporous expanded PTFE were introduced in 1975 for use in lower limb bypass surgery. There has been much interest in this material and it is estimated that over 200 000 expanded PTFE prostheses were implanted between 1976 and 1981 [79]. Figure 1.3 shows a scanning electron micrograph of the inner surface of an expanded PTFE prosthesis. The wall is composed of relatively large, circumferentially orientated

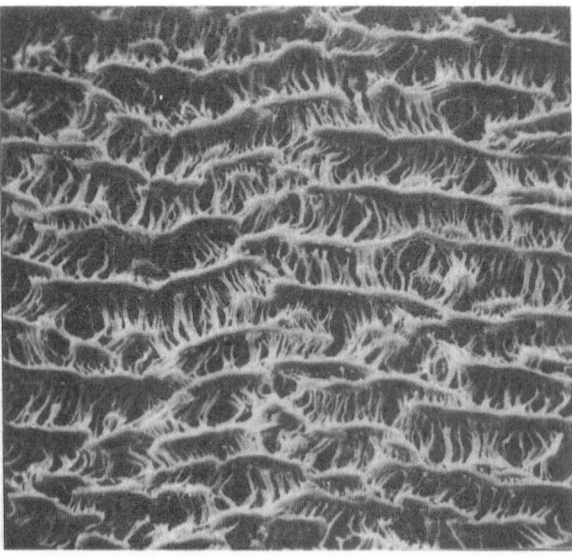

Fig. 1.3. Scanning electron micrograph of the internal surface of an expanded PTFE prosthesis (Gore-Tex).

nodes from which extend fine longitudinal fibrils. This inhomogeneous structure is responsible for the high degree of longitudinal compressibility. This, combined with the radial stiffness due to the nodes, results in a highly conformable and relatively kink-resistant conduit. Early designs of this prosthesis were susceptible to creep and dilatation. This problem was overcome by incorporating reinforcing layers of a fibrous expanded PTFE film on the outer surface [80] or using thicker wall grafts [79].

Mechanical Properties of PET and PTFE Prostheses

The mechanical properties of fabric prostheses have been investigated in vitro using both strips and cylindrical segments. Initial measurements were focused on tensile strength, as the major concern was the prevention of aneurysm and rupture. Tensile strength is defined as the maximum load per unit undeformed cross-sectional area applied to the strip to cause failure. Prostheses should have adequate strength to resist rupture or excessive dilatation when subjected to pulsatile pressures in vivo. They should also have stable mechanical properties during their expected life.

Harrison [81] reported on the rupture force (maximum load in pounds for standard 0.5-inch wide specimens) of various types of fabric prostheses, including PET and PTFE measured on an Instron tensile tester. Using his values of wall thickness, tensile strength can be calculated (Table 1.2). It would be expected, in a woven prosthesis, that tensile strength would be proportional to the number of yarns in the direction of the applied load [83]. Although this was the case with the PTFE prostheses, for reasons which are not clear it was not applicable to the PET prostheses. From Table 1.2, it can be seen that the tensile strength of both PET and PTFE prostheses is very much greater than that of aortic tissue. After implantation, Harrison [81] observed a reduction in rupture force of 17–21% in PET after 128 days and 1.7–3% in PTFE prostheses after 113–358 days. The loss in the strength of the material was probably underestimated, especially in PET prostheses, since the contribution of the fibrous tissue ingrowth to the rupture force was not taken into account.

A measure of the strength of the prosthesis can also be obtained by measuring the pressure at which a cylindrical specimen ruptures. From the magnitude of this pressure and the dimensions of the prosthesis, a burst strength can be calculated. Using Laplace's law [84], the burst strength may be derived from tensile strength if the prosthesis can be assumed to be isotropic and thin-

Table 1.2. Tensile strength of Dacron no. 14 and Teflon TF-208 vascular prostheses compared with that of canine aorta

Material	Circumferential (MPa)	Longitudinal (MPa)	Reference
Dacron no. 14	128	139	81
Teflon TF-208	85.2	66.7	81
Thoracic aorta	0.73	0.32	82
Abdominal aorta	1.47	5.29	89

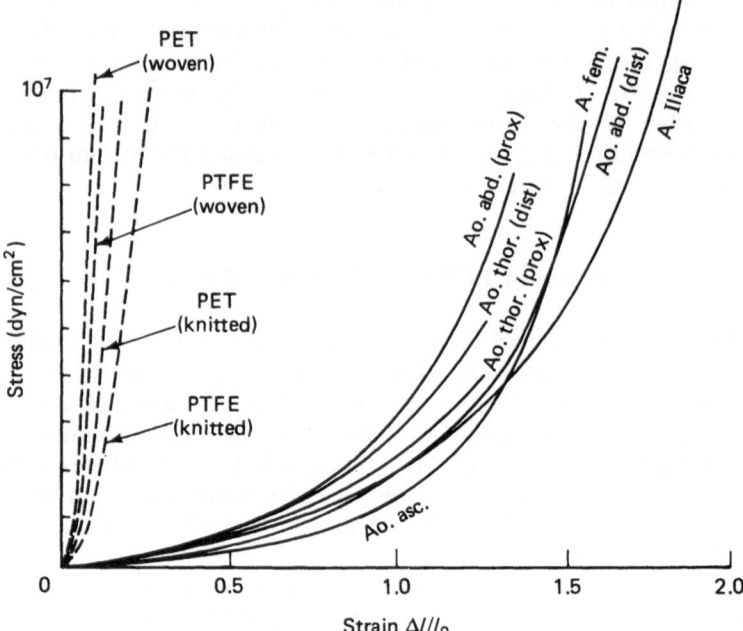

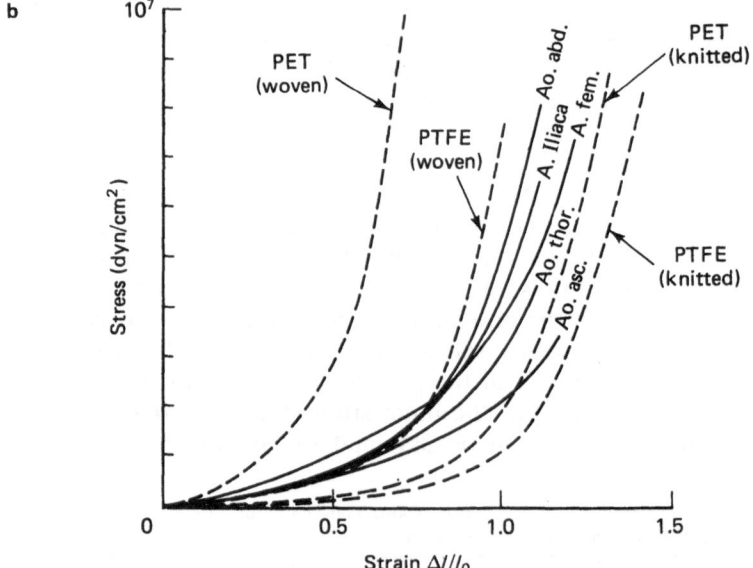

Fig. 1.4. a Circumferential stress–strain curves of woven and knitted PET and PTFE prostheses. Data for the following arteries are also plotted on the same graph: ascending aorta (Ao.asc); proximal (Ao.thor.prox) and distal (Ao.thor.dist) portions of the thoracic aorta; proximal (Ao.abd.prox) and distal (Ao.abd.dist) portions of the abdominal aorta; the iliac (A.iliaca) and femoral (A.fem) arteries. **b** Longitudinal stress–strain curves for woven and knitted PET and PTFE prostheses. Data for canine arteries are also included for comparison. Abbreviations as in **a**. (Reprinted with permission from the *Journal of Biomechanics* [86]. © 1979 Pergamon Press.)

walled. A large variety of textile prostheses are currently available in different constructions using different types of PET and PTFE yarns. It is therefore expected that they would display a wide range of properties. For example, in a survey of 26 PET prostheses in clinical use, burst strength ranged from 2.6 to 4.9 MPa for woven and from 1.1 to 3.8 MPa for knitted constructions [85].

There have been few studies of the uniaxial stress–strain behaviour of fabric prostheses. Hasegawa and Azuma [86] carried out quasi-static measurements on circumferential and longitudinal strips of woven and knitted PET and PTFE prostheses. Specimens, 5 mm wide, were tested in physiological saline at 30°C. Figure 1.4 shows typical stress–strain curves of circumferential and longitudinal specimens. Data for aortic specimens are plotted on the same graphs for comparison. The circumferential tensile moduli calculated from Fig. 1.4a are 18 MPa and 14 MPa for woven PET and PTFE prostheses, respectively. These values are considerably lower than those measured by Paasche et al. [87] who quoted 733 MPa for PET and 320 MPa for PTFE prostheses.

Due to the presence of crimps the longitudinal specimens exhibited apparently high extensibility, at lower strains, comparable with that of aortic tissue, but as the strain was gradually increased the crimps straightened out, leading to a progressive greater stiffness.

Viscoelastic properties were investigated in terms of stress relaxation and it was observed that the relaxation strength (expressed as the percentage change in stress between $t = 0$ and $t = 300$s) was greater in PTFE than in PET specimens [88]. Moreover, the relaxation strength was a function only of the material and was independent of the type of construction or the direction of the specimens.

Compliance

Compliance has been defined [89] as the change in volume, V, of a vessel segment per unit pressure change ($\Delta V/V\ \Delta P$) and is usually expressed as a percentage value. Assuming that the length of the vessel remains unchanged, $\Delta V/V$ can be expressed in terms of internal diameter D_i as:

$$\frac{\Delta V}{V} = \frac{(D_i + \Delta D_i)^2 - D_i^2}{D_i^2} = \frac{2\Delta D_i}{D_i} + \frac{\Delta D_i^2}{D_i^2}. \tag{1.5}$$

Since $\Delta D_i^2/D_i^2$ may be neglected when ΔD_i is small, equation (1.5) can be approximated as $(2\Delta D_i/D_i\Delta P)$ [89]. Kidson and Abbot [90] used this expression for compliance but omitted the factor of 2. Since internal diameter is difficult to measure, especially in vivo, the compliance could be more usefully defined in terms of external diameter:

$$C = \frac{\Delta D_o}{D_o \Delta P}. \tag{1.6}$$

Comparing equations (1.6) and (1.2) it can be seen that compliance is the inverse of pressure–strain modulus E_p. Thus compliance calculated from equation (1.6) can be easily compared with published E_p values for natural arteries [91]. Table 1.3 lists some values of C and E_p of arteries and various

Table 1.3. Compliance C and pressure-strain modulus E_p of arteries and arterial grafts

Vessel	Diameter (mm)	C (%/mmHg)[a]	Mean E_p ($\times 10^5$ Pa)	Measurement of diameter[b]	Reference
In vitro					
Knitted PET crimped	8	0.075 (3)		c	75
Knitted PET non-crimped	8	0.055 (3)		c	75
Dacron velour		0.019 (1)	[7.02]	c	92
Expanded PTFE		0.016 (1)	[8.33]	c	92
Human saphenous vein		0.044 (1)	[3.03]	c	92
Human umbilical vein		0.037 (1)	[3.60]	c	92
Human femoral artery		0.059 (1)	[2.26]	c	92
In vivo					
Woven PET	10	0.0016(3)		a	88
Knitted PET	10	0.015 (3)		a	88
Dacron double velour	4	0.034 (2)	7.7	c	89
Woven PTFE	8	0.0018(3)		a	88
Knitted PTFE	9.5	0.0138(3)		a	88
Expanded PTFE	4	0.014 (4)		d	93
Expanded PTFE	6.06 (O.D.)	0.012 (1)	[11.11]	c	79
Expanded PTFE	6.24 (O.D.)	0.012 (1)	[11.11]	c	79
Replamineform Biomer	4	0.062 (4)		d	93
Human umbilical vein		0.049 (2)	5.4	c	89
Human femoral artery <35 years	11	0.0579(2)	2.64	b	15
Human femoral artery 35–60 years	11.1	0.04 (2)	3.88	b	15
Human femoral artery >60 years	12.1	0.0337(2)	6.28	b	15
Dog femoral vein		0.048 (2)	5.5	c	89
Dog femoral vein		0.033 (4)		d	93
Dog femoral artery		0.127 (3)	2.1	c	89
Dog femoral artery		0.084 (4)		d	93

[a] C was calculated from $[\Delta D_o/D_o\Delta P] \times 100$ (1), $[2\Delta D_i/D_i\Delta P] \times 100$ (2), $[\Delta V/V\Delta P] \times 100$ (3), and $[\Delta D_i/D_i\Delta P] \times 100$ (4).
[b] Various techniques were employed for measuring diameter: (a) mercury in silastic strain gauge, (b) ultrasonic pulsed echo tracker, (c) cantilever beam and (d) electromagnetic rheoangiometer.

types of vascular grafts reported in the literature. The E_p values in brackets are those derived from compliance measurements. The difference in the compliance for the same type of graft can be attributed to differences in the material as well as the variation in the construction, the definition of compliance and the method of its measurement, and, in the case of in vivo values, the variation in diastolic and pulse pressures. Table 1.3 should therefore serve only as a guide. Most grafts have anisotropic properties and their compliances are a function of axial strain. Unfortunately, in in vitro measurements, this is rarely specified.

Woven prostheses have the lowest compliance of all grafts listed in Table 1.3. They are virtually rigid since their diameter change ($\pm 3\,\mu$m for a 10-mm prosthesis) over the normal pulse pressure of 40 mmHg is at the limit of resolution of most diameter gauges. Because of their construction, knitted prostheses are less stiff than woven materials. Their compliance is similar in magnitude to that of expanded PTFE prostheses. With a mean C of 0.015%/mmHg, the diameter change for a normal pulse pressure of 40 mmHg is 24 μm for a 4-mm diameter prosthesis. This small change in diameter requires a stable and accurate diameter gauge to measure.

The compliance of vascular grafts measured in vivo is generally lower than that measured under static conditions in vitro because of viscoelastic behaviour. This is further altered after implantation when the prosthesis undergoes a process of healing and incorporation into the surrounding tissue; this has been described in detail by Burkel and Kahn [94]. In a healed PET prosthesis fibrin and whole blood thrombi, initially present in the interstices and on the surfaces, are ultimately replaced by connective tissue and fibroblast. On the inner surface, fibroblasts which have migrated from the outside spread randomly, forming an inner capsule. The thickness of this inner capsule is greater but is less uniform in crimped than in non-crimped prostheses [95]. A limited ingrowth, or pannus, occurs from the anastomosis and the endothelial cells in the host artery migrate across the anastomosis onto the luminal surface of the prosthesis. With time more of the luminal surface becomes endothelialized but the coverage is irregular and incomplete. As a result of the ingrowth of fibrous tissue in the wall and the presence of the inner and outer capsules, PET prostheses become stiffer both in the circumferential and longitudinal directions. Since the circular channels are filled with fibrin and fibrous tissue, crimped prostheses lose their axial extensibility and become more susceptible to kinking. The reduction in volume compliance of PET prostheses has been shown to be dependent on the elapsed time after implantation [96].

Long-Term Properties

PET and PTFE fabric prostheses have proved to be very successful for the replacement of medium and large arteries in man. Since they are being increasingly used in younger patients, their long-term stability in vivo becomes an important consideration. Although fabric grafts have very high strength, greater than 100 times the stresses encountered in vivo, there has been a number of documented cases of aneurysmal dilatation and fatal rupture in

PTFE [97] and PET [98–107] prostheses. Berger and Sauvage [106] reported that about 5% of PET prostheses implanted for periods greater than 3 years showed signs of dilatation, damaged yarn filaments and holes and tears in the prosthesis wall.

Since arterial prostheses in vivo are subjected to periodic stresses, their fatigue properties (due to material failure or degradation of mechanical properties under oscillatory stresses or deformation) should be characterized. Fatigue failure can be caused by the progressive growth of defects in the filaments or flaws in the prosthesis. Heat build-up and temperature increases may occur in the material due to viscous dissipation. Since the strength of polymers decreases with temperature, fatigue life (the number of cycles, at a given load, to cause failure) may be reduced. Fatigue life is a function of stress and it is greatly reduced as the applied stress is increased. Tensile strength and fatigue life can also be reduced by chemical degradation of the material in vivo and friction between filaments of adjacent yarns leading to abrasion and wear. Edwards et al. [108] and Marceau et al. [109] have developed fatigue testers which have been used for fabric prostheses. Both systems were designed to simulate physiological pressures as well as net flow through the prosthesis. Consequently their operating frequency was limited to 1–1.5 Hz. Four types of PET and PTFE prostheses were tested over a 24-week period by Edwards et al. [108]. The pressures were not specified. Diameter and tensile strength were measured on short segments obtained at 8-week intervals. In all prostheses, an increase in diameter and a reduction in length were reported. There was no significant change in the strength of PTFE fabric with time but the PET prostheses became weaker.

Biological Grafts

Vascular grafts of biological origin are classified as heterografts, homografts and autografts. The use of untreated homografts (e.g. umbilical vein graft) and heterografts (e.g. bovine carotid artery) can provoke immunological reactions in the host. Rosenberg et al. [110] developed a method for removing the immunoreactive smooth muscle and other cellular materials from the bovine carotid artery by digestion with ficin. The resulting collagen tube was tanned with dialdehyde starch to cross-link the collagen and increase the tensile strength of the graft. Elastic fibres were also removed when the artery was treated with ficin and consequently a bovine carotid artery segment increased in length and diameter by about 30–35%. The modified bovine artery graft has been extensively investigated both in experimental animals and in man. Although some have remained patent for periods over 10 years when placed in the iliac artery, where blood flow is relatively high, their performance when used for femoropopliteal bypass has been poor. A high incidence of aneurysm formation has been reported [111], probably due to a combination of fibre fatigue and degradation, and they are no longer recommended for use as bypass grafts.

Human Umbilical Vein Grafts

Human umbilical vein grafts can be rendered non-antigenic by tanning in 1% glutaraldehyde solution or in 1.3% dialdehyde starch after immersion in 95% ethanol. Since there is no enzymatic digestion, it is stated that the basic architecture of the vessel wall is preserved. Glutaraldehyde-stabilized human umbilical vein (HUV) grafts have been extensively used for arterial bypass in the lower limb. Although these grafts are provided with an outer support consisting of a coarse polyester mesh, several cases of aneurysm formation have been reported. Dardik et al. [112] observed a correlation between the incidence of graft aneurysm and the time of implantation. Mechanical fatigue, reversal of the aldehyde crosslink and immunological factors were thought to be responsible.

Weinberg et al. [113] carried out tensile tests on HUV grafts using a universal mechanical tester (the size, shape and orientation of the specimens were not specified). The elongation at break was typically about 35%. At strains ε of up to 0.15, the stress–strain relationship was modelled by: $\sigma = 5200 \, (e^{8\varepsilon} - 1)$ dynes cm^{-2}. The tensile modulus can be evaluated by differentiating the above expression with respect to ε. Thus at $\varepsilon = 0.15$ the tensile modulus was 1.38×10^5 dynes cm^{-2} and increased to 2.47×10^5 dynes cm^{-2} at $\varepsilon = 0.20$. Thereafter, it remained relatively constant up to failure. These figures show that the HUV graft has very low stiffness, being about two orders of magnitude smaller than the Young's moduli of peripheral arteries at in vivo strains.

Because of their relatively higher wall thickness to radius ratio the compliance of modified HUV grafts is lower than that of the host artery and the autologous saphenous vein grafts but greater than PTFE and PET prostheses. A large variation in individual values can be expected because the variation in wall thickness has been reported to lie between 0.5 to 2.0 mm for grafts of diameter from 4 to 7 mm [114]. After implantation, HUV grafts become stiffer as a result of encapsulation of the graft mesh by fibrous tissue, and the compliance is reduced to that of PET and PTFE prostheses [112]. Moreover, the wall density and the internal diameter increases as fluid is displaced from the wall by the transmural pressure.

Autogenous Vein Graft

The autogenous vein is widely accepted as the graft of choice for peripheral arterial reconstruction [115]. Compared with arteries of similar size, the walls of veins are much thinner. However, there are regional differences, with the wall thickness being generally greater in the lower limbs. Because of its relatively thick walls and its ability to withstand high hydrostatic pressure, the long saphenous vein is considered to be an ideal arterial substitute.

The basic structure of veins is similar to that of arteries. In veins greater than 2 mm diameter, the walls can be divided into the three characteristic layers observed in arteries although they are less distinct and have a looser texture [116]. The adventitia forms the bulk of the venous wall. It is composed mainly of collagen fibres but also contains some elastic fibres. The media is much thinner and consists mostly of circularly-arranged smooth muscle cells, collagen and some elastic fibres. The thin intima is made up of a layer of endothelium and a poorly-defined internal elastic lamina.

The venous wall contains relatively large amounts of collagen, the collagen to elastin ratio in the saphenous vein being more than $3:1$ [117]. There are differences in composition between upper and lower segments of the saphenous vein. In the lower segment, where hydrostatic pressure is higher, there is relatively more smooth muscle but less connective tissue than in the upper segment.

The mechanical properties of veins are, in general, similar to those of arteries but there are important differences associated with the large changes in cross-sectional area and shape at low transmural pressure. The uniaxial stress–strain curves of veins are highly non-linear and are dependent upon the angle of the strip specimens to the longitudinal axis, indicating anisotropic properties [118]. Attinger [119] has examined the elastic properties of canine vena cava and jugular vein and compared them with those of the descending aorta and carotid artery. Because of the relatively lower wall thickness to radius ratio of veins (0.03) compared with the descending aorta (0.10) and the carotid artery (0.14), he used a simplified formula for E_{inc} [equation (1.1)]:

$$E_{inc} = \frac{\Delta P R_o^2}{\Delta R_o h}(1 - \sigma^2) \qquad (1.7)$$

and showed that the relationship of pressure and E_{inc} for the veins was approximately linear when plotted on a log–log scale. Although the vena cava and jugular vein were very compliant at low pressures they became much stiffer at pressures above about 10 cm H_2O. Their elastic modulus was greater than that of the aorta and carotid artery, indicating that the collagen fibres play a major role in the stress–strain properties at a much lower pressure than in arteries. The increase in E_{inc} with pressure in the human saphenous vein appears to be monotonic as shown in Fig. 1.5.

The effect of venous smooth muscle tone on elastic properties is similar to that observed in arteries. That is, at the same transmural pressure, the elastic modulus is lower when smooth muscle is activated with norepinephrine than when it is relaxed. This has been confirmed by Morris et al. [120] who studied the pressure–diameter relationship of the canine femoral vein.

Wesly et al. [121] have studied the anisotropic properties of the human saphenous vein maintained at a constant longitudinal force of about 5 g. They found that below 5 kPa the ratio of circumferential to longitudinal elastic modulus was less than unity, but with increasing pressure it rose sharply and at arterial pressures the elastic modulus in the circumferential direction was about five times that in the longitudinal direction.

As the figures in Table 1.3 show, the human saphenous vein is only about one-third less compliant than the human femoral artery, despite the fact that it has an elastic modulus, at arterial pressure, one order of magnitude greater. This is due to the much thinner walls of veins compared with arteries of similar size.

Despite the superior long-term patency rates of the saphenous vein grafts compared with any other grafts in the femoropopliteal position, about one-

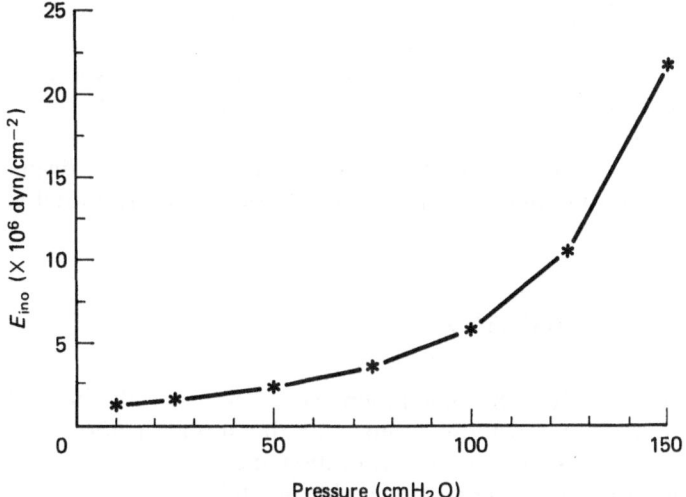

Fig. 1.5. Relationship between the incremental elastic modulus, E_{inc}, of the normal human saphenous vein and transmural pressure. E_{inc} was computed according to equation (1.1) (Data from Wesly et al. [121].)

third fail within 5 years of operation [122]. Early failures are generally attributed to problems of surgical technique or the use of poor quality veins [123,124]. Progression of atherosclerosis in the host artery and intimal hyperplasia are major causes of late failure of autogenous veins [125–127]. The exact cause of intimal thickening is not known. Graft handling and preparation [127,128], ischaemia [129] due to the interruption of blood supply to the vessel wall and proliferative repair of intima damaged by haemodynamic stresses [130,131] have been suggested as possible causes.

Intimal thickening seems to occur, in varying degrees, in all autogenous vein grafts and may be observed as early as 8 days after implantation [125]. Its effect on graft compliance has been examined by several authors; most studies have shown that vein grafts become stiffer. Waddell et al. [132] studied the changes in contractility and the load–deformation properties of saphenous vein grafts using helically-cut strips and observed only a slight increase in stiffness up to 7 months after the implantation. However, graft specimens tested after 1 year were between 40% and 45% stiffer than fresh saphenous vein. Similarly, after the same period the vein grafts showed marked reduction in, and in some cases complete absence of, contractility when stimulated with norepinephrine. This loss of contractility was to be expected since the destruction of smooth muscle cell was progressive with time. White et al. [93] using electromagnetic rheoangiometry to determine internal diameter changes in vivo, observed a reduction in mean compliance from 0.033%/mmHg at implantation to 0.016%/mmHg at 4 weeks and 0.015%/mmHg at 8 weeks. This has also been reported by Baird et al. [89] who noted a reduction in the mean compliance of femoral vein grafts from 0.048 to 0.033%/mmHg 3 months after surgery. They also observed a significant increase in diastolic diameter of the graft over this period. Lye et al. [91] measured the compliance and the pressure–strain modulus E_p of saphenous vein grafts in 19 patients non-invasively. Although the grafts had been implanted for periods ranging between 11 days and 128 months they found no correlation between compliance (mean value = 0.034%/mmHg) and age of vein graft. In contrast, jugular vein grafts placed in the carotid artery and aorto-mammary position were found to be essentially rigid 10 months after implantation [121]. All the jugular vein grafts displayed pronounced wall thickening due to intimal proliferation and adventitial scarring.

Elastomeric Prostheses

Over the past decade there has been increasing interest in the development of small diameter arterial prostheses. Much of the research effort has concentrated on the development of non-thrombogenic elastomeric polymers and novel techniques of fabricating porous or fibrous tubes.

Lyman et al. [133–135] produced 4 mm internal diameter prostheses from copolyether-urethane by precipitating a solution of the polymer by solvent–nonsolvent exchange. The resulting graft was described as being non-porous and having a controlled void structure similar to a spongy material. Being an elastomeric polymer the stiffness of the copolyether-urethane is lower than that of PET and PTFE. The stiffness is further reduced by the precipitation process as the wall density is decreased.

In a series of implants in dog femoral artery Seifert et al. [136] examined the effect of the compliance of 4 mm inner diameter (I.D.) copolyether-urethane prostheses on patency. Compliance was varied by changing the wall density. An "elastic index" (defined as the force per unit distance required to increase the cross-sectional area of the lumen by 20%) was measured for each prosthesis as well as the natural artery. The elastic index ranged from 21 to 45 × 10^4 dynes cm^{-2} for the prosthesis and 29.6 ± 4.4 × 10^4 dynes cm^{-2} for the femoral artery. They reported that the prostheses with elastic index which more closely matched that of the dog femoral artery had the best patency rate at 1 month. Recently these grafts have been available with a PET reinforcement. Stewart and Lyman [137] have reported the uniaxial and cylindrical elastic properties of 4 mm diameter reinforced grafts but did not compare their results with those of previous studies.

Hayashi et al. [138] have developed a small diameter polyurethane prosthesis of similar construction to those of Lyman's. The prostheses were produced by a phase separation technique and comprised a polyester outer mesh to prevent excessive dilatation. The mechanical properties of 3 mm I.D. specimens with 0.8 mm wall thickness were characterized using ring and tubular samples. The stress–strain relationship was approximately linear at strains of less than 1, and over this range the elastic moduli (secant moduli) were between 0.571 and 0.822 MPa. The pressure–radius relationship was modelled by the following equation:

$$\ln\left[\frac{P}{P_s}\right] = \beta\left[\frac{D_o}{D_s} - 1\right] \tag{1.8}$$

where P_s is an arbitrarily chosen pressure (e.g. 100 mmHg), D_s is the diameter at P_s and β is known as the stiffness parameter. The stiffness parameters for the polyurethane grafts were greater than those of the human femoral and common carotid arteries but lower than those of the coronary artery.

Kardos et al. [139] argued that the anisotropic properties of arteries should be replicated in the prosthesis design. They stated that a mismatch in anisotropic properties between the graft and the host artery can lead to torsional and buckling failure. Most prostheses are either isotropic or orthotropic, and when they are subjected to physiological loads only normal strains are present. Torsional strains are negligible if no permanent twisting is applied when the graft is sutured onto the host artery. Buckling can occur with orthotropic prostheses because of the length changes accompanying pressurization. However, if the mechanical properties are properly characterized the changes in length can be predicted and allowance made for at implantation. Kardos et al. constructed anisotropic prostheses using a 0.16 mm thick laminated sheet consisting of four segmented polyurethane films. Anisotropy was induced in each film by hot-stretching it to known elongations. The films were stacked in a cross-wise fashion with the direction of stretch of adjacent films being at right angles. The resulting prostheses were therefore orthotropic. Uniaxial tensile properties showed that the prostheses were anisotropic only at strains greater than about 20% (the ratio of longitudinal to circumferential stiffness was 1.45 at 30% strain). Below strains of 20% the prostheses were essentially isotropic.

White et al. [140,141] have developed a novel process – termed replamineform – for fabricating microporous polyurethane prostheses. The process is based on replicating the microporous calcite structure of sea urchin spines. The spines are treated in a 5% sodium hypochlorite solution to remove all organic materials. They are then machined into tubes of the required dimensions, typically 4 mm I.D. and 1 mm wall thickness. Polyurethane solution is injected into the calcite structure and after polymerization the calcite is dissolved in hydrochloric acid leaving a microporous polyurethane tube with pore size between 15 and 20 µm. Despite their relatively thick walls, the replamineform prostheses made from Biomer polyurethane had a mean compliance of 0.083%/mmHg. Compliance was determined from internal diameter measurement using electromagnetic rheoangiometry [93]. When implanted, the prostheses were gradually incorporated with a dispersed fibrohistiocytic cellular infiltrate resulting in a gradual decrease in compliance 3 weeks after implantation. At 8 weeks the compliance was reduced to 0.027%/mmHg.

Three techniques of manufacturing microfibrous polyurethane prostheses have been reported recently. The fibres are formed from the polymer solution by electrostatic spinning [142], extrusion under pressure through an orifice [143] or by suction through a nozzle [144], the negative pressure being produced by air flow around the nozzle. The fibres are wound onto a rotating mandrel and layers of fibres gradually collected. When the required wall thickness is attained the process is stopped and the fibrous tube is removed from the mandrel.

Using a 200 µm orifice Leidner et al. [143] were able to produce fibres of diameter in the range 10–30 µm. These fibres could be wound at different angles to the mandrel axis. The winding angle, α, is an important process

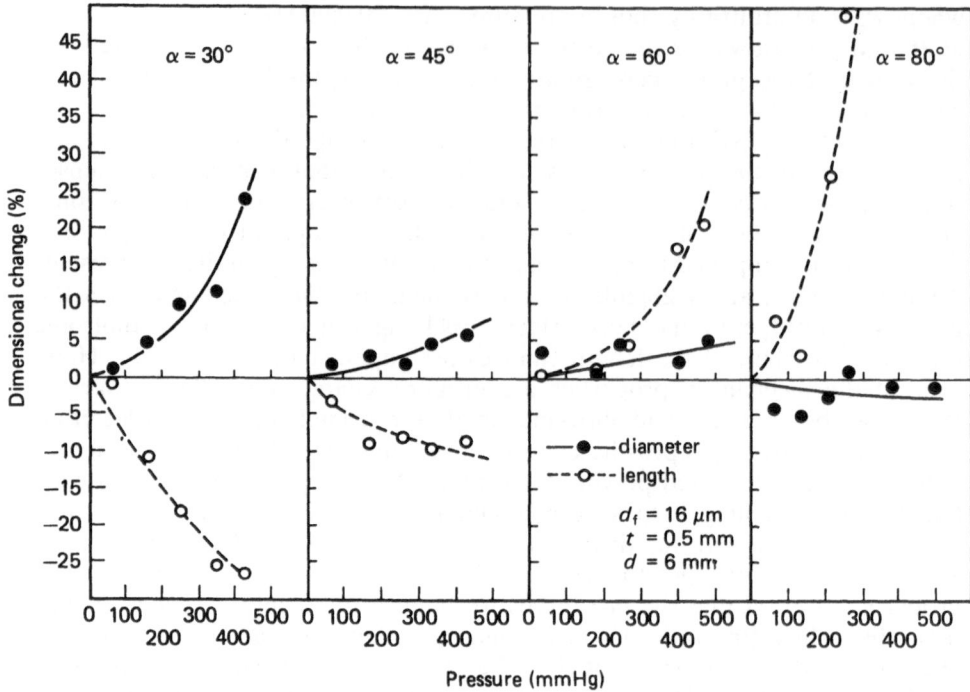

Fig. 1.6. Pressure–diameter and pressure–length curves of polyurethane prosthesis of internal diameter 6 mm and wall thickness 0.5 mm with various winding angles α. (Reprinted with permission of John Wiley from the *Journal of Biomedical Materials Research* [143].)

parameter since it affects the kinking properties of the prosthesis; the prosthesis becoming more kink resistant with increasing winding angle. The compliance and the anisotropic properties are also dependent on α. Figure 1.6 shows the response of a prosthesis of 6 mm I.D. and 0.5 mm wall thickness as a function of α. Although the dimensions were measured approximately with calipers, the decrease in compliance with increasing α is clearly demonstrated. The effect of α on anisotropy can be seen from the length changes with increasing pressure. For α of less than 45°, the prosthesis is stiffer longitudinally, and it retracts when the internal pressure is increased. At higher values of α the prosthesis becomes less stiff longitudinally and consequently elongates with pressure. Uniaxial tensile properties of these polyurethane prostheses with α between 45° and 75° were measured and compared with those of the iliac vessels and other synthetic prostheses [145]. The cylindrical properties were examined using a two-dimensional incremental model [146]. An expression was derived relating compliance with internal and external radii, circumferential elastic modulus and the Poisson's ratios. The polyurethane graft with a 45° angle was shown to have incremental moduli and Poisson's ratios closely matched to those of canine iliac arteries.

The fibres produced by electrostatic spinning are much finer, being between 1 and 2 µm in diameter (Fig. 1.7). Although under high magnification the fibres appear to be randomly orientated the prosthesis behaves, macroscopically,

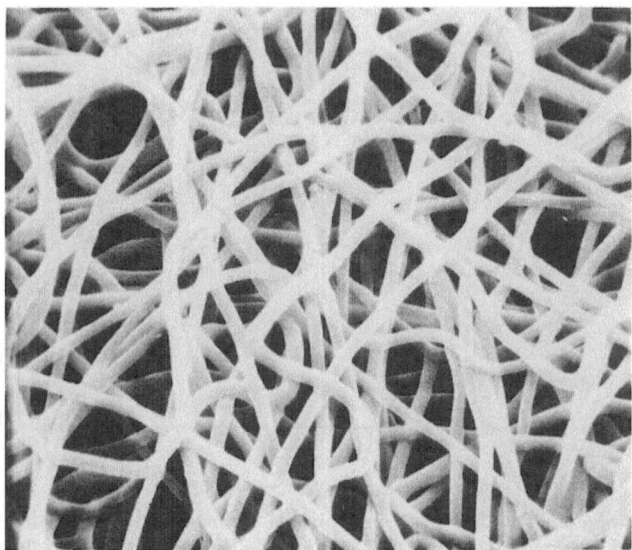

Fig. 1.7. Scanning electron micrograph of the internal surface of an electrostatically spun polyurethane prosthesis. The fibre diameters are about $1-2\,\mu$m.

as an anisotropic cylinder. Control of the anisotropic properties is achieved principally by varying the rotation speed of the mandrel [147]. This is demonstrated in Fig. 1.8 which shows that the ratio of circumferential to longitudinal elastic modulus increases with rotation speed. In order to determine whether electrostatically spun prostheses are orthotropic, strips obtained at various angles to the horizontal axis were tested on an Instron tensile tester and the stress–strain curves were plotted (Fig. 1.9). The stress–strain relationship can be seen to be non-linear and may be represented by a third order polynomial of the form:

$$\sigma = a_o + a_1\lambda + a_2\lambda^2 + a_3\lambda^3 \tag{1.9}$$

where σ is the stress and λ the extension ratio. Since the stress–strain curves for the 45° and 135° specimens are almost coincident it can be concluded that orthotropic symmetry exists.

The cylindrical properties have been investigated by How and Clarke [148] using electrostatically spun polyurethane prostheses of 4 mm I.D. The pressure–diameter relationship of prostheses of different wall thickness were obtained under quasi-static loading and at longitudinal extensions between 6% and 12%. The mathematical model used to analyse the experimental data was based on the model proposed by Vaishnav et al. [32]. They adopted a continuum mechanical approach to analyse the two-dimensional elastic behaviour of arteries. By treating the arterial segment as an incompressible orthotropic cylinder a non-linear theory for large elastic deformation was developed. They assumed a strain energy density function for arterial tissue approximated by the polynomial:

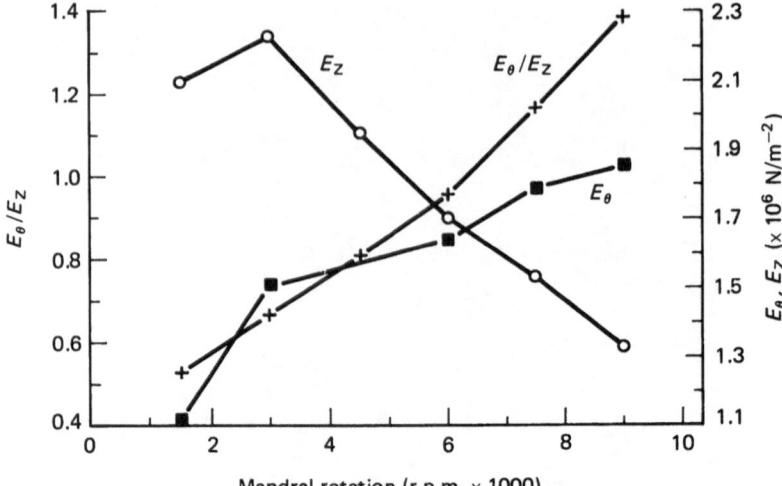

Fig. 1.8. Effect of mandrel rotation speed on the initial tensile modulus in the circumferential (E_θ) and longitudinal (E_z) directions. At about 6000 r.p.m. $E_\theta/E_z = 1$ indicating isotropic behaviour.

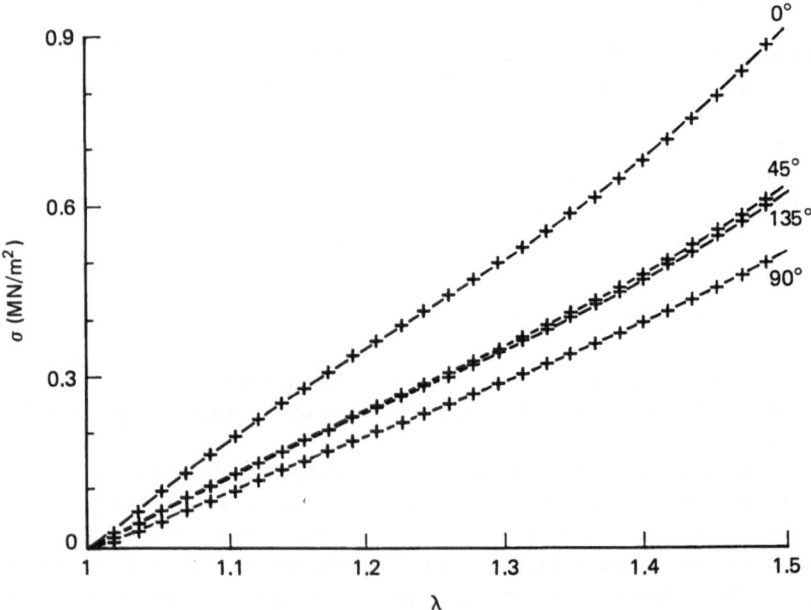

Fig. 1.9. Uniaxial tensile properties of electrostatically spun polyurethane prosthesis. Specimens were obtained at different angles to the longitudinal axis. Note that 45° and 135° specimens have similar stress–strain relationship indicating orthotropic symmetry. (Reprinted with permission from the *Journal of Biomechanics* [148]. © 1984 Pergamon Press.)

$$W = Aa^2 + Bab + Cb^2 + Da^3 + Ea^2b + Fab^2 + Gb^3 \tag{1.10}$$

where $A, B, \ldots, G$ are the constitutive constants which are determined from experimental data. a and b are the Green–St. Venant strains given below, in terms of the graft length L and mid-wall radius R (the mid-wall radius is the external radius minus half the wall thickness) (subscript i indicates the initial undeformed dimensions):

$$a = \frac{1}{2}\left[\left(\frac{R}{R_i}\right)^2 - 1\right] \qquad b = \frac{1}{2}\left[\left(\frac{L}{L_i}\right)^2 - 1\right]. \tag{1.11}$$

From the stress–strain relationship for a thin-wall cylinder subjected to an internal pressure and a longitudinal extension, the following equations can be derived which relate pressure P, and longitudinal force T, with the graft dimensions and the constitutive constants [148]:

$$P = \frac{H}{R}[Da^3 + (4A + 3D + 4Eb)a^2 + 2(A + Bb + Eb + Fb^2)a$$
$$+ (Bb + Fb^2)] \tag{1.12}$$

$$T = 2\pi RH\left[(6Gb^3 + (4C + 4aF + 3G)b^2 + 2(aB + C + a^2E)b \right.$$
$$\left. + (ab + a^2E) - \frac{PR}{2H}\right] \tag{1.13}$$

Assuming that the material is incompressible, that is, the volume of the material remains constant during deformation, the deformed wall thickness H, is given by:

$$H = \frac{V}{2\pi LR} \tag{1.14}$$

where V is the volume of a segment of graft of length L_i, initial mid-wall radius R_i and wall thickness H_i.

A typical set of curves of outer diameter and longitudinal force plotted against pressure at λ_z of 1.06 is shown in Fig. 1.10. These data, together with those of prostheses of the same diameter but different wall thicknesses were used to calculate the material constants A–G (Table 1.4). Prostheses made from different polyurethanes or fabricated under different spinning conditions have been shown to have different values of constants [149]. Equations (1.11) to (1.14) can be used to predict the behaviour of prostheses (3.4–3.8 mm I.D.) of any wall thickness and for any combination of internal pressure and

Table 1.4. The mean, standard error (SE) and coefficient of variation (CV) of the constitutive constants of electrostatically spun polyurethane prostheses

	A	B	C	D	E	F	G
				($\times 10^5$ N m^{-2})			
Mean	3.30	1.98	7.31	−1.38	1.23	0.43	−11.98
SE	0.14	0.13	0.20	0.30	0.34	0.36	0.58
CV	0.13	0.19	0.08	0.61	0.82	2.47	0.14

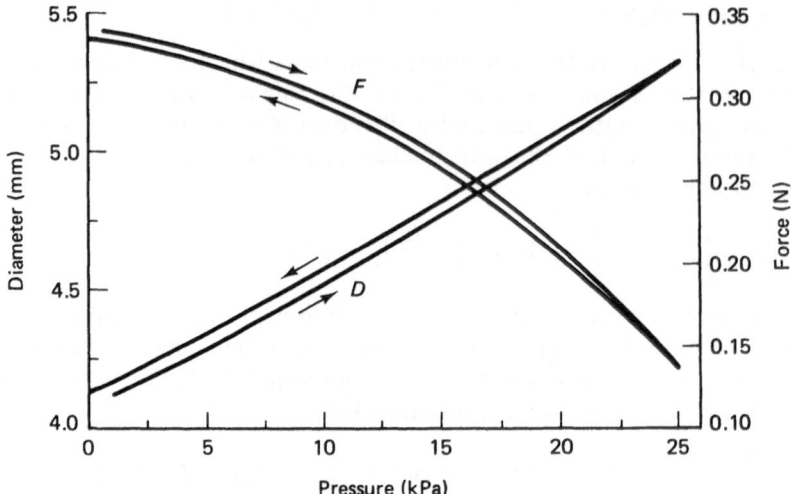

Fig. 1.10. Typical pressure–diameter and pressure–longitudinal force curves of an electrostatically spun prosthesis under quasi-static loading.

longitudinal extension, provided these are not beyond the range over which the constants were derived. For the values given in Table 1.4 the ranges are: wall thickness 0.25–0.55 mm; internal pressure 0–26 kPa (200 mmHg); longitudinal extension 4–10%. Thus the relationship between compliance C and wall thickness for a 3.7 mm I.D. polyurethane prosthesis can be readily determined. This is shown in Fig. 1.11 for longitudinal extension ratios λ_z ($\lambda_z = L/L_i$) of 1.04 and 1.10. C was calculated at a mean pressure of 13.33 kPa. This type of analysis is useful in the design of electrostatically-spun prostheses and is applicable to a wide range of materials. Recently, the same method was

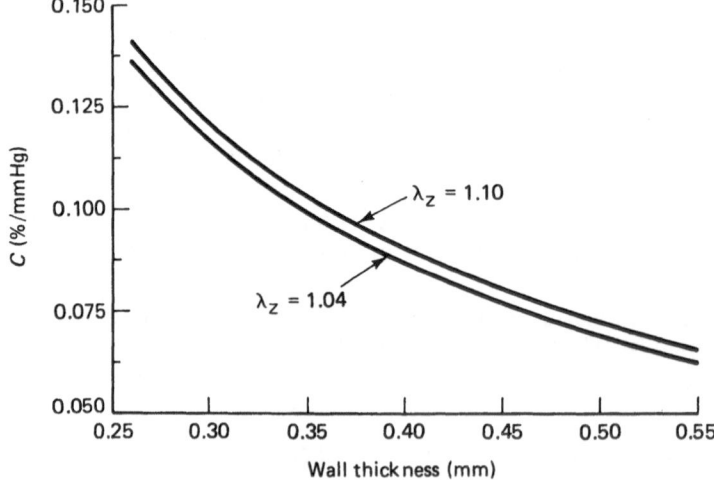

Fig. 1.11. The relationship between the compliance of electrostatically spun prostheses and wall thickness for λ_z of 1.04 and 1.10.

applied to the study of the elastic properties of tapered polyurethane prostheses [150].

The viscoelastic properties of electrostatically-spun prostheses have been studied by performing dynamic mechanical tests on cylindrical specimens [149]. The pressure signal consisted of a sinusoidal component of constant amplitude of 5.33 kPa peak-to-peak superimposed on a mean pressure of 13.33 kPa. The dynamic pressure was derived from an electromechanical shaker driven by a function generator and D.C.-coupled power amplifier. Pressure and diameter were measured over the frequency range 0.05–25 Hz, at constant longitudinal extensions of 4–10%. Diameter was measured by means of a non-contacting pulsed infrared diameter gauge having unity amplitude ratio of up to 50 Hz and resolution of 2 μm [151].

The diameter variation was sinusoidal with no observable distortion except in the more compliant thin-walled prostheses where high harmonics were present at the upper frequencies. The polyurethane prostheses may therefore be treated as linearly viscoelastic when they are subjected to small amplitude oscillatory deformations (<5%) superimposed on a finite mean deformation. However, when the amplitude of the sinusoidal strains was >5%, as in the thin-walled prostheses, non-linear behaviour was observed. The results of the dynamic tests are presented as the ratio of dynamic compliance C_{dyn} to static compliance C_{stat} plotted against frequency for different λ_z. Figure 1.12a shows C_{dyn}/C_{stat} decreasing with frequency (i.e. the prosthesis appears to become stiffer with increasing frequency). When plotted against the logarithm of frequency the curve can be approximated by a straight line. At frequencies above 1 Hz the phase lag of diameter behind pressure, shown in Fig. 1.12b, increases almost linearly with frequency, at a rate of 0.017 rad/Hz. In the natural arteries this was 0.0004 rad/Hz and there was no significant difference in phase response of the various arteries examined [49].

Longitudinal extension appears to have very little effect on either the amplitude or phase responses. This was also found to be the case with the wall thickness when the dynamic compliance was normalized with respect to the quasi-static compliance. These findings suggest that the viscoelastic properties of the polyurethane prosthesis may be a function of the polymer only. Studying the relaxation properties of PET and PTFE prostheses Hasegawa and Azuma [86] also observed that these were independent of the types of construction of the prostheses and were dependent only on the polymer.

The dynamic elastic modulus, E_{dyn}, of a 3.7 mm diameter polyurethane prosthesis was determined from equations (1.1) and (1.4) and plotted as E_{dyn}/E_{stat} against frequency (Fig. 1.13). The data of Bergel [49] for canine carotid and femoral arteries are plotted on the same graph for comparison. This shows that the dynamic mechanical behaviour of the polyurethane prostheses more closely matches that of the canine femoral arteries than the carotid arteries. It is frequency dependent but between 4–18 Hz, E_{dyn} can be considered to be constant. The heart rate in the dog lies within the region where compliance is frequency dependent and therefore the compliance of the prosthesis will vary as the heart rate changes. This is also the case when the prosthesis is used in man, where the heart rate lies between 1 and 2 Hz.

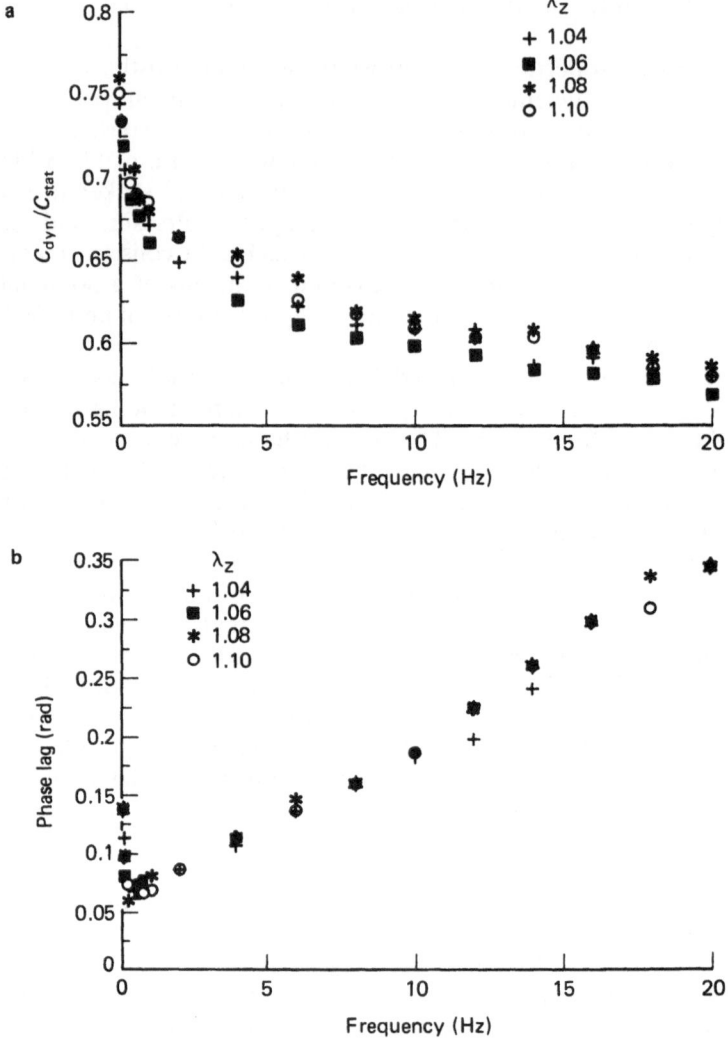

Fig. 1.12. a Ratio of dynamic to static compliance (C_{dyn}/C_{stat}) of electrostatically spun polyurethane prosthesis for different values of longitudinal extension ratios. **b** Phase lag of diameter signal with respect to pressure signal plotted against frequency.

Conclusions

The study of the properties of arteries has been the subject of intensive research over the past two decades. As a result, more sophisticated and realistic mathematical models are now available for the analysis of their non-linear anisotropic viscoelastic properties. In order to obtain the data necessary to validate these models, improved experimental techniques and more accurate instrumentation have been developed. Although much information

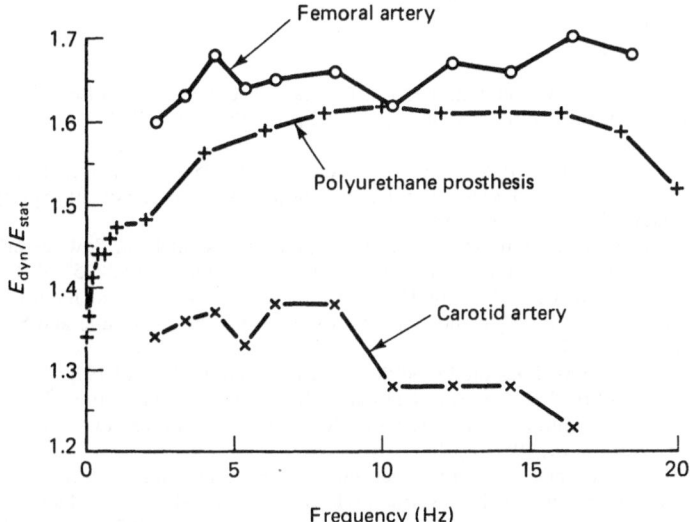

Fig. 1.13. Plot of E_{dyn}/E_{stat} against frequency for an electrostatically spun prosthesis. Data of Bergel [49] for the canine carotid and femoral arteries are included for comparison. The viscoelastic properties of the polyurethane prosthesis are more closely matched to those of the femoral artery.

is now available on the properties of large and medium-size arteries in vitro, uncertainties still exist as to whether results obtained from excised vessels can be used to predict the properties in vivo. The main difficulty is that the smooth muscle is relaxed in isolated segments of arteries whereas its degree of activity in vivo is not known. The effect of arterial disease and ageing on mechanical properties is important in the design of arterial prostheses. This information is still lacking and should perhaps be obtained by non-invasive techniques.

The mathematical models and experimental techniques developed for blood vessels have not been widely adopted for studying the properties of vascular prostheses. Compliance is a parameter widely used to characterize the elasticity of arterial grafts. Since it is a one-dimensional quantity, its limitation for describing the distensibility of vessels which may have non-linear anisotropic viscoelastic behaviour must be appreciated. Although it is now possible to design prostheses with mechanical properties similar to those of the artery, over a limited range of strain at least, these properties will change with time after implantation. There is a lack of data on the changes in mechanical properties of elastomeric prostheses following implantation. When available, they have been obtained in insufficient numbers of specimens and over relatively short periods. The question remains as to whether the properties to be matched should be based on those of the virgin prosthesis or those at a specific time after implantation.

References

1. Womersley JR. Oscillatory flow in arteries. II: The reflection of the pulse wave at junctions and rigid inserts in the arterial system. Phys Med Biol 1956;2:313–332
2. Daly BJ. Pulsatile flow through a tube containing rigid and distensible sections. In: van de Vooren AJ, Zandbergen PJ (eds) Proceedings of the 5th international conference on numerical methods in fluid dynamics: Lecture notes in physics, vol 59. Springer, Berlin Heidelberg New York, 1976, pp 153–158
3. Miyawaki F, How TV, Annis D. Effect of compliance mismatch on flow disturbances in a model of an arterial graft replacement. Med Biol Eng Comput 1990;28:457–464
4. Karino T, Motomiya M, Goldsmith HL. Flow patterns in model and natural vessels. In: Stanley JC et al. (eds) Biologic and synthetic vascular prostheses. Grune and Stratton, New York, 1982, pp 153–178
5. Baird RN, Abbott WM. Pulsatile blood-flow in arterial grafts. Lancet 1976;2:948–950
6. Abbott WM, Cambria RP. Control of physical characteristics (elasticity and compliance) of vascular grafts. In: Stanley JC et al. (eds) Biologic and synthetic vascular prostheses. Grune and Stratton, New York, 1982, pp 189–220
7. Glagov S. Haemodynamic risk factors: mechanical stress, mural architecture, medial nutrition and the vulnerability of arteries to atherosclerosis. In: Wissler RW, Geer JC (eds) The pathogenesis of atherosclerosis. Williams and Wilkins, Baltimore, 1971, pp 164–199
8. Patel DJ, Fry DL. In situ pressure–radius–length measurements in ascending aorta of anaesthetized dogs. J Appl Physiol 1964;19:413–416
9. Arndt JO, Klauske J, Mersch F. The diameter of the intact carotid artery in man and its change with pulse pressure. Pflugers Archiv 1968;301:230–240
10. Patel DJ, De Freitas FM, Greenfield JC, Fry DL. Relationship of radius to pressure along the aorta in living dogs. J Appl Physiol 1963;18:1111–1117
11. Barnett GO, Mallos AJ, Shapiro A. Relationship of aortic pressure and diameter in the dog. J Appl Physiol 1961;16:545–548
12. Luchsinger PC, Sachs M, Patel DJ. Pressure–radius relationship in large blood vessel of man. Circ Res 1962;11:885–888
13. Olson RM, Shelton DK. A nondestructive technique to measure wall displacement in the thoracic aorta. J Appl Physiol 1972;32:147–151
14. Greenfield JC, Tindall GT, Dillon ML, Mahaley MS. Mechanics of the human common carotid artery in vivo. Circ Res 1964;15:240–246
15. Mozersky DJ, Sumner DS, Hokanson DE, Strandness DE. Transcutaneous measurement of the elastic properties of the human femoral artery. Circulation 1972;46:948–955
16. Arndt JO, Stegall HF, Wicke HJ. Mechanics of the aorta in vivo. A radiographic approach. Circ Res 1971;28:693–704
17. Carton TW, Dainauskas J, Clark JW. Elastic properties of single elastic fibres. J Appl Physiol 1962;17:547–551
18. Benedict JV, Walker KB, Harris EH. Stress–strain characteristics and tensile strength of unembalmed human tendon. J Biomechanics 1968;1:53–63
19. Roach MR, Burton AC. The reason for the shape of the distensibility curves of arteries. Can J Biochem Physiol 1957;35:681–690
20. Roy CS. The elastic properties of the arterial wall. J Physiol 1880;37:125–159
21. Attinger FML. Two-dimensional in-vitro studies of femoral arterial walls of the dog. Circ Res 1968;22:829–840
22. Tanaka T, Fung YC. Elastic and inelastic properties of the canine aorta and their variation along the aortic tree. J Biomechanics 1974;7:357–370
23. Cox RH. Comparison of arterial wall mechanics using ring and cylindrical segments. Am J Physiol 1983;244:H298–H303
24. McDonald DA. Blood flow in arteries. Edward Arnold, London, 1974
25. Carew TE, Vaishnav RN, Patel DJ. Compressibility of the arterial wall. Circ Res 1968;22:61–68
26. Bergel DH. The static elastic properties of the arterial wall. J Physiol 1961;156–445–457
27. Cox RH. Anisotropic properties of the canine carotid artery in vivo. J Biomechanics 1975;8:239–300

28. Peterson LH, Jensen RE, Parnell J. Mechanical properties of arteries in vivo. Circ Res 1960;8:622–639
29. Patel DJ, Fry DL. The elastic symmetry of arterial segments in dogs. Circ Res 1969;24:1–8
30. Vaishnav RH, Vossoughi J. Incremental formulations in vascular mechanics. J Biomech Eng 1984;106:105–111
31. Patel DJ, Janicki JS, Carew TE. Static anisotropic elastic properties of the aorta in living dogs. Circ Res 1969;25:765–779
32. Vaishnav RN, Young JT, Janicki JS, Patel DJ. Nonlinear anisotropic elastic properties of the canine aorta. Biophys J 1973;12:1008–1027
33. Cox RH, Jones AW, Fisher GM. Carotid artery mechanics, connective tissue and electrolyte changes in puppies. Am J Physiol 1974;227:563–568
34. Cox RH. Passive mechanic and connective tissue composition of canine arteries. Am J Physiol 1978;234:H533–541
35. Patel DJ, Janicki JS. Static elastic properties of the left coronary circumflex artery and the common carotid artery in dogs. Circ Res 1970;27:149–158
36. Weizsacker HW, Lambert H, Pascale K. Analysis of the passive mechanical properties of the rat carotid arteries. J Biomechanics 1983;16:703–715
37. Tickner EG, Sacks AH. A theory for the static elastic behaviour of blood vessels. Biorheology 1967;4:151–168
38. Fung YC, Fronek K, Patitucci P. Pseudoelasticity of arteries and the choice of its mathematical expression. Am J Physiol 1979;237:H620–H631
39. Patel DJ, Vaishnav RN. The rheology of large blood vessels. In: Bergel DH (ed) Cardiovascular fluid dynamics, vol 2. Academic Press, London, 1972.
40. Wurzel M, Cowper GR, McCook JM. Smooth muscle contraction and viscoelasticity of arterial wall. Can J Physiol Pharmacol 1970;48:510–523
41. Azuma T, Hazegawa M. A rheological approach to the architecture of arterial walls. Jap J Physiol 1971;21:27–47
42. Zatzman M, Stacy RW, Randal J, Eberstein A. Time course of stress relaxation in isolated arterial segments. Am J Physiol 1954;177:299–302
43. Mikami T, Attinger EO. Stress relaxation of blood vessels. Angiologica 1968; 5:281–292
44. Wiederhielm CA. Distensibility characteristics of small blood vessels. Fed Proc 1965; 24:1075–1084
45. Bagshaw RJ, Attinger FML. Longitudinal stress relaxation in the canine aorta. Experientia 1974;30:1046–1047
46. Apter JT, Marquez E. Correlation of viscoelastic properties of large arteries with microscopic structure. V. Effects of sinusoidal forcings at low and at resonance frequencies. Circ Res 1968; 22:393–404
47. Goedhard WJA, Knoop AA. A model of the arterial wall. J Biomechanics 1973;6:281–288
48. Yin FCP, Spurgeon HA, Kallman CH. Age-associated alteration in viscoelastic properties of canine aortic strips. Circ Res 1983;53:464–472
49. Bergel DH. The dynamic elastic properties of the arterial wall. J Physiol 1961; 156:458–469
50. Cox RH. A model for the dynamic mechanical properties of arteries. J Biomechanics 1972; 5:135–152
51. Gow BS, Schonfeld D, Patel DJ. The dynamic elastic properties of the canine left circumflex coronary artery. J Biomechanics 1974;7:389–395
52. Gow BS, Taylor MG. Measurement of viscoelastic properties of arteries in the living dog. Circ Res 1968;23:111–122
53. Gow BS. Viscoelastic properties of conduit arteries. Circ Res 1970 Suppl II:26–27:II-113-II-122
54. Patel DJ, Janicki JS, Vaishnav RN, and Young JT. Dynamic anisotropic viscoelastic properties of the aorta in living dogs. Circ Res 1973;32:93–107
55. Barbenel JC. The arterial wall. In: Rodkiewicz CM (ed) Arteries and arterial blood flow. International Centre for Mechanical Science, courses and lectures no. 270. Springer, Berlin Heidelberg New York, 1984.
56. Dobrin PB. Mechanical properties of arteries. Physiol Rev 1978;58:397–460
57. Saxton JA. Elastic properties of the rabbit aorta in relation to age. Arch Pathol 1942;34:262–274

58. Band W, Goedhard WJA, Knoop AA. Effects of ageing on dynamic viscoelastic properties of the rat's thoracic aorta. Pflugers Arch 1972;331:357–364
59. Roach MR, Burton AC. The effect of age on the elasticity of human iliac arteries. Can J Biochem Physiol 1959;37:557–570
60. Learoyd BM, Taylor MG. Alteration with age in the viscoelastic properties of human arterial walls. Circ Res 1966;28:278–292
61. Bader H. Dependence of wall stress in the human thoracic aorata on age and pressure. Circ Res 1967;20:354–361
62. Nakashima T, Tanikawa J. A study of human aortic distensibility with relation to atherosclerosis and aging. Angiology 1971;22:477–490
63. Gozna ER, Marble AE, Shaw A, Holland JG. Age related changes in the mechanics of the aorta and pulmonary artery of man. J Appl Physiol 1974;36:407–411
64. Hallock P. Arterial elasticity in man in relation to age as evaluated by the pulse wave velocity method. Arch Intern Med 1934;54:770–798
65. O'Rourke MF, Blazek JV, Morreels CL, Krovetz LJ. Pressure wave transmission along the human aorta. Changes with age and in arterial degenerative disease. Circ Res 1968;23: 567–579
66. Miller CW, Nealeigh RC, Crowder ME. Evaluation of the cardiovascular changes associated with ageing in a colony of dogs. ISA BM 1976;76320:107–110
67. Newman DL, Gosling RG, Bowden NLR. Changes in aortic distensibility and area ratio with the development of atherosclerosis. Atherosclerosis 1971;14:231–240
68. Band W, Goedhard WJA Knoop AA. Comparison of effects of high cholesterol intake on viscoelastic properties of the thoracic aorta in rats and rabbits. Atherosclerosis 1973;18: 163–171
69. Haut RC, Garg BD, Metke M, Josa M, Kaye MP. Mechanical properties of the canine aorta following hypercholesterolemia. J Biomech Eng 1980;102:98–102
70. Butcher HR, Newton WT. The influence of age, arteriosclerosis and homotransplantation upon the elastic properties of major human arteries. Ann Surg 1958;148:1–19
71. Moncrieff RW. Man-made fibres, 5th edn. Heywood Books, London, 1970
72. Brydson JA. Plastics materials, 4th edn. Butterworths, London, 1982
73. Maarek JM, Guidoin R, Aubin A, Prud'homme RE. Molecular weight characterisation of virgin and explanted polyester arterial prostheses. J Biomed Mater Res 1984;18:881–894
74. Guidoin R, Martin L, Marois, M, Gosselin C, King M, Gunasekera K, Domurado D, Sigot-Luizard MF, Sigot M, Blais P. Polyester prostheses as substitutes in the thoracic aorta of dogs. II. Evaluation of albuminated polyester grafts stored in ethanol. J Biomed Mat Res 1984;18:1059–1072
75. Cengiz M, Sauvage LR, Berger K, Robel SB, Robel V, Wu HD, Walker M, Appleyard RF, Wood SJ. Effects of compliance alteration on healing of a porous Dacron prosthesis in the thoracic aorta of the dog. Surg Gynecol Obstet 1984;158:145–151
76. Charlesworth D. Arterial replacements. In: Taylor S (ed) Recent advances in surgery, vol 10. Churchill Livingstone, Edinburgh, 1980, pp 93–111
77. Kenney DA, Sauvage LR, Wood SJ, Berger K, Davis CC, Smith JC, Rittenhouse EA, Hall DG, Mansfield PB. Comparison of noncrimped, externally supported (EXS) and crimped, nonsupported Dacron prostheses for axillofemoral and above-knee femoropopliteal bypass. Surgery 1982;92:931–946
78. Geiger G, Hoevels J, Storz L, Bayer HP. Vascular grafts in below-knee femoro-popliteal bypass: a comparative study. J Cardiovasc Surg 1984;25:523–524
79. Hanel KC, McCabe C, Abbott WM, Fallon J, Megerman J. Current PTFE grafts. A biomechanical, scanning electron, and light microscopic evaluation. Ann Surg 1982; 195: 456–463
80. Boyce B. Physical characteristics of expanded polytetrafluoroethylene grafts. In: Stanley JC et al. (eds) Biologic and synthetic vascular prostheses. Grune & Stratton, New York, 1982, pp 553–560
81. Harrison JH. Synthetic materials as vascular prostheses. Am J Surg 1958;95:16–24
82. Cohen J, Litwin SB, Aaron A, Fine S. The rupture force and tensile strength of canine aortic tissue. J Surg Res 1972;13:321–333
83. Snyder RW, Botzko KM. Woven, knitted and externally supported Dacron vascular prostheses. In: Stanley JC et al. (eds) Biologic and synthetic vascular prostheses. Grune and Stratton, New York, 1982, pp 485–494

84. Oka S. Cardiovascular hemorheology. Cambridge University Press, Cambridge, 1981
85. Guidoin R, King M, Gosselin C, Blais P, Gunasekera K, Marois M, Cardou A. Les prothèses arterielles en polyester. Rev Biotech Med 1982;4:13-25
86. Hasegawa M, Azuma T. Mechanical properties of a synthetic arterial grafts. J Biomechanics 1979;12:509-517
87. Paasche PE, Kinley CE, Dolan FG, Gozna ER, Marble AE. Consideration of suture-line stresses in the selection of synthetic grafts for implantation. J Biomechanics 1973;6:253-259
88. Hokanson DE, Strandness DE. Stress-strain characteristics of various arterial grafts. Surg Gynecol Obstet 1968;127:57-60
89. Baird RN, Kidson IG, L'Italien GJ, Abbott WM. Dynamic compliance of arterial grafts. Am J Physiol 233:H568-H572
90. Kidson IG, Abbott WM. Low compliance and arterial graft occlusion. Cardiovasc Surg 1978, Suppl I, 58:I1-I4
91. Lye CR, Sumner DS, Hokanson DE, Strandness DE. The transcutaneous measurement of the elastic properties of the human saphenous vein femoropopliteal bypass graft. Surg Gynecol Obstet 1975;141:891-895
92. Walden R, L'Italien GJ, Megerman J, Abbott WM. Matched elastic properties and successful arterial grafting. Arch Surg 1980;115:1166-1169
93. White R, Goldberg L, Hirose F, Klein S, Bosco P, Miranda R, Long J, Nelson R, Shors E. Effect of healing on small internal diameter arterial graft compliance. Biomater Med Devices Artif Organs 1983;11:21-29
94. Burkel WE, Kahn RH. Biocompatibility of prosthetic grafts. In: Stanley JC et al. (eds) Biologic and synthetic vascular prostheses. Grune & Stratton, New York, 1982, pp 221-247
95. Herring H, Dilley R, Gardner A, Glover J. The effect of crimping on the healing of prosthetic arterial grafts. J Cardiovasc Surg 1980;21:596-603
96. Newton WT, Stokes JM, Butcher HR. Changes in the elasticity of arterial substitutes following implantation. Surgery 1959;46:579-587
97. Hayward RH, White RR. Aneurysm in a woven Teflon graft. Angiology 1971;22:188-190
98. Cooke PA, Nobis PA, Stoney RJ. Dacron aortic graft failure. Arch Surg 1974;108:101-103
99. Ottinger LW, Darling RC, Wirthlin LS, Linton RR. Failure of ultraweight knitted Dacron grafts in arterial reconstruction. Arch Surg 1976;111:146-149
100. Hayward RH, Korompai FL. Degeneration of knitted Dacron grafts. Surgery 1976;79:581-583
101. Blumenberg RM, Gelfand ML. Failure of knitted Dacron as an arterial prosthesis. Surgery 1977; 81:493-496
102. Yashar JJ, Richman MH, Dyckman J, Witoszka M, Burnard RJ, Weyman AK, Yashar J. Failure of Dacron prostheses caused by structural defect. Surgery 1978;84:659-663
103. May J, Stephen M. Multiple aneurysms in Dacron velour grafts. Arch Surg 1978;113:320-321
104. Nunn DB, Freeman MH, Hudgins PC. Postoperative alterations in size of Dacron aortic grafts. Ann Surg 1979;189:741-745
105. Kim GE, Imparato AM, Nathan I, Riles TS. Dilation of synthetic grafts and junctional aneurysms. Arch Surg 1979;114:1296-1303
106. Berger K, Sauvage LR. Late fiber deterioration in Dacron arterial grafts. Ann Surg 1981; 193:477-491
107. Batt M, King M, Guidoin R, Goeau-Brissonierc O, Michetti C, Marois M, Gosselin C, Garton A, Le Bas P. Fatigue mécanique d'une prothèse arterielle. Presse Med 1984;13:1997-2000
108. Edwards WS, Snyder RW, Botzko K, Larking J. Comparison of durability of tensile strength of Teflon and Dacron grafts. In: Dardik H (ed) Graft materials in vascular surgery. Symposia Specialists Inc., Miami, 1978, pp 169-183
109. Marceau D, Cardou A, Guidoin R. Developpement d'un systeme pour l'essai dynamique des prothèses arterielles alloplastiques: le Vivocycleur. In: Guidoin R (ed) Proc 4th Annual Meeting, Canadian Biomaterials Society, June 22-23 1983, Quebec, pp 32.1-32.5
110. Rosenberg N, Gaughran ERL, Henderson J, Lord GH, Douglas JF. The use of segmental arterial implants prepared by enzymatic modification of heterologous blood vessels. Surgical Forum 1982;6:242-246
111. Dale WA, Lewis MR. Further experience with bovine arterial grafts. Surgery 1976;80:711-721

112. Dardik H, Ibrahim IM, Sussman B, Kahn M, Sanchez M, Klausner S, Baier RE, Meyer AE, Dardik II. Biodegradation and aneurysm formations in umbilical vein grafts. Ann Surg 1984;199:61–68

113. Weinberg SL, Cipolletti GB, Turner RJ. Human umbilical vein grafts: Physical evaluation criteria. In: Stanley JC (ed) Biologic and synthetic vascular prostheses. Grune and Stratton, New York, 1982, pp 433–444

114. Guidoin R, Marois M, Martin L, Noel HP, Laroche F, Gosselin CO, Cote R, Benichoux R, Blais P. Processed human umbilical veins as arterial substitutes evaluation in canine models. Biomaterials 1980;1:82–88

115. Kakkar VV. The cephalic vein as a peripheral vascular graft. Surg Gynecol Obstet 1969; 124:551–556

116. Caro CG, Pedley TJ, Schroter RC, Seed WA. The mechanics of the circulation. Oxford University Press, Oxford, 1978

117. Svejcar J, Prerovsky I, Linhart J, Kruml J. Content of collagen, elastin and water in walls of the internal saphenous vein in man. Circ Res 1962;11:296–300

118. Vonderlage M. Untersuchungen uber die mechanischen Eigenschaften von streifenpraparaten verschiedener Schnittrichtung aus der Vena cava abdominalis des Kaninchens. Pflugers Arch 1968;303:71–80

119. Attinger EO. Wall properties of veins. IEEE Trans Biomed Eng BME 1969;16:253–261

120. Morris TW, Abbrecht PH, Leverett SD. Diameter–pressure relationships in the unexposed femoral vein. Am J Physiol 1974;227:782–788

121. Wesly RLR, Vaishnav RN, Fuchs JCA, Patel DJ, Greenfield JC. Static linear and nonlinear elastic properties of normal and arterialized venous tissue in dog and man. Circ Res 1975; 37:509–520

122. Brewster DC, LaSalle AJ, Robinson JG, Strayhorn EC, Darling RC. Factors affecting patency of femoropopliteal bypass grafts. Surg Gynecol Obstet 1983;175:437–447

123. Ramos JR, Berger K, Mansfield PB, Sauvage LR. Histologic fate and endothelial changes of distended and nondistended vein grafts. Ann Surg 1976;183:205–228

124. Szilagyi DE, Hageman JH, Smith RF, Elliott JP, Brown F, Dietz P. Autogenous vein grafting in femoropopliteal atherosclerosis: the limits of its effectiveness. Surgery 1979;86:836–851

125. McCabe M, Cunningham GJ, Wyatt AP, Rothrie NG, Taylor GW. A histological and histochemical examination of autogenous vein grafts. Br J Surg 1967;54:147–155

126. Brody WR, Angell WW, Kosek JC. Histologic fate of the venous coronary artery bypass in dogs. Am J Pathol 1972;66:111–119

127. Abbott WM, Wieland S, Austen WG. Structural changes during preparation of autogenous venous grafts. Surgery 1974;76:1031–1040

128. Imparato AM, Bracco A, Kim GE, Zeff R. Intimal and neointimal fibrous proliferation causing failure of arterial reconstructions. Surgery 1972;72:1007–1017

129. Brody WR, Kosek JC, Angell WW. Changes in vein grafts following aorto-coronary bypass induced by pressure and ischemia. J Thorac Cardiovasc Surg 1972;64:847–854

130. Rittgers SE, Karayannacos PE, Guy JF, Nerem RM, Shaw GM, Hostetler JR, Vasko JS. Velocity distribution and intimal proliferation in autologous vein grafts in dogs. Circ Res 1978;42:792–801

131. Karayannacos PE, Rittgers SE, Kakos GS, Williams TE, Meckstroth CV, Vasko JS. Potential role of velocity and wall tension in vein graft failure. J Cardiovasc Surg 1980;21: 171–178

132. Waddell WG, Vogelfanger IJ, Bosc M, Malik KU, MacConaill M, Ling G. Changes in contractility, compliance and elasticity in experimental arterial vein autografts. Can J Surg 1973;16:252–260

133. Lyman DJ, Albo DJr, Jackson R, Knutson K. Development of small diameter vascular prostheses. Trans Am Soc Artif Intern Organs 1977;23:253–261

134. Lyman DJ, Fazzio J, Voorhees H, Robinson G, Albo DJr. Compliance as a factor affecting the patency of a copolyurethane vascular graft. J Biomed Mater Res 1978;12:337–345

135. Lyman DJ. Synthetic elastomers in vascular surgery. In: Dardik E (ed) Graft materials in vascular surgery. Symposia Specialists, Miami, 1978, pp 213–224

136. Seifert KB, Albo D, Knowlton H, Lyman DJ. Effect of elasticity of prosthetic wall on patency of small diameter arterial prostheses. Surg Forum 1979;30:206–208

137. Stewart SFC, Lyman DJ. Finite elasticity modelling of the biaxial and uniaxial properties of compliant vascular grafts. ASME J Biomech Eng 1988;110:344–348

138. Hayashi K, Takamizawa K, Saito T, Kira K, Hiramatsu K, Kondo K. Elastic properties and strength of a novel small-diameter, compliant polyurethane vascular graft. J Biomed Mater Res 1989;23:229–244

139. Kardos JL, Mehta BS, Apostolou SF, Thies C, Clark RE. Design, fabrication and testing of prosthetic blood vessels. Biomater Med Devices Artif Organs 1975;2:387–396

140. White RA, Weber JN, White EW. Replamineform: a new process for preparing porous ceramic, metal and polymer synthetic materials. Science 1972;176:922–924

141. White RA, White EW, Hanson EL, Rohner RF, Webb WR. Preliminary report: Evaluation of tissue ingrowth into experimental Replamineform vascular prostheses. Surgery 1976;79: 229–232

142. Annis D, Bornat A, Edwards RO, Higham A, Loveday B, Wilson J. An elastomeric vascular prosthesis. Trans Am Soc Artif Intern Organs 1978;24:209–214

143. Leidner J, Wong EWC, MacGregor DC, Wilson GJ. A novel process for the manufacturing of porous grafts: process description and product evaluation. J Biomed Mater Res 1983;17: 229–247

144. Blood vessel prostheses, UK Patent GB 2015118B, 1982, H. Planck and P. Ehrler (Inventors)

145. Lee JM, Wilson GJ. Anisotropic tensile viscoelastic properties of vascular graft materials tested at low strain rates. Biomaterials 1986;7:423–431

146. Nahon D, Lee JM, Wilson GJ. A two-dimensional incremental study of the static mechanical properties of vascular grafts. Clin Mater 1986;1:177–197

147. How TV, Clarke RM, Annis D. Uniaxial tensile properties of the Liverpool artificial artery. In: Proceedings of the international conference on biomedical polymers, 12–15 July 1982, Durham, UK, Biological Engineering Society, pp 171–179

148. How TV, Clarke RM. The elastic properties of a polyurethane arterial prosthesis. J Biomechanics 1984;17:597–608

149. How TV, Annis D. Viscoelastic behaviour of polyurethane vascular prostheses. J Biomed Mater Res 1987;21:1093–1108

150. How TV. Elastic deformation of a tapered vascular prosthesis. Submitted for publication to J Mater Sci: Materials in Medicine.

151. How TV, Bhuvaneshwar GS, Annis D. Infrared diameter gauge for in vitro mechanical testing of vascular grafts. J Biomed Eng 1984;6:195–199

Chapter 2

Blood Compatibility in Cardiopulmonary Bypass

J.M. Courtney, L. Irvine, J.D.S. Gaylor, C.D. Forbes and K.M. Taylor

Introduction

The purpose of this chapter is to consider blood compatibility in cardiopulmonary bypass, where compatibility is related to alterations in blood constituents resulting both from the procedure and from contact with the biomaterials utilized.

This association of blood compatibility with the clinical procedure applies to all biomaterials and is particularly relevant in cardiopulmonary bypass, where a range of devices, differing in design, operation, and influence on the blood, may be used.

The principal application of cardiopulmonary bypass [1–3] involves the use of devices in cardiothoracic surgery, where the natural heart and lungs are bypassed via an extracorporeal circuit. The basic features of the circuit are shown in Fig. 2.1. Blood is drained by gravity from the vena cava and passes through a heat exchanger to regulate the temperature of the bypass. Cardiotomy blood, removed by suction from the surgical area and filtered, is also delivered to the heat exchanger. Blood from the heat exchanger passes to a gas exchange section, where the addition of oxygen and the removal of carbon dioxide take place. The oxygenated blood passes to a reservoir from which it is elevated to arterial pressure by a mechanical pump and may be filtered to remove emboli prior to return to the arterial circulation via the aortic arch. The heat exchanger, gas exchanger and reservoir are integrated into the devices used for the majority of cardiopulmonary bypass procedures.

The original concept of the cardiopulmonary bypass procedure, first demonstrated successfully on a human by Gibbon [4], was that of total replacement of heart and lung in acute situations, with the duration of bypass normally in the range 1–3 hours. The majority of procedures are performed with devices utilizing direct blood–gas interfaces, with oxygen bubbled through the blood.

An alternative to direct contact gas exchange emerged with the development of membrane-based devices [5–8]. Separation of the blood and gas phases by a gas-permeable membrane reduced trauma and extended the bypass procedure into the area of long-term assist and also to the application of artificial lungs in the treatment of potentially reversible lung disease.

In addition to the influence on blood compatibility of the direct or indirect devices, other factors have to be taken into account. The biological responses during bypass can be altered by the use of pulsatile flow [9,10] and in the clinical application of prolonged extracorporeal membrane oxygenation (ECMO), there are potential advantages in substituting the normal veno-arterial mode of perfusion by arteriovenous perfusion [11,12].

The strong dependence of compatibility on the nature of the procedure means that, with respect to blood compatibility, cardiopulmonary bypass cannot be treated in an analogous manner to other extracorporeal applications such as the artificial kidney. Present artificial kidneys are almost exclusively membrane-based [13,14] and consideration of blood compatibility is normally focused on membrane properties. This is not wholly possible in the case of cardiopulmonary bypass.

A further factor, common to extracorporeal applications, is that acceptable clinical performance requires operation of the device in association with an

Table 2.1. The physiology and pharmacology of extracorporeal circulation (ECC) compared to normal cirulation and pulmonary function

Normal function	Physiological changes with ECC	Mechanical factors	Pharmacological factors
	↑ Total flow	Venous cannula size	Steroids
	↓ Negative venous P		
	↑ Adrenergic response		Adrenergic blockers
	↑ Renin–angiotensin	Arterial cannula size	
	Abnormal distribution		Diuretics
Blood flow	Non-pulsatile	Pump characteristics	
	Non-servo		Volume expanders
	↓ Tissue washout		
	↓ Oxygen delivery	Heat exchanger	Hypothermia
	Acidosis		Buffers-tris
			HCO^-_3
	O_2–CO_2 exchange	Oxygenator	
	requires large	Bubble	
	blood volume	Membrane	
Gas exchange	Microbubbles		Defoamer ?
	Emboli & aggregates	Reservoirs	Platelet-active drugs
		connectors, tubing	
Blood– endothelial interface	Stagnant zones		
	Anticoagulant	Surface coating	Heparin
	↑ Fibrinolytic activity		Priming solutions
	↓ Platelet function	Coronary suction	
Reticulo endothelial function			Haemodilution
	Blood dilution		
	Tissue histocytes	Filters	
	loaded		
	↓ Phagocytes		

Reproduced with permission from Bartlett RA, Gazzaniga AB. In: Ionescu MI (ed) *Techniques in extracorporeal circulation*, 2nd edn. Butterworths, London, 1981, p 1.

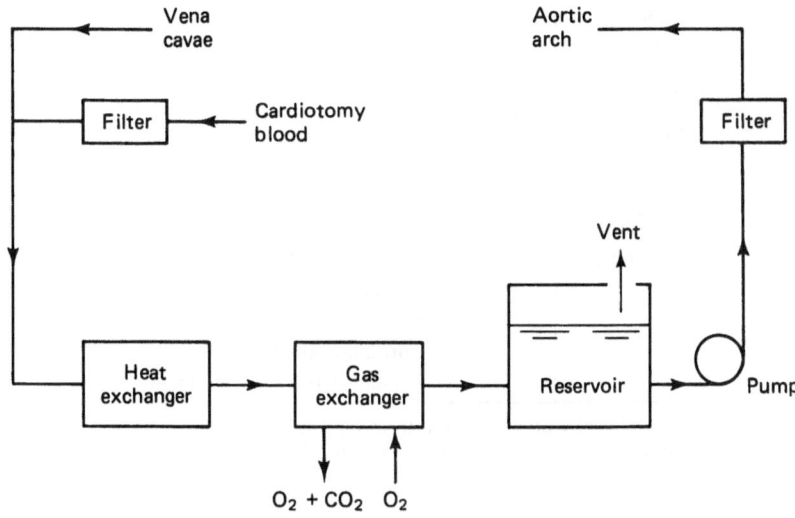

Fig. 2.1. Basic features of the cardiopulmonary bypass extracorporeal circuit.

antithrombotic agent, usually the anticoagulant heparin, perhaps in combination with an antiplatelet agent such as prostacyclin.

In summary, the changes in blood constituents during cardiopulmonary bypass are a consequence of a complex extracorporeal process (Table 2.1) and blood compatibility may be influenced by materials, device design, mode of operation, and the nature of antithrombotic agents. Prior to an examination of the changes occurring in cardiopulmonary bypass, it is convenient to consider relevant features of blood–material interactions and gas exchange devices.

Blood–Material Interactions

Knowledge of blood–material interactions [15–19] indicates that contact of blood with an artificial surface will induce protein adsorption, which may be followed by the reaction of cellular and protein blood components leading to the formation of a thrombus. Alterations to blood components are inevitable. An understanding of these alterations is assisted by first examining reactions occurring in the constituent parts of the processes of haemostasis and thrombosis.

Haemostasis and Thrombosis

The processes of haemostasis and thrombosis include the complex reactions between the endothelium, blood platelets, the coagulation system and the fibrinolytic system [20,21].

Table 2.2. Contents of platelet dense granules and alpha granules

Dense granules	Alpha granules
ADP	Fibrinogen
ATP	Factor V
5-Hydroxytryptamine	Factor VIII: vWF
Calcium	Platelet factor 4
Pyrophosphate	β-thromboglobulin
	Albumin
	Fibronectin
	Thrombospondin
	Platelet-derived growth factor

Reproduced with permission from Ogston D. *The physiology of hemostasis.* Croom Helm, London, 1983.

Blood coagulation occurs as a result of a series of reactions of soluble inactive proteins present in plasma. These proteins (coagulation factors) are pro-enzymes, which are activated in a sequential manner to convert the soluble plasma protein fibrinogen to insoluble fibrin. An integral aspect of blood coagulation and fibrin formation is the role of platelets.

Platelets

The action of platelets in thrombosis can be considered in terms of platelet adhesion, the platelet release reaction and platelet aggregation.

Platelets do not normally adhere to the luminal surface of endothelial cells [22–26] but following vascular injury, platelet adhesion occurs, with the interaction of subendothelial collagen, a platelet membrane glycoprotein and plasma von Willebrand factor (vWF) [27–29]. Adhesion initiates a series of complex, interactive reactions, leading to platelet secretion, with the specific discharge of the contents of the platelet granules in what is termed the platelet release reaction [30]. The contents of the platelet granules are listed in Table 2.2.

A consequence of platelet adhesion and the platelet release reaction is the synergistic action of released adenosine diphosphate (ADP) and synthesized thromboxane A2 (TXA2) in causing the attachment of circulating platelets to each other and to platelets already adhering to the injured surface. The mechanism of platelet aggregation is complex and involves a platelet membrane–fibrinogen receptor complex and calcium-dependent interplatelet bridging by fibrinogen [31–33], with the possibility of this bridging reaction involving other platelet proteins such as fibronectin and thrombospondin [34,35].

Platelet adhesion, release and aggregation act to prevent continuing blood loss and form a temporary haemostatic plug. Formation of a mechanically stable thrombus involves participation of blood coagulation factors. Platelets contribute significantly to the reactions of the coagulation factors by the provision of membrane phospholipids (platelet factor 3) and platelets play an early

Table 2.3. Nomenclature of blood coagulation factors

Factor	Other common names
I	Fibrinogen
II	Prothrombin
III	Tissue thromboplastin
IV	Calcium
V	Proaccelerin, Plasma Ac-globulin, Labile factor
VII	Proconvertin, Stable factor, SPCA
VII	Antihaemophilic factor, AHF, Antihaemophilic globulin, AHG, Antihaemophilic factor A
IX	Plasma thromboplastin component, PTC, Christmas factor, Antihaemophilic factor B
X	Stuart–Prower factor
XI	Plasma thromboplastin antecedent, PTA
XII	Hageman factor, HF
XIII	Fibrin stabilising factor, Fibrinase, Laki–Lorand factor
3	Platelet phospholipid clotting activity
4	Platelet antiheparin activity

Reproduced with permission from Szycher M. In: Szycher M (ed) *Biocompatible polymers, metals, and composites.* Technomic, Lancaster, Pennsylvania, 1983, p 1.
Note: The coagulation factors are all proteins with the exception of factor IV (Ca^{2+}). Factors VI, 1 and 2 are omitted since they were found to be impure macromolecules.

role in these reactions by means of a process involving a factor XI receptor and high molecular weight kininogen (HMWK).

Blood Coagulation Factors

The reactions of the blood coagulation factors (Table 2.3) are conveniently summarized in terms of the intrinsic, extrinsic and common pathways. The routes to thrombus formation utilizing platelets and coagulation factors are depicted in Fig. 2.2.

The intrinsic pathway is initiated by contact of blood with a foreign surface. The activation of factor XII in the presence of kallikrein and HMWK transforms factor XII to the activated form XIIa. This converts factor XI into its activated form, XIa, which in turn activates factor IX. Subsequently factor X is converted to Xa in the presence of a complex consisting of factor IXa, factor VIII, calcium ions and platelet factor 3 (PF3).

The extrinsic pathway is initiated when blood contacts an injured vessel and activation of factor X takes place by the reaction of tissue factor and factor VII in the presence of calcium ions.

In the common pathway, factor Xa, in the presence of PF3, calcium ions and factor V, catalyzes the transformation of prothrombin to thrombin.

The progression to the formation of the fibrin clot involves thrombin, fibrinogen and factor XIII. The conversion of fibrinogen by thrombin into soluble

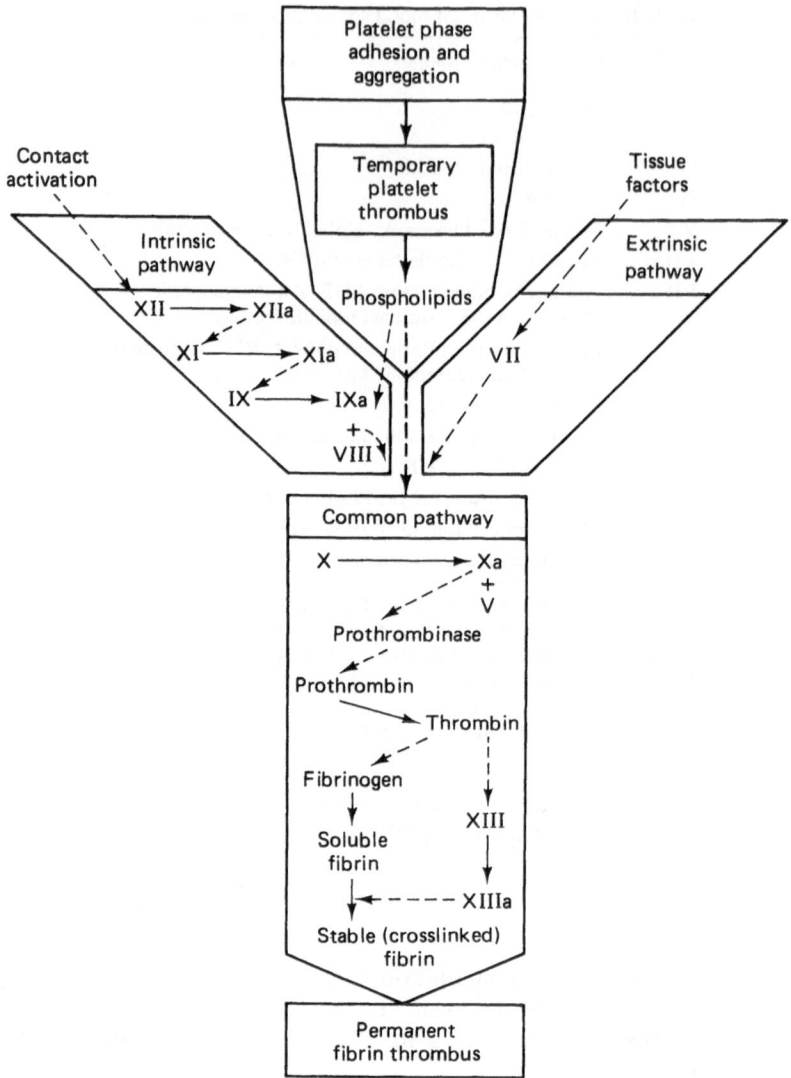

Fig. 2.2. Routes to thrombus formation utilizing platelets and blood coagulation factors. (Reproduced with permission from [17].)

fibrin is followed by the formation of a polymeric fibrin and, under the influence of factor XIIIa, the formation of a cross-linked, insoluble or stabilized fibrin.

Fibrinolysis

The activity of the blood coagulation process in promoting the conversion of soluble fibrinogen to insoluble fibrin is offset by the ability of the fibrinolytic system to dissolve formed fibrin [36]. The fibrinolytic system is a multi-component enzymatic system [37,38], with the enzyme plasmin the essential

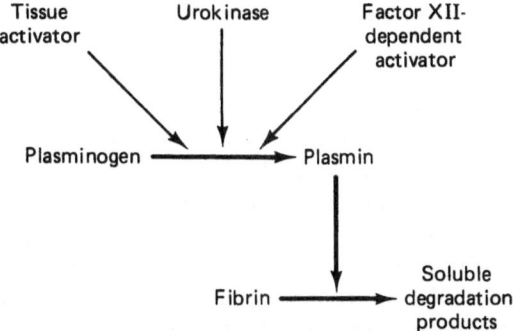

Fig. 2.3. Outline of the fibrinolytic system. (Reproduced with permission from Ogston D. *The physiology of hemostasis.* Croom Helm, London, 1983.)

end product. The key reaction of the fibrinolytic system (Fig. 2.3) is the conversion of plasminogen by plasminogen activators into the protease plasmin, which acts within the thrombus, digesting fibrin to produce thrombus dissolution.

There are different routes to plasminogen activation. In the intrinsic pathway, all the components involved are present in precursor form in the blood. In the extrinsic pathway, the activator originates from tissue or vessel wall and is released into the blood by certain stimuli or trauma. In an exogenous pathway, activating substances such as urokinase or streptokinase are infused for therapeutic purposes.

Regulation and Control

The regulation and control which promote localized thrombus and inhibit extension of a thrombus, are achieved by interactions of the endothelium, the platelets, the coagulation process and the fibrinolytic system.

The endothelium can limit thrombus formation by the release of the platelet anti-aggregating substance prostacyclin (PGI$_2$) [39], the secretion of a plasminogen activator that initiates the fibrinolytic system as well as an inhibitor of plasminogen activation [40,41], the metabolism of proaggregatory ADP released during platelet activation [42], the uptake and degradation of pro-aggregatory vasoactive amines [43], the complexing of thrombin with the glycoprotein antithrombin III [44], and activation of protein natural inhibitors of the blood coagulation system.

Circulating plasminogen may be converted to plasmin by blood components involved in the intrinsic pathway [45] and the release of tissue plasminogen activator is markedly increased by activated protein C generated by the action of thrombin and an endothelial cofactor [46].

Complement System

If it is assumed that body systems involved in the defensive responses to injury function in an integrated manner, consideration should be given to interactions between the haemostatic and complement systems [20,47].

The complement system consists of a group of circulating precursor plasma proteins numbered C1 to C9. These components interact sequentially to bring about systems of inflammation. Complement activation is a series of enzymatic reactions, similar to the coagulation cascade, that results in the cleavage of components leading to the generation of new enzymatic activities and to the formation of complement complexes with additional biological activities [20,48].

Complement activation (Fig. 2.4) takes place via one of two pathways, the classical and the alternative, of which C3 is the pivotal component. The classical pathway is activated by antigen–antibody complexes, including IgG and IgM. Activators of the alternative pathway are primarily polysaccharides but also immune complexes of IgA and IgD as well as endotoxins. The classical pathway is initiated by the activation of C1, a macromolecular complex of the three proteins C1q, C1r and C1s. Activated C1s hydrolyses C2 and C4 to produce C2a, C2b, C4a and C4b respectively. C4b and C3a form a complex known as C3 convertase, a primary activator of C3 [49,50]. The alternative pathway is activated via C3 independently of C1, C2 and C4.

An important feature is that although some components, such as C3b, become bound to the activating surface, the molecules C3a, C4a and C5a are released into the liquid phase. Anaphylatoxins C3a, C4a and C5a are low

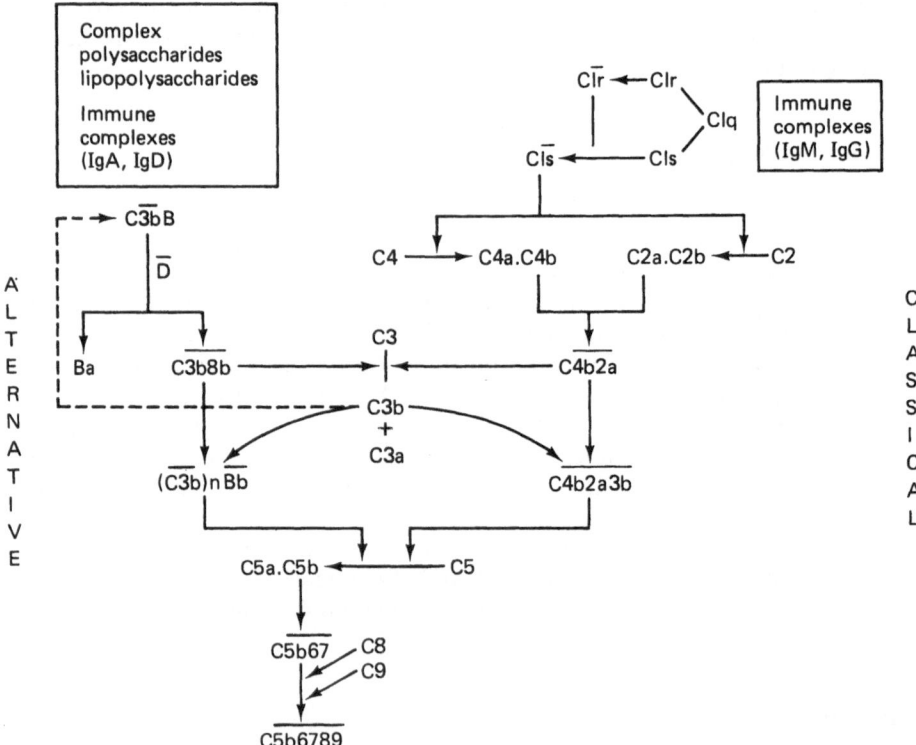

Fig. 2.4. The complement pathways. (Reproduced with permission from Ogston D. in *The physiology of hemostasis.* Croom Helm, London, 1983.)

molecular weight cleavage products which act as inflammatory molecules. They induce degranulation of the mast cells resulting in histamine release. In plasma, C3a and C5a are rapidly transformed to stable des Arg derivatives and may stimulate interleukin 1 release from monocytes.

The complement system interacts with the endothelium, the platelets, the coagulation process and the fibrinolytic system.

Endothelial cells contain receptors for complement components [25,51], there is a possible involvement of complement components in the platelet release reaction [52] and complement may have a role in normal platelet function [20]. The inhibitory effect of C1q on platelet aggregation and adhesion to collagen [53] has been attributed to the collagen-like structure of the sub-component enabling it to compete with collagen for sites on the platelet surface. C1q has an important influence on normal haemostasis by regulating platelet reactivity to collagen. Platelet aggregation and adhesion to collagen are also inhibited by the C1s subcomponent [54].

With respect to an inter-relationship between the complement system and the coagulation process, a possible role for factor XII in complement activation has been raised [55]. The factor XII influence may be indirect and stem from its interaction with kallikrein and plasmin which may themselves activate complement [56] or the influence may be direct, since there is evidence that a factor XII fragment can activate C1 directly rather than through the formation of kallikrein or plasmin [57].

Regarding the fibrinolytic system, it has been suggested that complement components contribute to normal fibrinolysis [58] and that complement activation may induce the formation of plasmin [59]. Interactions between the fibrinolytic and complement systems are further supported by in vitro studies indicating that plasmin is capable of activating C1s [60], C1r [61] and possibly the alternative pathway [62].

Natural and Artificial Surfaces

In a consideration of blood–material interactions, a strong contrast between the behaviour of the natural endothelium and that of artificial surfaces must be expected.

The most important function of the endothelium may be to offer a blood compatible surface [63]. The fundamental observation that platelets, erythrocytes and leucocytes do not adhere to endothelial cells suggests that the endothelium is able to present a non-attractive surface to blood cells [25]. By a variety of mechanisms, endothelial cells prevent adhesion of cells and activation of clotting factors and ensure the removal of thrombus already formed, thereby providing the most compatible surface for blood [24,25,51].

In considering haemostasis, thrombosis and the endothelium, the complex nature of the processes involved [64–66] can be conveniently examined in terms of particular aspects such as platelet activation, intrinsic and extrinsic coagulation, thrombolysis and complement activation. It is possible to adopt a similar approach when considering the events following contact of blood with an artificial surface provided two important distinctions are realized [19,67]:

1. Artificial surfaces cannot perform an active role similar to that achieved by the endothelium through the synthesis and release of specific substances.

2. Artificial materials cannot provide a non-attractive surface comparable to that of the endothelium.

The inability of artificial surfaces to perform an active role means that the application of such surfaces may require simultaneous therapy with anti-coagulants, platelet aggregation inhibitors or plasminogen activators, the utilization of such substances bound to the surface, or the controlled release of such substances from the surface. The failure to provide a non-attractive surface means that platelet adhesion, which is likely on cell surfaces other than endothelial, must be anticipated with artificial materials [68]. In addition, while the endothelium does not appear to adsorb proteins under physiological conditions [16], protein adsorption is a very important feature of the interaction of blood with artificial surfaces [17].

Consequences of Blood Contact with Artificial Surfaces

Protein Adsorption

There is rapid adsorption to artificial surfaces from protein solutions [69–72], plasma [73] or whole blood [74]. Therefore, protein adsorption, which is promoted by the amphipathic (polar/non-polar) character of protein molecules and their limited solubility [75], is inevitable during cardiopulmonary bypass.

While the critical role of the adsorbed protein in blood–material interactions has led to the term "conditioning" layer [18,75,76], the adsorbed protein should not be considered passive [16]. There is the possibility of transient adsorption, denaturation or changes in configuration [77,78].

Blood–material interactions subsequent to protein adsorption are strongly influenced by the composition of the adsorbed protein layer [79,80]. In relation to the influence on platelets, the proteins albumin, fibrinogen and gamma globulin have been most widely studied, with the consensus that platelet adhesion to surfaces is inhibited by prior adsorption of albumin and promoted by prior adsorption of fibrinogen or gamma globulin [81–89]. This beneficial property of albumin has been utilized in the preparation of artificial surfaces with enhanced blood compatibility [19,90].

There is a close relationship between fibrinogen and platelets and information derived from defibrinated or afibrinogenaemic plasma [83,91], ADP-induced platelet aggregation [92], and ADP-stimulated fibrinogen receptors [93–95] supports the possibility that the deposition of fibrinogen on artificial surfaces is associated with specific receptors on adherent platelets and is not independent of platelet deposition [96]. The importance of fibrinogen adsorption for blood–material interactions is emphasized by the following:

1. The replacement of adsorbed fibrinogen by HMWK [97], a protein involved in the activation of the intrinsic coagulation.

2. The possible interaction of fibrinogen with leucocytes [17].

3. The view that the timing of fibrinogen deposition and of its removal from artificial surfaces by blood may have important clinical implications [98].

Adsorption of gamma globulin on artificial surfaces has been reported to promote platelet adhesion and stimulate the platelet release reaction [99] and gamma globulin adsorption may be followed by leucocyte adhesion [100].

The focus on albumin, fibrinogen and gamma globulin is probably too narrow and further investigations of protein–artificial surface interactions are necessary with respect to the composition of the adsorbed protein layer and the possible influence of trace proteins [75]. A protein recommended for further study is fibronectin [17], which can be adsorbed from plasma onto artificial surfaces [101,102]. Although fibronectin may not be involved in platelet adhesion and aggregation [103,104], it has a possible involvement in leucocyte adhesion [98].

Regarding the blood coagulation factors, the extrinsic pathway is usually not activated by the exposure of a biomaterial to blood [17] but intrinsic pathway activation, which is determined by protein adsorption, must be considered. The proteins involved in the activation of the intrinsic pathway are factor XII, factor XI, HMWK and prekallikrein [105]. A sequence of enzymatic reactions is initiated by the adsorption of factor XII and HMWK. A complex formed between bound HMWK and prekallikrein activates factor XII to factor XIIa, which catalyzes the conversion to kallikrein of the prekallikrein involved in the complex with HMWK. Since kallikrein activates factor XII, a cycle of reactions leads to the rapid production of factor XII on or near the artificial surface. The ability of HMWK to form a complex with factor XI makes factor XI available to factor XIIa and ensures the continuation of the coagulation cascade.

Platelet Reactions

The exposure of blood to an artificial surface invariably leads to the adhesion and aggregation of platelets [106,107], with the platelet adhesion strongly influenced by protein adsorption. Platelet interaction with adsorbed fibrinogen or gamma globulin has been attributed to the formation of a complex between incomplete heterosaccharides of these proteins and glycosyl transferases located in the platelet membrane [99,108,109]. This mechanism is similar to that proposed for the platelet–collagen reaction [110]. The inhibition of platelet adhesion by adsorbed albumin might result from the absence of saccharide chains. The adherence of circulating platelets to fibrinogen-covered surfaces leads to a change in platelet shape, coalescence of platelets into an irregular monolayer and, as more platelets adhere, the formation of mounds with erythrocytes and leucocytes entrapped in fibrin [111]. Platelet adhesion to an artificial surface is likely to be followed by the platelet release reaction [30] taking place in the adhering platelets and then platelet aggregation occurring on the surface [112]. Platelet constituents of interest to a study of blood–material interactions [19] include serotonin [5-hydroxytryptamine (5-HT)], beta thromboglobulin (BTG), platelet factor 4 (PF4), TXB2, ADP, and thrombospondin (glycoprotein G).

An interaction between platelets and the intrinsic pathway is likely if blood clotting on an artificial surface proceeds [15]. Intrinsic coagulation may be initiated by thromboplastins liberated from platelets [113,114] or by factor XII activation resulting from platelets stimulated by released ADP. Thrombin formation resulting from intrinsic pathway activation leads to the rapid production of a fibrin monolayer on an artificial surface and the enhancement of platelet adhesion and aggregation [115,116]. Thrombin generation may also induce the platelet release reaction with the secretion of PF4, thromboxane and thrombospondin [117–119].

The platelet response in blood–material contact is influenced by diffusion [120] and shear forces [121], with the shear rate and contact time critical factors for platelet adhesion [122].

Erythrocytes

Erythrocytes can adhere to the adsorbed protein layer [15] and under certain conditions haemolysis occurs, with the platelet release reaction induced by released ADP and erythrocyte ghosts [123]. Erythrocytes may also influence protein adsorption [124,125]. This influence appears to be primarily membrane-related or particle-related, although there is the possibility of an effect arising from the competitive adsorption of released haemoglobin.

In blood–material interactions, promotion by red cells of platelet adhesion is normally assigned to the hydrodynamic behaviour of the cells but contributory factors may be a reduction in the adsorption of platelet-protective proteins or the deposition by the red cells of an adhesive substance [75].

Significant changes in the metabolism of erythrocyte membranes can be caused by blood–material contact; shear-induced haemolysis is possible and in coagulation under low shear forces, entrapped erythrocytes and fibrin form the so-called red thrombus [16].

Leucocytes

In thrombus formation on artificial surfaces, the action of leucocytes differs markedly from the primarily passive role of the erythrocytes [17]. Leucocytes are attracted to the thrombus and in the thrombosis process, leucocytes may contribute to platelet recruitment and fibrin formation by enzymatic release and then participate in fibrinolysis. Consequently, white cell adhesion and function are important topics in blood–material interactions, particularly in extracorporeal applications [126]. Leucocyte adhesion to artificial surfaces has been long recognized [127] and the preferential adsorption of polymorphonuclear leucocytes or granulocytes in comparison to lymphocytes is supported by evidence from leucopheresis [128] and in vitro studies [129,130]. There is an apparent similarity between leucocytes and platelets with respect to sensitivity to mechanical trauma [131]. Leucocyte damage and aggregation are influenced by shear stress and the incorporation of leucocytes into platelet microaggregates [132]. A direct role of leucocytes in thrombus formation resulting from granulocyte adhesion and its effect on platelet aggregation [133] is supported by granulocyte possession of endogenous procoagulant activity and proaggregatory activity [134–136].

Blood–material interactions may induce changes in leucocyte function. White cell damage as a result of blood exposure to artificial surfaces [127] leads to an impairment of phagocytic activity and a reduced ability to combat infection [16].

In recent years, investigation of the response of white blood cells to artificial surfaces in extracorporeal circulation has been linked with the concomitant behaviour of the complement system.

Complement Activation

Activation of the complement system during extracorporeal passage of blood has become a topic of major importance. This has encouraged study of complement activation by surfaces in blood–material interactions, although such study is recent in comparison to that of surface-induced complement activation in immunology [48]. While the focus of interest has been on the relationship between complement activation and the leucopenia occurring in haemodialysis with cellulose membranes [137], complement activation is also relevant for cardiopulmonary bypass [138–148].

Activation of complement components mediates the chemotactic, adhesive and phagocytic responses of polymorphonuclear leucocytes in the inflammatory process, with the anaphylatoxin molecules, C3a, C4a and C5a of particular interest. Leucocyte adhesion to artificial surfaces may also be mediated by the activation of complement components [149].

With haemodialysis, the fact that polysaccharides are known alternative pathway activators supports the view that complement activation by cellulose membranes is via the alternative pathway. There is also evidence that complement activation during cardiopulmonary bypass is initiated by the alternative pathway. However, leucopheresis studies [150] have indicated artificial surfaces may activate complement by a process similar to that of the classical pathway and classical pathway involvement in cardiopulmonary bypass is a possibility [145].

Role of Antithrombotic Agents

Antithrombotic agents are directed towards specific areas of thrombosis. The three types of antithrombotic agents of interest to cardiopulmonary bypass (Table 2.4) are anticoagulants, platelet aggregation inhibitors (antiplatelet agents) and plasminogen activators.

The most widely used antithrombotic agent in extracorporeal processes is the anticoagulant heparin, which operates by potentiating the influence of antithrombin III. By forming a complex with antithrombin III, heparin catalyzes the action of antithrombin III on thrombin [151] and thereby inhibits thrombin, the aggregation of platelets by thrombin, the thrombin-mediated conversion of

Table 2.4. Antithrombotic agents

Type	Example	Action
Anticoagulant	Heparin	Enhances inhibition of proteases by antithrombin III
	Warfin	Vitamin K antagonist
Antiplatelet	Aspirin, sulphinpyrazone	Decreases platelet aggregation and release
	Dipyridamole	Decrease platelet adhesion
	Ticlopidine	Blocks ADP-induced platelet interactions with fibrinogen and von Willebrand factor
	PGI2	Activates adenyl cyclase
Fibrinolytic	Urokinase, streptokinase	Activates plasminogen

fibrinogen to fibrin, and factors Xa, IXa, XIa and XIIa. In order to enhance the blood compatibility of artificial materials, heparin has been ionically and covalently bonded to surfaces and heparin-like materials have been prepared [19,90].

Platelet aggregation inhibitors may be used as a replacement for heparin or in association with heparin during extracorporeal blood circulation. With artificial materials, such agents have been used in immobilized form [152–154] or in controlled release form [155,156].

Fibrinolytic therapy can be achieved by the administration of the plasminogen activators streptokinase and urokinase. Binding of urokinase to artificial materials has been reported [157–159].

Blood Gas Exchange in Extracorporeal Devices

The objective of extracorporeal circulation in cardiac surgery is to provide suitable conditions for intracardiac surgical operations, while maintaining essential physiological tissue and organ perfusion and oxygenation for limited periods of time, with complete return of functional integrity of all parameters of homeostasis after the procedure [160]. The objective is attained by the use of a gas exchange device placed in an extracorporeal blood flow circuit.

Gas Exchange

The achievement of satisfactory gas exchange during extracorporeal circulation has not proved difficult [2]. When flowing blood is exposed to an oxygen-rich gas phase, either directly or through a gas-permeable membrane, oxygen diffuses into the blood plasma under the action of the partial pressure gradient between oxygen in the gas phase and oxygen in the venous blood. This is followed by diffusion of oxygen from the plasma through the red cell membrane to combine with unsaturated haemoglobin. Since the chemical binding of oxygen to haemoglobin is rapid, the limiting factor in oxygenation of flowing blood is the rate of oxygen diffusion through plasma [161] and this rate is dependent on the thickness of the blood film existing in the exchange device.

Carbon dioxide diffuses out of the flowing blood in the gas exchange device as a result of the partial pressure gradient of carbon dioxide between the venous blood and the gas phase. While this gradient is relatively low, the mass flux of carbon dioxide through plasma is so rapid because of its high solubility that carbon dioxide removal always proceeds more efficiently than oxygenation.

Blood Flow

An important consideration for blood flow in cardiopulmonary bypass is that of selecting pulsatile or non-pulsatile perfusion [162]. Since blood flow is normally pulsatile, it would seem advantageous to utilize this mode of flow in extracorporeal circulation. However, the selection of pulsatile or non-pulsatile flow has been controversial (2). Published studies comparing the influence of pulsatile and non-pulsatile flow have been confusing [9], although the apparent inconsistencies in the results obtained can be explained by consideration of the flow rates used during perfusion.

There is evidence [9,163,164] that differences between the effects of pulsatile and non-pulsatile perfusion only become obvious at flow rates less the $100 \, \text{ml} \, \text{kg}^{-1} \, \text{min}^{-1}$. When flow rates of this order have been used in experimental animals [165–168] and in humans [169], differences between pulsatile and non-pulsatile flow have been demonstrated, with pulsatile flow desirable for the preservation of normal function of various organs and systems of the body [9].

Device Utilization

The choice of an oxygenator is related to the ease of application and the possible damage to blood components [2]. There are two basic types of gas exchange device utilized in extracorporeal circuits, viz. direct contact devices, and membrane-based devices. Generally, in direct contact devices oxygen is bubbled directly through blood which is then debubbled through a settling or filtering chamber. In membrane-based devices, a gas exchange membrane is interposed between the gas and blood phases. Examples of both types have been described elsewhere [3].

Direct Contact Devices

At present, bubble oxygenators are widely used because of their ease of assembly and priming and relatively low cost. The traumatic mode of operation of direct contact devices has been linked with damage to blood elements, microemboli formation and protein denaturation, with the effects possibly caused more by the repeated renewal of the interface [170] than by the nature of the interface itself [171,172].

Membrane-Based Devices

The initial impetus to the utilization of membrane oxygenators arose from the belief that an improved physiological response would be achieved by devices operating on the same principle as the human lung. A direct blood–gas contact is avoided by the presence of a permeable membrane between blood and gas phases [173].

Evidence emerged [174] indicating that membrane-based devices were less traumatic to the blood than direct contact devices. This encouraged device design and development [6], and the eventual clinical use of membrane oxygenators for prolonged extracorporeal circulation [170,175], where the less traumatic influence on blood constituents was advantageous [176,177].

Membrane Selection

Membranes in current use or under development may be considered under three categories. These are (a) homogeneous, (b) microporous and (c) composites of types (a) and (b).

Homogeneous membranes have been dominated by the use of polysiloxane or silicone rubber. Prior to the introduction of polysiloxane membranes, the use of crystalline homogeneous polymers such as polyethylene and polytetrafluoroethylene meant that large membrane areas were essential for adequate gas exchange [178] and machines were cumbersome and unreliable [179].

Polysiloxane possesses oxygen and carbon dioxide permeability coefficients several orders of magnitude greater than other homogeneous membranes, primarily because of a lack of crystallinity [178]. The greater solubility of carbon dioxide in polysiloxane in comparison to oxygen leads to a correspondingly higher permeability and a compensation for the disparity in available partial pressure gradients.

The beneficial gas permeability of polysiloxane is offset by poor mechanical strength, which necessitates incorporation of a reinforcing silica filler or casting the membrane onto a reinforcing fabric. Incorporation of carbonate groups in polysiloxane also improves mechanical strength but at the expense of reduced permeability.

Microporous membranes are those having permanent pores (>5 nm diameter) which are deliberately introduced into the membrane during manufacture. Hydrophobic polymers such as polypropylene and polytetrafluoroethylene are selected and the pores permit gas transfer but preclude blood leakage because of surface tension effects. When interposed between two gaseous phases, microporous membranes show little selectivity towards oxygen and carbon dioxide, since these gases are of similar molecular size. However, there is evidence to suggest that diffusion in the pores is altered by the presence of a liquid phase in contact with the membrane [180].

Laboratory and clinical results [181–183] have encouraged the use of micro-porous membranes. The surface of such membranes is a hybrid [179] in that most of the surface is direct gas interface and the remainder hydrophobic polymer. From the blood compatibility aspect, an important question is whether microporous membranes resemble more closely homogeneous membranes or direct blood contact devices [179].

Although not evident in short duration cardiac surgery, problems may arise with the use of microporous membranes in long-term respiratory support. Higher water vapour fluxes may eventually result in the wetting of the pore structure, with consequent exudation of plasma. Reports vary with respect to the time course of such events, which will be dependent on the temperature, flow rate and relative humidity of the ventilating gas.

Composite membranes are produced by casting a layer of polymer onto a microporous membrane [178,184] or through deposition of polymer onto a microporous membrane by plasma polymerization techniques [185,186].

Influence of Cardiopulmonary Bypass on Blood Components

The cardiopulmonary bypass procedure exposes blood to artificial surfaces and the consideration of blood–material interactions and the influence on blood of artificial surfaces points to the inevitability of a platelet response and activation of the intrinsic coagulation. In order to avoid thrombosis, the use of an antithrombotic agent, usually the anticoagulant heparin, is essential. This means that the study of blood–material interactions during cardiopulmonary bypass is largely the study of heparinized blood within extracorporeal systems [187]. From knowledge of the interactions of blood with artificial surfaces (Fig. 2.5), it can be anticipated that such extracorporeal systems will induce damage to blood elements, the release of contents from platelets, erythrocytes and leucocytes and activation of the complement system.

In addition to the influence of artificial surfaces, it is necessary to consider other factors, and of relevance are the nature of the process, circuit priming and microemboli.

Nature of Process

Severe alterations in haemostasis are created by cardiopulmonary bypass pro-cedures [188] and the manner by which body homeostasis is deranged by extracorporeal perfusion is not completely understood [189]. The safety of cardiopulmonary bypass procedures has increased markedly in recent years [190] but in about 5% of patients, the risk of serious haemorrhage remains. The duration of the bypass procedure is a critical factor and recent reductions in the incidence of side effects from cardiopulmonary bypass may represent more efficient surgical techniques rather than improvement in machine design.

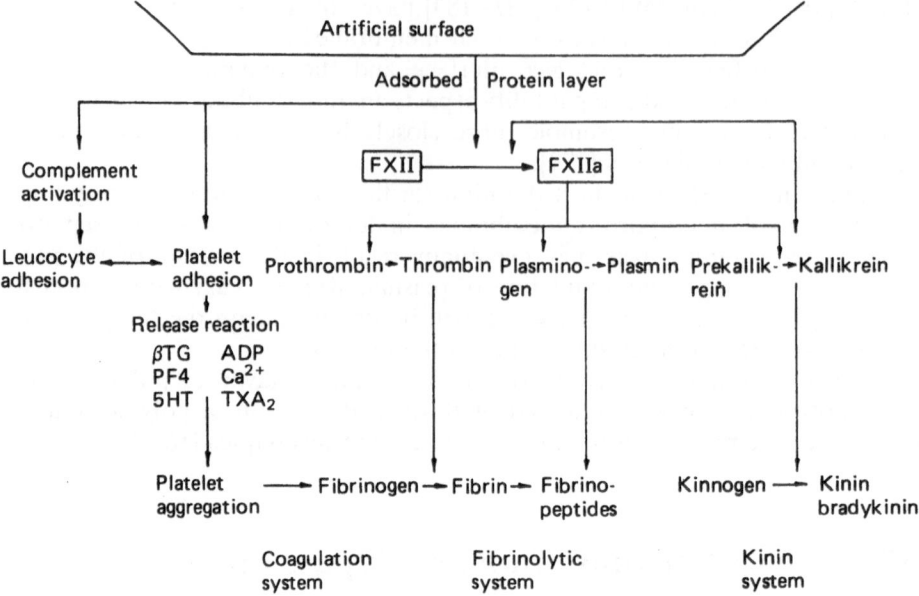

Fig. 2.5. Interactions of the haemostatic and complement systems following contact of blood with an artificial surface.

In addition to the surgical procedure, blood trauma and the reactivity of blood elements in the extracorporeal perfusion systems can be influenced by the following [189,191]:

1. Temperature gradients.
2. Mechanical trauma (shear stresses).
3. Mode of blood flow.
4. Drug administration.

Circuit Priming

The priming volume of the extracorporeal circuit is the summation of the volumes within the gas exchange device, the venous reservoir, connecting lines and circuit filters. The composition of the solution used to prime the circuit may contribute to haematological problems encountered during and after extracorporeal circulation [192].

During the early use of cardiopulmonary bypass, fresh heparinized homologous blood was used as the priming solution [193]. However, problems due to procurement and an incompatibility of pooled homologous blood elements [194] encouraged the use of alternative primes. These primes [160,193] have included acid citrate dextrose (ACD) blood, saline, saline-like solutions, dextrose solution, dextran solution and adjuvant solutions utilizing albumin and Pluronic F68. The addition of albumin has been suggested as a means of reducing platelet deposition [195] and Pluronic F68, an ethylene oxide–propylene oxide copolymer, as a means of reducing haemolysis [196].

An all blood prime provides normal haematocrit and oxygen-carrying capacity but these advantages are offset by increased viscosity, haemolysis and potential for transfusion reaction, hepatitis and blood interaction [2].

The haemodilution induced by the use of non-blood prime has been reported to cause no serious haematological derangement [197]. Haemodilution may offer benefits with respect to a reduction of blood viscosity and haemolysis, and improvement of the microcirculation and preservation of the blood coagulation mechanism [198], although it has been suggested that haemodilution should be recognized as one factor in the overall improvement in haematological alterations after cardiopulmonary bypass [193].

Microemboli

The production of particulate or gaseous microemboli is an important consideration in cardiopulmonary bypass [199] and the significance of emboli in the production of cerebral dysfunction is demonstrated in Table 2.5.

Attention has been drawn [200–202] to the role of microemboli in producing an alteration in cerebral physiology. Implicated in organ dysfunction following open heart surgery have been particulate emboli of aggregated blood elements [203], denatured proteins [204], fat [205,206], calcium [207] and antifoam [208].

Table 2.5. Aetiological factors in cerebal dysfunction during open-heart surgery

A. *Haemodynamic*
  Age of patient
  Duration of heart-lung bypass
  Systemic arterial pressure during heart-lung bypass
  Cerebral blood flow during heart-lung bypass
  Pulsatile versus non-pulsatile flow

B. *Embolic*
  Gaseous microemboli from   (i) heart and pulmonary veins
                             (ii) pump oxygenator

  Foreign material from   (i) oxygenator (cotton fibres, silicone, plastic chips)
                          (ii) pump (spallation of pump tubing)
                          (iii) operative equipment (talcum powder thread, dust, cloth particles)

Red cell, platelet and leucocyte aggregates

Fibrin

Calcium and arteriosclerotic debris

Denatured proteins

Fat globules

Reproduced with permission from: Pearson DT. In: Ionescu MI (ed) *Techniques in extracorporeal circulation*, 2nd edn. Butterworths, 1981, p 155.

Alterations in myocardial and cerebral physiology during cardiac surgery have been attributed to gaseous microemboli originating from the oxygenator, heart and pulmonary veins [209–213].

Particulate emboli can form in stored or donor blood [214,215], with the rate of formation dependent on storage duration and blood anticoagulation [216]. Such emboli may be derived from platelet-fibrin aggregates [217], leucocyte or platelet aggregates, fragmented erythrocytes and denatured proteins [199]. The particulate emboli in donor blood can affect cerebral function [218].

Microemboli produced by the oxygenator are influenced by the type of device. Gaseous microemboli, which are produced by bubble oxygenators [213,219], are believed to be less numerous with membrane oxygenators [176,220].

Particulate emboli may come from the formation of leucocyte and platelet aggregates [221–223], with aggregate formation reduced by the use of membrane oxygenators [223,224].

Cardiotomy suction has been identified as a potent source of particulate [176,225] and gaseous microemboli [213,219,226,227]. In addition, particulate emboli may arise from spallation of polymer tubing used in the circuit pumps [199] or from the use of polysiloxane antifoaming agents [208,228].

The problem of microemboli production during cardiopulmonary bypass has led to the study and utilization of filters [203,219,229–236]. An ideal filter should ensure elimination of aggregates of damaged or non-functional cells, while allowing the passage of normal platelets, erythrocytes and leucocytes [199]. In practice, filters may be regarded as screen filters or depth filters [199,237]. With a screen filter, filtration is mechanical and microemboli are trapped by passage through a mesh of known pore size. In contrast, a depth filter traps microemboli by adsorption. Combination filters have also been used, with blood passing in turn through a first screen filter, a depth filter and a second screen filter of lower porosity than the first [238].

While filtration is important, it is not always beneficial in that a reduction in platelet level may occur [239]. The requirements for a filter are dependent on the type of oxygenator, since certain membrane oxygenators, by virtue of their construction, act as coarse filters for large aggregates.

Alteration to Blood Components

Proteins

The evidence from studies of artificial surfaces in contact with blood [16,75] emphasizes that protein adsorption will be an inevitable consequence of cardiopulmonary bypass. However unlike other extracorporeal procedures such as haemofiltration where protein adsorption is of interest because of the possible influence on the effectiveness of the process [240], in cardiopulmonary bypass the interest in proteins has concentrated not on protein adsorption but on protein denaturation and the tendency to form emboli.

Blood trauma in cardiopulmonary bypass can lead to denaturation of plasma proteins [204] with an increase in circulating lipids [205] and this in turn augments the microemboli load to the patient. Denatured proteins constitute common emboli [192] and such emboli have been implicated in the causation of the widespread organ dysfunction which may follow open heart surgery [204].

Protein denaturation is dependent on the type of device and the denaturation of plasma proteins resulting from the large blood–gas interface area present in the early oxygenators determined the time limit of perfusion [241]. Denaturation of proteins by oxygenators in which there is a blood–gas interface has been demonstrated [204] and the bubble oxygenator has been incriminated in causing denaturation of proteins leading to pulmonary vasculitis with capillary leakage of plasma [242]. The membrane oxygenator, by eliminating the blood–gas interface, reduces protein denaturation and the tendency to form microaggregates. The nature of the membrane is likely to influence the pattern of protein adsorption (Fig. 2.6).

Platelets

The platelet response is a significant feature of blood–material interactions and platelets have been considered to be the most important haemostasis element influenced by cardiopulmonary bypass.

In an examination of the platelet response, both platelet number and platelet function are relevant. While emphasis has been placed on investigations regarding platelet number during cardiopulmonary bypass, the possibility of abnormalities in platelet function has been long recognized [243]. Platelet number and function are strongly influenced by cardiopulmonary bypass. Contact of blood with gaseous or solid surfaces during cardiopulmonary bypass may induce a fall in platelet count [244], the formation of circulating platelet aggregates [223], a loss of platelet sensitivity to activating agents [245,246] and the release of platelet contents [247,248].

There is firm documentation [192] of a decrease in platelet count during cardiopulmonary bypass, although there is uncertainty regarding the precise mechanism. A fall in platelet count occurring with the onset of extracorporeal circulation could result not only from platelet adhesion but also from the formation of platelet aggregates [2,222,249]. In addition, an investigation in dogs using radiolabelled platelets [249] demonstrated a reversible sequestration of platelets in the liver during extracorporeal circulation, thus indicating the possibility that a decrease in platelet count does not necessarily reflect damage induced by the oxygenator.

Platelets are activated and inhibited by cardiopulmonary bypass, with the loss of platelet function regarded as the most significant haematological consequence of cardiopulmonary bypass using bubble or membrane oxygenator systems [250].

Platelet function has been assessed by the determination of platelet adhesion and this determination is influenced by several factors which could be altered by cardiopulmonary bypass. These factors include pH [251], the presence of fibrin degradation products [252], drugs [253], haematocrit [254] and absolute platelet count [255]. Another possible cause of altered platelet function during cardiopulmonary bypass is platelet membrane damage due to contact with

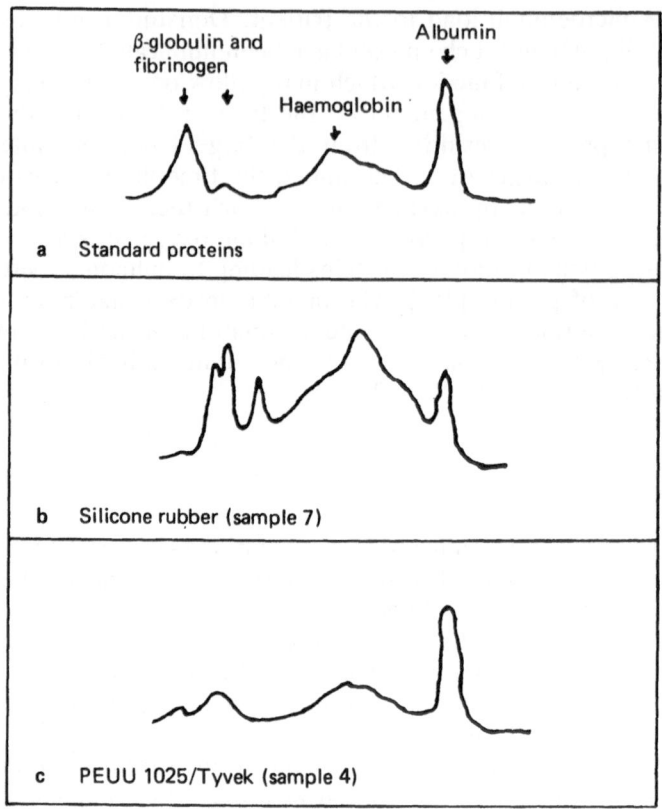

Fig. 2.6. Densitometer scans of three electrophopresis disc gels containing **a** protein standards, and proteins desorbed from **b** silicone rubber and **c** polyurethane membranes. (Reproduced with permission of the publishers, Raven Press, from Knight PM, Lyman DJ. *Artificial Organs*, 1985;9:28.)

artificial surfaces or the action of shear forces [188,250]. While knowledge of the mechanism is incomplete, studies have revealed that a significant platelet function defect is induced in all patients undergoing cardiopulmonary bypass [188].

Platelets release active substances during bypass either in response to activation or from cytolysis [256]. During cardiopulmonary bypass, there are increases in thromboxane B2 and prostacyclin metabolites (6 keto-PGFIa) and the platelets also release serotonin, catecholamines, acid hydrolases, a vascular permeability factor, a chemotactic factor and various coagulation factors.

The release of platelet alpha granules during cardiopulmonary bypass and the synthesis of thromboxane have been reported [246–248,257]. However, the marked increase in platelet factor 4 during bypass is believed to represent only a small amount of the total platelet factor 4 contained within platelets [250]. The evidence that platelets partially release stored dense granule contents with bubble oxygenators [258] led to the hypothesis that an acquired storage pool deficiency in platelets results in reduced platelet function. In contrast, other data [246,250] do not support the hypothesis that reduced platelet function during bypass is due to partial depletion of the contents of alpha granules or dense granules.

Another hypothesis is that a platelet inhibitory factor, capable of protecting platelets from further activation, appears in plasma shortly after blood contact with artificial surfaces in the extracorporeal circulation [250]. No inhibitor has yet been detected but the concept is supported by in vitro investigations [259].

Platelet activation following blood–artificial surface contact causes the formation of platelet aggregates [19]. The generation of platelet aggregate emboli has been considered a feature of the extracorporeal circulation [223]. This generation is followed by a breakdown into individual platelets [260] or disaggregation into the microcirculation [187], although platelet aggregate emboli have been observed in the central nervous system of patients who have died after open heart surgery [261].

Early studies of haemostasis during cardiopulmonary bypass observed significant thrombocytopenia in patients undergoing bypass surgery, with the degree of thrombocytopenia dependent on bypass time [188]. Other investigations [262–264] have failed to find significant thrombocytopenia during cardiopulmonary bypass. Accumulated data [250] indicate that the most profound changes in platelets take place immediately following contact of blood with the artificial surfaces of the extracorporeal circuit. While some continued platelet activation and destruction probably occur throughout bypass, particularly in bubble oxygenator systems, most platelets are not destroyed and do not participate in an irreversible release of contents. There is an inhibition of platelets during bypass and this persists for some hours after the cessation of the procedure. It is not certain whether the restoration of platelet function after bypass is due to the recovery of previously inhibited platelets or to the formation of new platelets. As a result of the platelet response to contact with artificial surfaces during cardiopulmonary bypass, bleeding times are prolonged and blood loss is increased.

Several factors other than the duration of the procedure may influence the platelet response. The surgery itself may cause disruption of blood vessels, with platelet adherence to the exposed subendothelial connective tissue resulting in the release of platelet contents and the promotion of platelet aggregation [176]. The utilization of filters designed to remove circulating platelet aggregates may actually induce platelet aggregation. Cardiotomy suckers, which provide a blood–gas interface, may cause platelet activation and thrombocytopenia [265], although this can be reduced by controlled suction [266].

Evidence [267–273] that platelet damage is less with membrane oxygenators is in agreement with the view [274] that the membrane oxygenator is less traumatic to blood elements. However a different view has been expressed by Edmunds et al. [250], who utilized previous data [223,244–248,257,259, 275], to provide a comparison of the platelet changes taking place during short-term cardiopulmonary bypass with membrane and bubble oxygenator systems. The conclusion drawn was that both systems induce qualitatively similar losses in sensitivity to ADP, similar increases in postoperative bleeding times and similar amounts of postoperative blood loss, thus contradicting the hypothesis that membrane oxygenator systems cause less trauma to patients during routine cardiopulmonary bypass.

With membrane oxygenators, platelet loss may also be reduced by selection of the priming procedure [276].

Different mechanisms for platelet activation by membrane and bubble oxygenators are supported by in vitro and experimental studies involving precoating surfaces with albumin or the addition of prostaglandin E_1 [277,278]. Such procedures have a much greater influence on the inhibition of platelet activation with membrane oxygenators than with bubble oxygenators. In addition, thromboxane synthesis begins immediately after blood contact in bubble oxygenator circuits but not in membrane oxygenator circuits [248,259]. Therefore, it is believed that direct blood contact with gas bubbles causes an additional platelet injury, possibly lysis of a small number of platelets.

Recent data [279] comparing the influence of membrane and bubble oxygenators on platelets are shown for platelet count and platelet release in Fig. 2.7 and Fig. 2.8 respectively.

Blood Coagulation Factors

The numerous studies which have examined and reported coagulation factor deficiencies during cardiopulmonary bypass have led to a wide variety of findings. These may reflect differences in surgical technique and preoperative medication, the selection of pulsatile or non-pulsatile flow, and the application of direct contact or membrane-based devices.

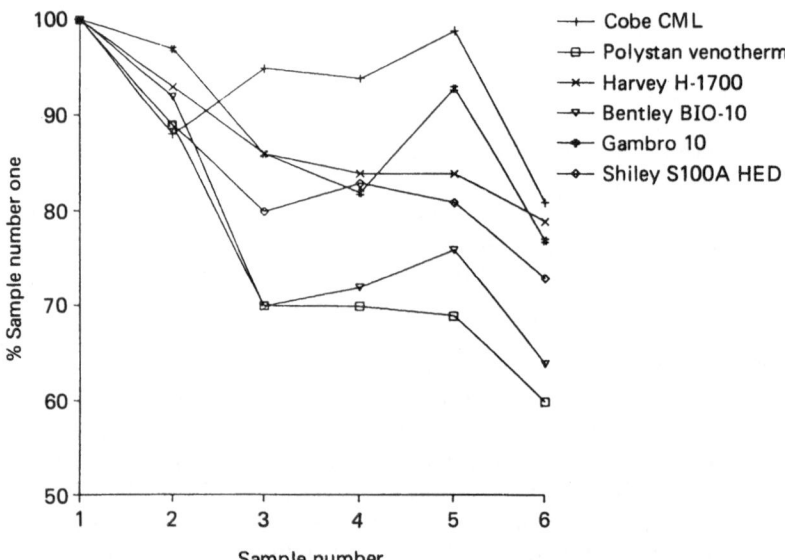

Fig. 2.7. Percentage change in haematocrit corrected mean oxygenator group platelet count (sample 1 = 100%) in five bubble oxygenators and one membrane (Cobe CML) oxygenator. (Reproduced with permission of the publishers, Edward Arnold, from [279].)

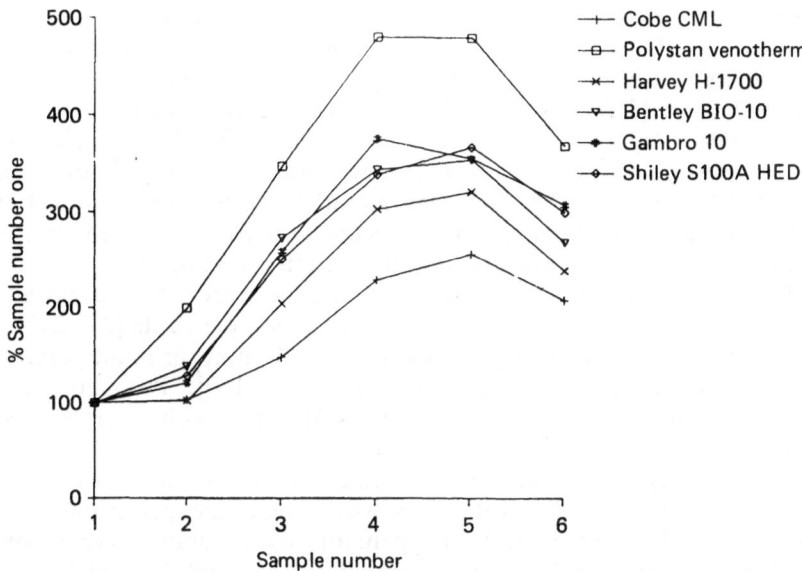

Fig. 2.8. Percentage change in haematocrit corrected mean oxygenator group beta thromboglobulin levels (sample 1 = 100%) in five bubble oxygenators and one membrane (Cobe CML) oxygenator. Reproduced with permission of the publishers, Edward Arnold, from [279].)

The haematological changes contributing to the deranged haemostasis and postoperative complications following open heart surgery include a deficiency of coagulation factors, although the relative importance of the induced deficiencies of the individual coagulation factors is controversial [160]. Blood contact induces adsorption of plasma proteins to the artificial surfaces of the extracorporeal circuit and, while coagulation factors are not selectively adsorbed, dilution and some adsorption routinely decrease factors II, V, VII, VIII, IX and X [246]. The reduction may be up to 20–60% of prebypass concentrations, returning to about 95% of prebypass levels within 20 minutes after bypass.

Determination of the clinical significance of the activity of factor XII (Hageman factor) during cardiopulmonary bypass revealed a gradual increase in factor XII activity, which was significant throughout the procedure [280]. Additionally, factor XII activity remained high during the postoperative period [281], gradually decreasing over 7 days. The pattern of factor XII activity was similar to that reported for the release of granulocyte elastase [282] and is a potential marker of postoperative complications [283].

Erythrocytes

Investigations have studied the mechanical and chemical factors influencing red cell fragility and haemolysis under conditions of gas exposure [284–286] and red cell lysis under controlled conditions [287] and it was shown that chemical factors are important for the predisposition of sensitized red cells to haemolysis. In addition to an immediate lysis of erythrocytes, perfusion can lead to increased cell fragility [288]. Postperfusion anaemia [289] and reduced red blood cell life [290] have been attributed to delayed haemolysis, with the sublethal trauma regarded as important as the immediate haemolysis [291].

Studies performed in relation to the factors influencing erythrocyte destruction in artificial organs [285,291] demonstrated the haemolytic effect of the shear forces and haemolysis can be expected in areas of high shear stresses, cavitation and turbulence. The cardiotomy suction is a major source of haemolysis [199] and aspiration of blood from the pericardium and intracardiac chambers induces microaggregation of formed blood elements [203,292].

Substances released from haemolysed red cells may promote aggregation [174,200] or enhance intravascular coagulability [160]. Probably the most thrombogenic substances released are ADP, red cell membranes and haemoglobin.

When erythrocyte damage was assessed by serum haemoglobin levels, comparisons demonstrated lower levels with membrane perfusions [293,294] and the superiority of membrane oxygenators over bubble oxygenators was also indicated when erythrocyte damage was assessed by red cell lactate dehydrogenase levels [294]. The more traumatic nature of direct contact means that haemolysis is an order of magnitude greater with bubble oxygenators than with membrane oxygenators [274]. Significant haemolysis can occur through mechanical stress during bubble collapse and this is reduced by membrane oxygenators [192].

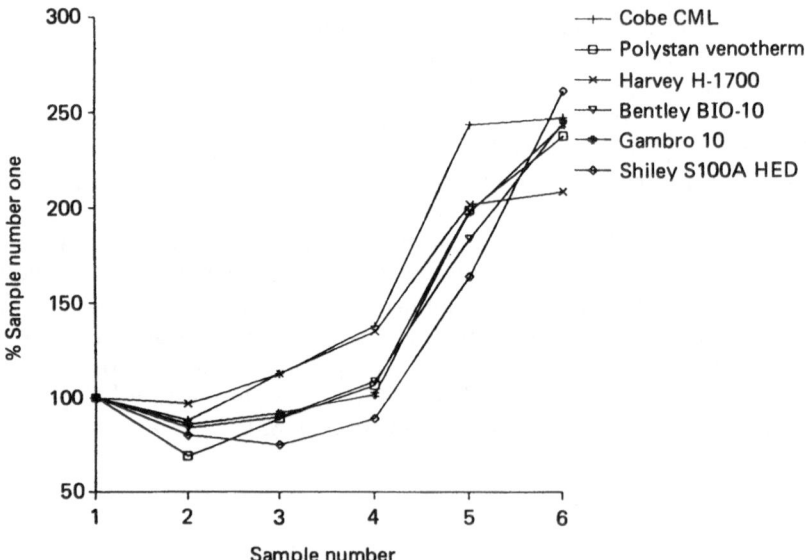

Fig. 2.9. Percentage change in haematocrit corrected mean oxygenator group leucocyte (WBC) count (sample 1 = 100%) in five bubble oxygenators and one membrane (Cobe CML) oxygenator. Reproduced with permission of the publishers, Edward Arnold, from [279].)

Investigations of prolonged extracorporeal circulation in animals [295–297] and in patients [298] indicate that haemolysis is negligible and the survival of radiolabelled red blood cells is not altered by prolonged exposure to artificial surfaces in systems without a gas interface. Haemolysis is an inevitable consequence of extracorporeal circulation for cardiac surgery involving a direct gas interface and coronary suction.

Leucocytes

White cells are activated during cardiopulmonary bypass and decrease in concentration with the onset of extracorporeal circulation [2,299]. This decrease takes place with both bubble and membrane oxygenators (Fig. 2.9). The decrease may be explained partly on the basis of dilution but aggregation and embolization may also occur [2,192].

Sequestration of leucocytes in the lungs has been reported [300] and aggregated leucocytes have been found in the lungs of dogs following cardiopulmonary bypass [139].

Leucocytes release active substances during bypass either in response to activation or from cytolysis [256] and the release of lysosomal enzymes may cause extravasation of plasma into surrounding tissues. Intrapulmonary leucocyte sequestration with release of lysosomal proteolytic enzymes, such as granulocyte elastase, and generation of oxygen-free radicals have been implicated in the mechanism of acute lung injury in the adult respiratory distress syndrome (ARDS) [301–305].

White blood cell count returns to normal by 2–4 hours after institution of bypass [2] but during and after bypass, white cells have reduced metabolism and phagocytosis. Decreased phagocytic function has been demonstrated in dogs [306] and clinically [307].

It has been suggested [299] that leucocyte behaviour during cardiopulmonary bypass is influenced by a plasma factor in a manner similar to the influence of complement component C5a on leucocytes during haemodialysis and C5a is known to activate neutrophils, altering their shape and motility [142,308].

Fibrinolytic System

There are several reports of activation of the fibrinolytic system during and after cardiopulmonary bypass [243,264,309–317].

Fibrinolytic activity, as measured by crosslinked fibrin degradation products (FDPs) has been monitored during cardiopulmonary bypass. FDPs increased steadily during bypass and fibrinolytic activity remained high for a postoperative period of 48 hours.

The generation of plasmin is accompanied by a non-competitive binding of plasmin by antiplasmin [318] and the scarcity of major haemorrhagic complications due to fibrinolysis after open-heart surgery is explained by the fact that the reserve of plasmin is not completely exhausted during bypass [319].

Activation of the fibrinolytic system may occur in the oxygenation procedure or pump-induced accelerated flow rates may activate the plasminogen-plasmin system or alter plasminogen activator activity [188]. However, the pathogenesis of fibrinolytic activation during cardiopulmonary bypass is unclear.

Complement System

It is now believed [320] that a wide variety of pathological events such as sepsis and trauma activate common humoral cascades leading to pulmonary membrane damage, with complement activation of high importance.

Activation of the complement system during cardiopulmonary bypass has been controversial [148], in that while a reduction of complement haemolytic activity has been demonstrated consistently, there has been uncertainty whether this was due to consumption through activation [138], denaturation [144] or interference with haemolytic activity by polyanions such as heparin [321]. The reported complement activation during bypass [141] has now been confirmed for bubble and membrane oxygenators [148] and is probably unrelated to pulsatile flow [146]. Current experiences in cardiopulmonary bypass [320] indicate that extracorporeal circulation itself activates complement and might increase damage in already affected lungs.

During cardiopulmonary bypass, contact of blood with artificial surfaces leads to the release of the anaphylatoxins C3a and C5a [141]. Based on the increase in C3a concentration, similar rates of complement activation have been found with bubble or membrane oxygenators [322], although silicone rubber may produce a shorter lasting complement activation than microporous polypropylene (Fig. 2.10) [320].

In the consideration of the influence of complement activation on cardiopulmonary bypass, comparison has been made with haemodialysis, where it has been demonstrated [323] that the sharp and profound leucopenia observed [324] is mediated by the anaphylatoxin C5a [325]. Interaction with polymorphonuclear leucocytes generates modification and activation of these cells which are then entrapped in the lung microvasculature [142] and this leuco-embolization is believed to cause some cardiac and lung complications of haemodialysis [325]. It is possible that the same pathogenesis is involved in some clinical consequences of cardiopulmonary bypass, in particular the "postperfusion syndrome" or multiorgan failure seen after uneventful bypass [140,141,147,326].

The view that leucopenia and pulmonary leucostasis during cardiopulmonary bypass result from complement activation with the leucopenia dependent on C5a-induced adhesiveness of granulocytes and trapping of cells within the pulmonary microcirculation [322] is supported by evidence from a study performed in sheep depleted of circulating complement prior to the initiation of ECMO [327]. It was also demonstrated that prior complement depletion prevented the acute thrombocytopenia that occurs at the initiation of bypass in normal sheep, thus suggesting that transient thrombocytopenia may be partially mediated by a complement-dependent mechanism analogous to that involved in bypass-induced leucopenia [327].

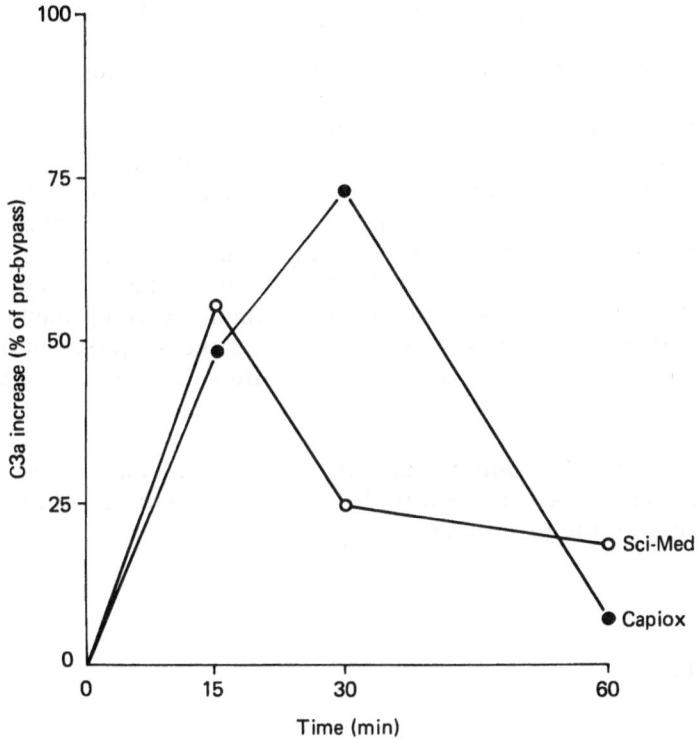

Fig. 2.10. C3a generation by a microporous polypropylene (Capiox) membrane and a silicone rubber (Sci-Med) membrane. Reproduced with permission of the publishers, W.B. Saunders, from [320].)

Modification by Antithrombotic Agents and Surface Treatment

The clinical utilization of cardiopulmonary bypass generally requires operation in association with heparin, an antithrombotic agent directed primarily towards inhibition of the intrinsic coagulation pathway. Extracorporeal circulation using high doses of heparin has been associated with the induction of platelet damage, with reduced platelet count and impaired function, and prolonged bleeding [328]. Possibilities exist for replacing the normal heparin preparation with a lower molecular weight fraction of greater anticoagulant activity [151] or with platelet aggregation inhibitors [328].

Investigations have been made on the use of prostaglandin E_1 or prostacyclin to inhibit platelets during extracorporeal circulation [329,330]. The evidence suggested that doses sufficient to achieve platelet inhibition also cause severe vasodilation and low blood pressures during bypass [329]. Since prostacyclin is not an anticoagulant, it appears preferable to use it in combination with some heparin to prevent activation of the intrinsic coagulation [328]. Another approach is to use a prostacyclin analogue with greater chemical stability and a low vasodilator effect [328].

In addition to selection of antithrombotic agents for influence on the coagulation system, agents with an influence on other body systems can be considered. In this respect, the possible application of a synthetic complement inhibitor has been reported [331].

A possible alternative to the use of antithrombotic agents is modification by surface treatment of the artificial surfaces of the circuit. One approach is protein coating and precoating surfaces with albumin has been shown to inhibit the initial activation of platelets [259]. The replacement of systemic heparinization by surface-bound heparin has been studied in a canine model of ECMO [332] and an evaluation has been made of the ability of heparinized surfaces to provide improved blood compatibility with minimally compromised support function [333]. Future success might depend on the successful utilization of covalent heparin attachment [334], which offers antithrombogenicity with minimal heparin elution.

Acknowledgement. The authors are grateful to Mrs Pauline Turner, Bioengineering Unit, for assistance with the drawings, and to Mrs Shona Ferguson for preparation of the manuscript.

References

1. Spaeth EE. Blood oxygenation in extracorporeal devices: theoretical considerations. Crit Rev Bioeng 1973;1:383
2. Bartlett RH. Gazzaniga AB. Physiology and pathophysiology of extracorporeal circulation. In: Ionescu MI (ed) Techniques in extracorporeal circulation. 2nd edn. Butterworths, London, 1981
3. Gaylor JDS. Artificial organs. In: Kenedi RM (ed) A textbook of biomedical engineering. Blackie, Glasgow, 1980, p 115
4. Gibbon JHJr. The application of a mechanical heart and lung apparatus to cardiac surgery. Minnesota Med 1954;37:171
5. Clowes JHAJr, Hopkins AL, Neville WE. An artificial lung dependent upon diffusion of oxygen and carbon dioxide through plastic membranes. J Thorac Cardiovasc Surg 1956; 32:630
6. Drinker PA. Progress in membrane oxygenator design, Anaesthesiology 1972;37:242
7. Galletti PM. Membrane oxygenation: an overview. In: Kenedi RM Courtney JM, Gaylor JDS, Gilchrist T (eds) Artificial organs. Macmillan, London, 1977, p 11
8. Eberhart RC, Dengle SK, Curtis RM. Mathematical and experimental methods for design and evaluation of membrane oxygenators, Artif Organs 1978;2:19
9. Bregman D, Marrin CAS, Spotnitz HM. Pulsatile flow in extracorporeal circulation. In: Ionescu MI (ed) Techniques in extracorporeal circulation, 2nd edn. Butterworths, London, 1981, p 601
10. Taylor KM. Pulsatile perfusion. In: Taylor KM (ed) Cardiopulmonary bypass principles and management. Chapman and Hall, London, 1986, P 85
11. Awad JA, Morin PJ. Arteriovenous partial perfusion. In: Zapol WM, Qvist J (eds) Artificial lungs for acute respiratory failure. Academic Press, New York, 1976, p 329
12. Borovetz HS, Hardesty RL, Griffith BP, Deeb GM, and Hung T-K. Arteriovenous extracorporeal membrane oxygenation for partial respiratory support. In: Ionescu MI (ed) Techniques in extracorporeal circulation, 2nd edn. Butterworths, London, 1981, p 643
13. Drukker W, Parsons FM, Maher JF. (eds) Replacement of renal function by dialysis. Martinus Nijhoff, The Hague, 1978

14. Courtney JM, Gaylor JDS, Klinkman H, Holtz M. Polymer membranes. In: Hastings GW, Ducheyne P. (eds) Macromolecular biomaterials. CRC Press, Boca Raton, 1984, p 143
15. Feijen J. Thrombogenesis caused by blood-foreign surface interaction. In: Kenedi RM, Courtney JM, Gaylor JDS, Gilchrist T (eds) Artificial organs. Macmillan, London, 1977, p 235
16. Bruck SD. Properties of biomaterials in the physiological environment. CRC Press, Boca Raton, 1980
17. Szycher M. Thrombosis hemostasis, and thrombolysis at prosthetic interfaces. In: Szycher M (ed) Biocompatible polymers, metals, and composites. Technomic, Lancaster, Pennsylvania, 1983, p 1
18. Klinkmann H. The role of biomaterials in the application of artificial organs. In: Paul JP, Gaylor JDS, Courtney JM, Gilchrist T (eds) Biomaterials in artificial organs. Macmillan, London, 1984, p 1
19. Forbes CD, Courtney JM. Thrombosis and artificial surfaces. In: Bloom AL, Thomas DP (eds) Haemostasis and thrombosis. Churchill Livingstone, Edinburgh, 1981, p 902
20. Ogston D. The physiology of hemostasis. Croom Helm, London, 1983
21. Sixma JJ. Role of blood vessel platelet and coagulation interactions in haemostasis. In: Bloom AL, Thomas DP (eds) Haemostasis and thrombosis. Churchill Livingstone, Edinburgh, 1981, 253
22. Spaet TH, Gaynor E. Vascular endothelial damage and thrombosis, Adv Cardiol, 1970;4:47
23. Danon D, Skutelsky E. Endothelial surface charge and its possible relationship to thrombogenesis, Ann NY Acad Sci 1976;275:47
24. Mason RG, Sharp DE. Chuang HYK, Mohammad SF. The endothelium: roles in thrombosis and hemostasis. Arch Pathol Lab Med 1977;101:61
25. Mason RG, Mohammad SF, Saba HI, Chuang HYK, Lee EL, Balis JU. Functions of endothelium. Pathobiol Ann 1979;9:1
26. Cazenave JP, Dejana E, Kinlough-Rathbone R, Packham MA, Mustard JF. Platelet interactions with the endothelium and the subendothelium: the role of thrombin and prostacyclin. Haemostasis 1979;8:183
27. Weiss HJ, Tschopp TB, Baumgartner HR, Sussman II, Johnson MM, Egan JJ. Decreased adhesion of giant (Bernard-Soulier) platelets to subendothelium. Further implications on the role of the von Willebrand factor in haemostasis. Am J Med 1974;57:920
28. Sakariassen KS, Bolhuis PA, Sixma JJ. Human blood platelet adhesion to artery subendothelium is mediated by factor VIII- von Willebrand factor bound to the subendothelium. Nature 1979;279:636
29. Nurden AT, Caen JP. The different glycoprotein abnormalities in thrombasthenic and Bernard-Soulier platelets. Semin Hematol 1979;16:234
30. Holmsen H, Day HJ, Stormorken J. The blood platelet release reaction. Scand J Haematol. Suppl 1969;8:1
31. Bennett JS, Vilaire G. Exposure of platelet fibrinogen receptors by ADP and epinephrine. J Clin Invest 1979;64:1393
32. Bennett JS, Vilaire G, Burch JW. A role for prostaglandins and thromboxanes in the exposure of platelet fibrinogen receptors. J Clin Invest 1981;68:981
33. Marguerie GA, Plow EF. Interaction of fibrinogen with its platelet receptor: kinetics and effect of pH and temperature. Biochemistry 1981;20:1074
34. Ginsberg MH, Painter RG, Forsyth J, Birdwell C, Plow EF. Thrombin increases expression of fibrinogen antigen on the platelet surface. Proc Natl Acad Sci USA 1980,77.1049
35. Jaffe EA, Leung LLK, Nachman RL, Levin RI, Mosher DF. Thrombospondin is the endogenous lectin of human platelets, Nature 1982;295:246
36. McNicol GP, Douglas AS. The fibrinolytic enzyme system. In: Biggs R (ed) Human blood coagulation, haemostasis and thrombosis, 2nd edn. Blackwell, Oxford 1976, p 399
37. Robbins KC, Summaria L. Biochemistry of fibrinolysis. Thromb Diath Haemorrh Suppl 1971;47:9
38. Collen D. On the regulation and control of fibrinolysis. Thromb Haemost 1980;43:77
39. Moncada S, Higgs EA, Vane JR. Human arterial and venous tissues generate prostacyclin (prostaglandin X), a potent inhibitor of platelet aggregation. Lancet 1977;i:18
40. Loskutoff DJ, Edgington TS. Synthesis of a fibrinolytic activator and inhibitor by endothelial cells. Proc Natl Acad Sci USA 1977;74:3903

41. Loskutoff DJ, Edgington, TS. An inhibitor of plasminogen activator in rabbit endothelial cells. J Biol Chem 1981;256:4142
42. Lieberman GE, Lewis GP, Peters TJ. A membrane-bound enzyme in rabbit aorta capable of inhibiting adenosine-diphosphate-induced platelet aggregation. Lancet 1977;ii:330
43. Johnson AR, Erdos EG. Metabolism of vasoactive peptides by human endothelial cells in culture: angiotensin I converting enzyme (kininase II) and angiotensinase. J Clin Invest 1977;59:684
44. Lollar P, Owen WG. Clearance of thrombin from circulation in rabbits by high-affinity binding sites on endothelium: possible role in the inactivation of thrombin by antithrombin III. J Clin Invest 1980;66:1222
45. Kaplan AP. Initiation of the intrinsic coagulation and fibrinolytic pathways of man: the role of surfaces, Hageman factor, prekallikrein, high molecular weight kininogen, and factor XI. Prog Hemost Thromb 1978;4:127
46. Comp PC, Esmon CT. Generation of fibrinolytic activity by infusion of activated protein C into dogs. J Clin Invest 1981;68:1221
47. Zimmerman TS. The coagulation mechanism and the inflammatory response. In: Miescher PA, Muller-Eberhard HJ (eds) Textbook of immunopathology, 2nd edn. Grune and Stratton, New York, 1976, p 95
48. Herzlinger GA. Activation of complement by polymers in contact with blood. In: Szycher M (ed) Biocompatible polymers, metals, and composites. Technomic, Lancaster, Pennsylvania 1983, p 89
49. Katzatchkine MD, Carreno MP. Activation of the complement system between blood and artificial surfaces. Biomaterials 1988;9:30
50. Katzatchkine MD. Mechanism of human alternative complement pathway activation. In: Polymers in medicine and surgery. Plastics and Rubber Institute, London, 1989, p 19/1
51. Thorgeirsson G, Robertson ALJr. The vascular endothelium – pathobiologic significance. Am J Pathol 1978;93:803
52. Chater BV. The role of membrane bound complement in the aggregation of mammalian platelets by collagen. Br J Haematol 1976;32:515
53. Wautier JL, Souchon H, Reid KBM, Peltier AP, Caen JP. Studies on the mode of reaction of the first component of complement with platelets: interaction between collagen-like portion of C1q and platelets. Immunochemistry 1977;14:763
54. Wautier JL, Legrand YJ, Fauvel F, Caen JP. Inhibition of platelet collagen interactions by the C1s subcomponent of the first component of complement. Thromb Res 1981;21:3
55. Donaldson VH. Mechanisms of activation of C1 esterase in hereditary angioneurotic edema plasma in vitro. The role of Hageman factor, a clot-promoting agent. J Exp Med 1968; 127:411
56. Gigli I, Mason JW, Colman RW, Austen KF. Interaction of kallikrein with C1 esterase inhibitor (C1aINH), J Immunol 1968;101:814
57. Ghebrehiwet B, Silverberg M, Kaplan AP. Activation of the classical pathway of complement by Hageman factor fragment, J Exp Med 1981;153:665
58. Moroz LA, Gilmore NJ. Fibrinolysis in normal plasma and blood: evidence for significant mechanisms independent of the plasminogen-plasmin system. Blood 1976;48:531
59. Sundsmo JS, Wood LM. Activated factor B (Bb) of the alternative pathway of complement activation cleaves and activates plasminogen. J Immunol 1981;127:877
60. Ratnoff OD, Naff GB. The conversion of C1s to C1 esterase by plasmin and trypsin. J Exp Med 1967;125:337
61. Cooper NR, Miles LA, Griffen JH. Activation of C1, the first complement component, by purified plasma kallikrein and plasmin. Thromb Haemost 1979;42:251
62. Brade V, Nicholson A, Bitter-Suermann D, Hadding U. Formation of the C3-cleaving properdin enzyme on zymosan. Demonstration that factor D is replaceable by proteolytic enzymes. J Immunol 1974;113:1735
63. Mohammad SF, Mason RGJr, Eichwald EJ, Shively JA. Healthy and impaired vascular endothelium. In: Lasslo A (ed) Blood platelet function and medicinal chemistry. Elsevier Biomedical, New York, 1984, p 129
64. Mustard JF, Packham MA. Normal and abnormal haemostasis. Br Med Bull 1977;33:187
65. Ratnoff OD. The surface-mediated initiation of blood coagulation and related phenomena. In: Ogston D, Bennett B (eds) Haemostasis. Biochemistry physiology and pathology. Wiley, London, 1977, p 25

66. Ratnoff OD, Forbes CD. (eds) Disorders of haemostasis, Grune and Stratton, London, 1984
67. Forbes CD, Prentice CRM. Thrombus formation and artificial surfaces. Br Med Bull 1978; 34:201
68. Spaet TH. Blood and biomaterials: a glimpse at the elephant, Ann NY Acad Sci 1977;283:2
69. Brash JL, Lyman DJ. Adsorption of plasma proteins in solution to uncharged hydrophobic polymer surfaces. J Biomed Mater Res 1969;3:175
70. Berger S, Salzman EW. Thromboembolic complication of prosthetic devices. Prog Hemost Thromb 1974;2:273
71. Bagnall RD. Adsorption of plasma proteins on hydrophobic surfaces. II. Fibrinogen and fibrinogen-containing protein mixtures. J Biomed Mater Res 1978;12:203
72. Chan BMC, Brash JL. Adsorption of fibrinogen on glass: reversibility aspects. J Coll Int Sci 1981;82:217
73. Vroman L, Adams AL, Klings M, Fischer GC, Munoz PC, Solensky RP. Reactions of formed elements of blood with plasma proteins at interfaces. Ann NY Acad Sci 1977; 283:65
74. Gendreau RM, Winters S, Leininger RI, Fink D, Hassler CR, Jakobsen RJ. Fourier transform infrared spectroscopy of protein adsorption from whole blood: ex vivo dog studies. Appl Spectros 1981;35:353
75. Brash JL. Protein adsorption and blood interactions. In: Szycher M (ed) Biocompatible polymers metals and composites. Technomic, Lancaster, Pennsylvania 1983, p 35
76. Baier RE. The organization of blood components near interfaces. Ann NY Acad Sci 1977; 283:17
77. Lee WH Jr. Hairston P. Structural effects on blood proteins at the gas-blood interface. Fed Proc 1971;30:1615
78. Ihlenfeld JV, Cooper SL. Transient in vivo protein adsorption onto polymeric biomaterials. J Biomed Mater Res 1979;13:577
79. Baier RE, Loeb GI, Wallace GT. Role of an artificial boundary in modifying blood proteins. Fed Proc 1971;30:1523
80. Lyman DJ, Metcalf LC, Albo DJr, Richards KF, Lamb J. The effect of chemical-structure and surface properties of synthetic polymers on the coagulation of blood. III. In vivo adsorption of proteins on polymer surfaces. Trans Am Soc Artif Intern Organs 1974;20:474
81. Packham MA, Evans G, Glynn MF, Mustard JF. The effect of plasma proteins on the interaction of platelets with glass surfaces. J Lab Clin Med 1969;73:686
82. Salzman EW, Merrill EW, Binder A, Wolf CRW, Ashford TP, Austen WJ. Protein-platelet interaction on heparinized surfaces. J Biomed Mater Res 1969;3:69
83. Zucker MB, Vroman L. Platelet adhesion by fibrinogen adsorbed onto glass. Proc Soc Exp Biol Med 1969;131:318
84. Lyman DJ, Klein KG, Brash JL, Fritzinger BK. The interaction of platelets with polymer surfaces. Thromb Diath Haemorrh 1970;23:120
85. Jenkins CSP, Packham MA, Guccione MA, Mustard JF. Modification of platelet adherence to protein-coated surfaces. J Lab Clin Med 1973;81:280
86. Whicher SJ, Brash JL. Platelet-foreign surface interactions: release of granule constituents from adherent platelets J Biomed Mater Res 1978;12:181
87. Neumann AW, Moscarello MA, Zingg W, Hum OS, Chang SK. Platelet adhesion from human blood to bare and protein coated polymer surfaces. J Pol Sci Pol Symp 1979;66:391
88. Adams GA, Feuerstein IA. Visual fluorescent and radio-isotopic evaluation of platelet accumulation and embolization. Trans Am Soc Artif Intern Organs 1980;26:17
89. Absolom DR, Zingg W, Policova Z, Neumann AW. Determination of the surface tension of protein coated materials by means of the advancing solidification front technique. Trans Am Soc Artif Intern Organs 1983;29:146
90. Fougnot C, Labarre D, Jozefonwicz J, Jozefowicz M. Modifications to polymer surfaces to improve blood compatibility. In: Hastings GW, Ducheyne P (eds) Macromolecular biomaterials CRC Press. Boca Raton, 1984, p 215
91. Mason RG, Read MS, Brinkhous KM. Effect of fibrinogen concentration on platelet adhesion. Proc Soc Exp Biol Med 1971;137:680
92. Mustard JF, Perry DW, Ardie NG, Packham MA. Preparation of suspensions of washed platelets from humans. Br J Haematol 1972;22:193
93. Plow EF, Marguerie GA. Participation of ADP in the binding of fibrinogen to thrombin-stimulated platelets. Blood 1980;56:553

94. Kornecki E, Niewiarowski S, Morinelli TA, Kloczewiak M. Effects of chymotrypsin and adenosine diphosphate on the exposure of fibrinogen receptors on normal and Glanzmann's thrombasthenic platelets. J Biol Chem 1981;256:5696

95. Di Minno G, Thiagarajan P, Perussia B, Martinez J, Shapiro S, Trinchieri G, Murphy S. Exposure of platelet fibrinogen-binding sites by collagen, arachidonic acid, and ADP: inhibition by a monoclonal antibody to the glycoprotein 11b-111a complex. Blood 1983;61:140

96. Young BR, Lambrecht LK, Albrecht RM, Mosher DF, Cooper SL. Platelet-protein interactions at blood-polymer interfaces in the canine test model. Trans Am Soc Artif Intern Organs 1983;29:442

97. Vroman L, Adams AL, Fischer GC, Munoz PC. Interaction of high molecular wieght kininogen, factor XII, and fibrinogen in plasma at interfaces. Blood 1980;55:156

98. Vroman L, Protein/surface interaction. In: Szycher M (ed) Biocompatible polymers metals and composites. Technomic, Lancaster, Pennsylvania 1983, p 81

99. Evans G. Mustard JF. Platelet-surface reaction and thrombosis. Surgery 1968;64:273

100. Adams AL, Fischer GC, Vroman L. The complexity of blood at simple interfaces. J Coll Int Sci 1978;65:468

101. Adams GA, Feurstein IA. How much fibrinogen or fibronectin is enough for platelet adhesion? Trans Am Soc Artif Intern Organ 1981;27:219

102. Grinnell F, Feld MK. Adsorption characteristics of plasma fibronectin in relationship to biological activity. J Biomed Mater Res 1981;15:363

103. Harfenist EJ, Izzotti MJ, Packham MA, Mustard JF. Plasma fibronectin is not involved in ADP-induced aggregation of rabbit platelets. Thromb Haemost 1980;44:108

104. Sochynsky RA, Boughton BJ, Burns J, Sykes BC, McGee JO'D. The effect of human fibronectin on platelet collagen adhesion. Thromb Res 1980;18:521

105. Griffin JH, Cochrane SG. Recent advances in the understanding of contact activation reactions. Sem Thromb Hemost 1979;5:254

106. Mason RG. The interaction of blood hemostatic elements with artificial elements. Prog Hemost Thromb 1972;1:141

107. Mason RG, Mohammad SF, Chuang HYK, Richardson PD. The adhesion of platlelets to subendothelium, collagen and artificial surfaces. Sem Thromb Hemost 1976;3:98

108. Kim SW, Lee RG, Oster H, Coleman D, Andrade JD, Lentz DJ, Olsen, D. Platelet adhesion to polymer surfaces. Trans Am Soc Artif Intern Organs 1974;20:449

109. Lee RG, Kim SW. The role of carbohydrate in platelet adhesion to foreign surfaces. J Biomed Mater Res 1974;8:393

110. Jamieson GA. Role of glycoproteins in platelet function. In: Gerlach E, Moser K, Deutsch E, Wilmanns W (eds) Erythrocytes, thrombocytes, leukocytes: recent advances in membrane and metabolic research. Thieme, Stuttgart, 1973, p 209

111. Salzman EW, Lindon J, Brier D. Merrill EW, Surface-induced platelet adhesion, aggregation, and release. Ann NY Acad Sci 1977;283:114

112. Baumgartner HR, Muggli R, Tschopp TB, Turitto VJ. Platelet adhesion release and aggregation in flowing blood: effects of surface properties and platelet function. Thromb Haemost 1976;35:124

113. Walsh PN. Platelet-coagulant protein interactions. In: Colman RW, Hirsh J, Marder VJ, Salzman EW (eds) Hemostasis and thrombosis: basic principles and clinical practice. Lippincott, Philadelphia 1982, p 404

114. Needleman SW, Hook JC. Platelets and leukocytes. In: Colman RW, Hirsh J, Marder VJ Salzman EW (eds) Hemostasis and thrombosis: basic principles and clinical practice. Lippincott, Philadelphia, 1982, p 716

115. Waugh DF, Baughman DJ. Thrombin adsorption and possible relations to thrombus formation. J Biomed Mater Res 1969;3:145

116. Chuang HYK, Crowther PE, Mohammad SF, Mason RG. Interactions of thrombin and antithrombin III with artificial surfaces. Thromb Res 1979;14:273

117. Shuman MA, Levine SP. Relationship between secretion of platelet factor 4 and thrombin generation during in vitro blood clotting. J Clin Invest 1980;65:307

118. Patrono C, Ciabattoni G, Pinca E, Pugliese F, Castrucci G, De Salvo A, Satta MA, Peskar BA. Low dose aspirin and thromboxane B_2 production in healthy subjects. Thromb Res 1980;17:317

119. Phillips DR, Jennings LK, Prasanna HR. Ca^{2+}-mediated association of glycoprotein G (thrombin-sensitive protein, thrombospondin) with human blood. J Biol Chem 1980;255: 11629
120. Feuerstein IA, Brophy JM, Brash JL. Platelet transport and adhesion to reconstituted collagen and artificial surfaces. Trans Am Soc Artif Intern Organs 1975;21:427
121. Richardson PD, Mohammad SF, Mason RG. Flow chamber studies of platelet adhesion at controlled, spatially varied shear rates. Proc Europ Soc Artif Organs 1977;4:175
122. Rieger H. Dependency of platelet aggregation (PA) in vitro on different shear rates. Thromb Haemost 1980;44:166
123. Stormorken H. Platelets, thrombosis and hemolysis. Fed Proc 1971;30:1551
124. Brash JL, Uniyal S. Adsorption of albumin and fibrinogen to polyethylene in presence of red cells. Trans Am Soc Artif Intern Organs 1976;22:253
125. Uniyal S, Brash JL, Degterev IA. Influence of red blood cells and their components on protein adsorption. Am Chem Soc Adv Chem 1982;199:277
126. Lindsay RM, Mason RG, Kim SW, Andrade JD, Hakim RM. Blood surface interactions. Trans Am Soc Artif Intern Organs 1980;26:603
127. Kusserow B, Larrow R, Nichols J. Perfusion-and surface-induced injury in leucocytes. Fed Proc 1971;30:1516
128. Wright DJ, Kauffman JC, Terpstra GK, Graw RG, Deisseroth AB, Gallin JI. Mobilization and exocytosis of specific (secondary) granules by human neutrophils during adherence to nylon wool in filtration leukapheresis (FL). Blood 1978;52:770
129. Lederman DM, Cumming RD, Petschek HE, Levine PH, Krinsky NI. The effect of temperature on the interaction of platelets and leukocytes with materials exposed to flowing blood. Trans Am Soc Artif Intern Organs 1978;24:557
130. Absolom DR, Neumann AW, Zingg W, van Oss CJ. Thermodynamic studies of cellular adhesion. Trans Am Soc Artif Intern Organs 1979;25:152
131. Dewitz TS, Hung TC, Martin RR, McIntire LV. Mechanical trauma in leukocytes. J Lab Clin Med 1977;90:728
132. Dewitz TS, Martin RR, Solis RT, Hellums JD, McIntire LV. Microaggregate formation in whole blood exposed to shear stress. Microvasc Res 1978;16:263
133. Cumming RD. Important factors affecting initial blood-material interactions. Trans Am Soc Artif Intern Organs 1980;26:304
134. Niemitz J. Coagulant activity of leukocytes. Tissue factor activity. J Clin Invest 1972;51:307
135. Saba HJ, Herion JC, Walker RI, Roberts HR. The procoagulant activity of granulocytes. Proc Soc Exp Biol Med 1973;142:614
136. Harrison MJ, Emmons PR, Mitchell JR. The effect of white cells on platelet aggregation. Thromb Diath Haemorrh 1966;16:105
137. Farrell PC. Biocompatibility aspects of extracorporeal circulation. In: Paul JP, Gaylor JDS, Courtney JM, Gilchrist T (eds) Biomaterials in artificial organs. Macmillan, London, 1984, p 342
138. Parker DJ, Cantrell JW, Karp RB, Stroud RM, Digerness SB. Changes in serum complement and immunoglobulins following cardiopulmonary bypass. Surgery 1972;71:824
139. Ratliff NB, Young WG Jr, Hackel DB, Mikat E, Wilson JW. Pulmonary injury secondary to extracorporeal circulation: an ultrastructural study. J Thorac Cardiovasc Surg 1973;65:425
140. Haslam PL, Townsend PJ, Branthwaite MA. Complement activation during cardiopulmonary bypass. Anaesthesia 1980;35:22
141. Chenoweth DE, Cooper SW, Hugli TE, Stewart RW, Blackstone EH, Kirklin JW. Complement activation during cardiopulmonary bypass: evidence for generation of C3a and C5a anaphylatoxins. N Engl J Med 1981;304:497
142. Hammerschmidt DE, Stroncek DF, Bowers TK, Lammi-Keefe CJ, Kurth DM, Ozalins A, Nicoloff DM, Lillehei RC, Craddock PR, Jacob HS. Complement activation and neutropenia during bypass. J Thorac Cardiovasc Surg 1981;81:370
143. White JV. Complement activation during cardiopulmonary bypass. N Engl J Med 1981;305:51
144. Boralessa H, Shifferli JA, Zaimi F, Watts E, Whitwam JG, Rees AJ. Perioperative changes in complement associated with cardiopulmonary bypass. Br J Anaesth 1982;54:1047
145. Jones HM, Mathews N, Vaughan RS, Stark JM. Cardiopulmonary bypass and complement activation. Involvement of classical and alternative pathways. Anaesthesia 1982;37:629

146. Boscoe MJ, Yewdall VMA, Thompson MA, Cameron JS. Complement activation during cardiopulmonary bypass: quantitative effects of methylprednisolone and pulsatile flow. Br Med J 1983;287:1747

147. Westaby S. Complement and the damaging effects of cardiopulmonary bypass. Thorax 1983;38:321

148. Collett B, Alhaq A, Abdullah NB, Korjtsas L, Ware RJ, Dodd NJ, Alimo E, Ponte J, Vergani D. Pathways to complement activation during cardiopulmonary bypass. Br Med J 1984;289:1251

149. Herzlinger GA, Cumming RD. Role of complement activation in cell adhesion to polymer blood contact surfaces. Trans Am Soc Artif Intern Organs 1980;26:165

150. Nusbacher J, Rosenfeld SJ, Macpherson JL, Thiem PA, Leddy JP. Nylon fiber leukapheresis: associated complement component changes and granulocytopenia. Blood 1978;51:359

151. Rosenberg RD. Heparin-antithrombin system. In: Colman RW, Hirsh J, Marder VJ, Salzman EW (eds) Hemostasis and thrombosis: basic principles and clinical practice. Lippincott, Philadelphia, 1982, p 962

152. Grode GA, Pitman J, Crowley JP, Leininger RI, Falb RD. Surface-immobilized prostaglandin as a platelet protective agent. Trans Am Soc Artif Intern Organs 1974;20:38

153. Marconi W, Bartoli F, Mantovani E, Pittalis F, Settembri L, Cordova C, Musca A, Alessandri C. Development of new antithrombogenic surfaces by enploying platelet anti-aggregating agents: preparation and characterization. Trans Am Soc Artif Intern Organs 1979;25:280

154. Ebert CD, Lees ES, Kim SW. The antiplatelet activity of immobilized prostacyclin. J Biomed Mater Res 1982;16:629

155. McRea JC, Kim SW. Characterization of controlled release of prostaglandin from polymer matrices for thrombus prevention. Trans Am Soc Artif Intern Organs 1978;24:746

156. McRea JC, Ebert CD, Kim SW. Prostaglandin releasing polymers – stability and efficacy. Trans Am Soc Artif Intern Organs 1981;27:511

157. Kusserow BK, Larrow RW, Nichols JE. The surface bonded, covalently crosslinked urokinase synthetic surface. In vitro and chronic in vivo studies. Trans Am Soc Artif Intern Organs 1973;19:8

158. Sugitachi A, Tanaka M, Kawahara T, Takagi K. Antithrombogenicity of UK-immobilized polymer surfaces. Trans Am Soc Artif Intern Organs 1980;26:274

159. Ohshiro T, Kosaki G. Urokinase immobilized on medical polymeric materials: fundamental and clinical studies. Artif Organs 1980;4:58

160. Ionescu MI, Tandon AP, Roesler MF, Mary DAS. Blood loss following extracorporeal circulation for heart valve surgery. In: Ionescu MI (ed) Techniques in extracorporeal circulation. 2nd edn. Butterworths, London, 1981, p 345

161. Bartlett RH, Kittredge D, Noyes BSJr, Willard RH III, Drinker PA. Development of a membrane oxygenator: overcoming blood diffusion limitation. J Thorac Cardiovasc Surg 1969;58:795

162. Mavroudis C. To pulse or not to pulse. Ann Thorac Surg 1978;25:259

163. Harrison TS, Chawla RC, Seton JF, Robinson BH. Carotid sinus origin of adrenergic responses compromising the effectiveness of artificial circulatory support. Surgery 1970;68:20

164. Harrison TS, Seton JF. An analysis of pulse frequency as an adrenergic excitant in pulsative circulatory support, Surgery 1973;73:868

165. Replogle R, Levy M, Dewall RA, Lillehei RC. Catecholamine and serotonin response to cardiopulmonary bypass. J Thorac Cardiovasc Surg 1962;44:638

166. Shepard RB, Kirklin JW. Relation of pulsatile flow to oxygen consumption and other variables during cardiopulmonary bypass. J Thorac Cardiovasc Surg 1969;58:694

167. Sanderson JM, Wright G, Sims FW. Brain damage in dogs immediately following pulsatile and non-pulsatile flows in extracorporeal circulation. Thorax 1972;27:275

168. Dunn J, Kirsch MM, Harness J, Carroll M, Straker J, Sloan H. Hemodynamic, metabolic, and hematologic effects of pulsatile cardiopulmonary bypass. J Thorac Cardiovasc Surg 1974;68:138

169. Trinkle JK, Helton NE, Wood RE, Bryant LR. Metabolic comparison of a new pulsatile pump and a roller pump for cardiopulmonary bypass. J Thorac Cardiovasc Surg 1969;58:562

170. Bartlett RH, Gazzaniga AB. Extracorporeal circulation for cardiopulmonary failure. Curr Prob Surg 1978;15:1

171. Kayser KL. Blood-gas interface oxygenators versus membrane oxygenators: what are the proved differences? Ann Thorac Surg 1974;17:459
172. Peirce ECII. Is the blood-gas interface of clinical importance? Ann Thorac Surg 1974;17: 526
173. Bramson ML, Osborn JJ, Gerbode F. The membrane lung. In: Ionescu MI (ed) Techniques in extracorporeal circulation. 2nd edn. Butterworths, London, 1981, p 63
174. Lee WHJr, Krumbaar D, Derry G, Sachs D, Lawrence SH, Clowes GHAJr, Maloney JVJr. Comparison of the effects of membrane and non-membrane oxygenators on the biochemical and biophysical characteristics of blood. Surg Forum 1961;12:200
175. Zapol WM. Qvist J (eds) Artificial lungs for acute respiratory failure, Academic Press, New York, 1976
176. Solis RT, Kennedy PS, Beall ACJr, Noon GP, DeBakey ME. Cardiopulmonary bypass: microembolization and platelet aggregation. Circulation 1975;52:103
177. Beall ACJr, Solis RT, Kakvan M, Morris GCJr, Noon GP, DeBakey ME. Clinical experience with the Teflon disposable membrane oxygenator. Ann Thorac Surg 1976;21:144
178. Courtney JM, Gaylor JDS. Artificial membranes, In: McAinsh TF (ed) Physics in medicine & biology encyclopedia. Medical physics, bioengineering and biophysics. Pergamon Press, Oxford, 1985, p 21
179. Cosgrove DM, Loop FD. Clinical use of the Travenol TMO membrane oxygenator. In: Ionescu MI (ed) Techniques in extracorporeal circulation. 2nd edn. Butterworths, London, 1981, p 83
180. Gilroy K, Brighton E, Gaylor JDS. Fluid vortices and mass transfer in a curved channel artificial membrane lung. Am Inst Chem Eng J 1977;23:106
181. Gille JP, Trudell L, Snider MT, Borsanyi AS, Galletti PM. Capability of the microporous, membrane-lined, capillary oxygenator in hypercapnic dogs. Trans Am Soc Artif Intern Organs 1970;16:365
182. Eiseman. B, Birnbaum D, Leonard R, Martinez FJ. A new gas permeable membrane for blood oxygenators. Surg Gynecol Obstet 1972;135:732
183. Murphy W, Trudell LA, Friedman LI, Kakvan M, Richardson PD, Karlson K, Galletti PM. Laboratory and clinical experience with a microporous membrane oxygenator. Trans Am Soc Artif Intern Organs 1974;20:278
184. Ketteringham J, Zapol W, Birkett J, Nelsen L, Massucco A, Raith C. A high permeability, nonporous, blood compatible membrane for membrane lungs: in vivo and in vitro performance. Trans Am Soc Artif Intern Organs 1975;21:224
185. Chawla AS. Preparation of silicone coated biomaterials using plasma polymerizations and their preliminary evaluations. Trans Am Soc Artif Intern Organs 1979;25:287
186. Piskin E, Evren V. Composite membranes for extracorporeal gas exchange. Life Support Systems 1986;4, Suppl 1:2
187. Uziel L, Colombo A, Cacciabue E, Cugno M, Agostini A. Extracorporeal circulation. Problems and answers. In: Dawids S, Bantjes A (eds) Blood compatible materials and their testing. Martinus Nijhoff, Hingham, MA, 1986, p 29
188. Bick RL. Alterations of hemostasis associated with surgery, cardiopulmonary bypass surgery, and prosthetic devices. In: Ratnoff OD, Forbes CD (eds) Disorders of hemostasis. Grune & Stratton, London, 1984, p 379
189. Edmunds LHJr, Stephenson LW. Cardiopulmonary bypass for open heart surgery. In: Glenn WWL, Baue AA, Lindskog BS (eds) Thoracic and cardiovascular surgery. Appleton-Century-Crofts, New York, 1982, p 1091
190. Forbes CD. Thrombosis and artificial surfaces. In: Bloom AC, Thomas DP (eds) Haemostasis and thrombosis. Churchill Livingstone, Edinburgh, 1981, p 761
191. Edmunds LHJr. Pulseless cardiopulmonary bypass. J Thorac Cardiovasc Surg 1982;84:800
192. de Leval MR, Hill JD, Mielke CH. Haematological aspects of extracorporeal circulation. In: Ionescu, M (ed) Techniques in extracorporeal circulation. 2nd edn. Butterworths, London, 1981, p 369
193. Edie RN, Haubert SM, Malm JR. The use of haemodilution and a non-haemic prime for cardiopulmonary bypass. In: Ionescu MI (ed) Techniques in extracorporeal circulation. 2nd edn. Butterworths, London, 1981, p 179
194. Gadboys HL, Slonim R, Litwak RS. Homologous blood syndrome. I. Preliminary observations on its relationship to clinical cardiopulmonary bypass. Ann Surg 1962;156:793

195. Landé AJ, Edwards L, Bloch JH, Carlson RG, Subramanian VA, Ascheim RS, Scheidt S, Fillmore S, Killip T, Lillehei CW. Clinical experience with emergency use of prolonged cardiopulmonary bypass with a membrane pump oxygenator. Ann Thorac Surg 1970;10:409

196. Vasko KA, Riley AM, DeWall RA, Poloxalkol (Pluronic F68): a priming solution for cardiopulmonary bypass. Trans Am Soc Artif Intern Organs 1972;18:526

197. Hara M, Maris M, Crumpler J, Corn B, Perkins WH. Effect of various priming solutions upon red cell mass. plasma volume, and extracellular fluid volume of dogs following hemodilution technique of extracorporeal circulation. J Thorac Cardiovasc Surg 1967;53:354

198. Peirce EC II. Extracorporeal circulation for open-heart surgery. Thomas, Springfield, 1969

199. Pearson DT. Cardiotomy reservoirs and blood filters. In: Ionescu MI (ed) Techniques in extracorporeal circulation, 2nd edn. Butterworths, London, 1981, p 155

200. Allardyce DB, Yoshida SH, Ashmore PG. The importance of microembolism in the pathogenesis of organ dysfunction caused by prolonged use of the pump oxygenator. J Thorac Cardiovasc Surg 1966;52:706

201. Patterson RH, Kessler J. Microemboli during cardiopulmonary bypass detected by ultrasound. Surg Gynec Obstet 1969;129:505

202. Solis RT, Noon GP, Beall AC, DeBakey ME. Particulate microembloism during cardiac operation. Ann Thorac Surg 1974;17:332

203. Osborn JJ, Swank RL, Hill JD, Aguilar MJ, Gerbode F, Clinical use of a Dacron wool filter during perfusion for open-heart surgery. J Thorac Cardiovasc Surg 1970;60:575

204. Lee WHJr. Krumharr D, Fonkalsrud EW, Schjeide OA, Maloney JVJr. Denaturation of plasma proteins as a cause of morbidity and death after intracardiac operations. Surgery 1961: 50I 29

205. Caguin F, Carter MG. Fat embolization with cardiotomy with the use of cardiopulmonary bypass. J Thorac Cardiovasc Surg 1963;46:665

206. Evans EA, Wellington JS, Emboli associated with cardiopulmonary bypass. J Thorac Cardiovasc Surg 1964;48:323

207. Baglio CM, Hunter WC. Calcific arterial embolization accompanying commisurotomy. J Thorac Cardiovasc Surg 1959;37:490

208. Cassie AB, Riddell AG, Yates PO. Hazard of antifoam emboli from a bubble oxygenator. Thorax 1960;15:22

209. Starr A. The mechanism and prevention of air embolism during correction of congenital cleft mitral valve. J Thorac Cardiovasc Surg 1960;39:808

210. Groves LK, Effler DB. A needle-vent safeguard against systemic air embolism in open-heart surgery. J Thorac Cardiovasc Surg 1964;47:349

211. Fishman NH, Carlsson E, Roe BB. The importance of the pulmonary veins in systemic air embolism following open-heart surgery. Surgery 1969;66:655

212. Lawrence GH, McKay HA, Sherensky RT. Effective measures in the prevention of intra-operative aeroembolus. J Thorac Cardiovasc Surg 1971;62:731

213. Gallagher EG, Pearson DT. Ultrasonic identification of sources of gaseous microemboli during open heart surgery. Thorax 1973;28:295

214. Moseley RV, Doty DB. Changes in the filtration characteristics of stored blood. Ann Surg 1970;171:329

215. Wright G, Sanderson JM. Cellular aggregation and destruction during blood circulation and oxygenation. Thorax 1976;31:405

216. Swank RL. Alteration of blood on storage: measurement of adhesiveness of "aging" platelets and leucocytes and their removal by filtration. N Engl J Med 1961;265:728

217. McNamara JJ, Boatright F, Burran EL, Molot MD, Summers E, Stremple JF. Changes in some physical properties in stored blood. Ann Surg 1971;174:58

218. Patterson RHJr. Wasser JS, Porro RS. The effect of various filters on microembolic cerebro-vascular blockade following cardiopulmonary bypass. Ann Thorac Surg 1974;17:464

219. Loop FD, Szabo J, Rowlinson RD, Urbanek K, Events related to microembolism during extracorporeal perfusion in man: effectiveness of in-line filtration recorded by ultrasound. Ann Thorac Surg 1976;21:412

220. Karlson KE, Murphy WR, Kakvan M, Anthony P, Cooper GN, Richardson PD, Galletti PM. Total cardiopulmonary bypass with a new Teflon membrane oxygenator. Surgery 1974; 76:935

221. Ashmore PG, Svitek V, Ambrose P. The incidence and effects of particulate aggregation and microembolism in pump-oxygenator systems. J Thorac Cardiovasc Surg 1968;55:691

222. Dutton RC, Edmunds LHJr. Measurement of emboli in extracorporeal perfusion systems. J Thorac Cardiovasc Surg 1973;65:523
223. Dutton RC, Edmunds LHJr, Hutchison JC, Roe BB. Platelet aggregate emboli produced in patients during cardiopulmonary bypass with membrane and bubble oxygenators and blood filters. J Thorac Cardiovasc Surg 1974;67:258
224. Subramanian VA, Berger RL. Comparative evaluation of a new disposable rotating membrane oxygenator with bubble oxygenator. Ann Thorac Surg 1976;21:48
225. Clark RE, Dietz DR, Miller JG. Continuous detection of microemboli during cardiopulmonary bypass in animals and man. Circulation 54, (6 Suppl. 3) 1976;111:74
226. Solis RT, Scott MA, Kennedy PS, Wilson RK. Filtration of cardiotomy reservoir blood. J Extracorporeal Tech 1976;8:69
227. Pearson DT, Watson BG, Waterhouse PS. An ultrasonic analysis of the comparative efficiency of various cardiotomy reservoirs and micropore blood filters. Thorax 1978;33:352
228. Valentin N, Vilhelmsen R. Blood and tissue silicone in extracorporeal circulation. J Cardiovasc Surg 1976;17:20
229. Swank RL, Porter JA. Disappearance of micro-emboli transfused into patients during cardiopulmonary bypass. Transfusion 1963;3:192
230. Patterson RHJr, Twichell JB. Disposable filter for \microemboli: use in cardiopulmonary bypass and massive transfusion. J Am Med Assoc 1971;215:76
231. Patterson R, Kessler J, Bergland RM. A filter to prevent cerebral damage during experimental cardiopulmonary bypass. Surg Gynec Obstet 1971;132:71
232. McNamara JJ, Burran EL, Suehiro G. Effective filtration of banked blood. Surgery 1972; 71:594
233. Solis RT, Gibbs MB. Filtration of the microaggregates in stored blood. Transfusion 1972; 12:245
234. Ashmore PG, Swank RL, Gallery R, Ambrose P, Pritchard KH. EFfect of Dacron wool filtration on the microembolic phenomenon in extracorporeal circulation. J Thorac Cardiovasc Surg 1972;63:240
235. Egeblad K, Osborn JJ Burns W, Hill JD, Gerbode F. Blood filtration during cardiopulmonary bypass. J Thorac Cardiovasc Surg 1972;63:384
236. Guidoin R, Laperche Y, Martin L, Awad J, Winchester J. Disposable filters for microaggregate removal from extracorporeal circulation. J Thorac Cardiovasc Surg 1976;71:502
237. Roesler MF, Tandon AP, Ionescu MI. Clinical use of the Shiley oxygenating system. In: Ionescu MI (ed) Techniques in extracorporeal circulation. 2nd edn. Butterworths, London, 1981, p 129
238. Marshall BE, Wurzel HA, Neufed GR, Klineberg PL. Effects of Intersept micropore filtration of blood on microaggregates and other constituents. Anaethesiology 1976;44:525
239. Barrett J, Dhurandhar HN, Miller E, Litwin MS. A comparison in vivo of Dacron wool (Swank) and polyester mesh (Pall) micropore blood transfusion filters in the prevention of pulmonary microembolism associated with massive transfusion. Ann Surg 1975;182:690
240. Lehmann HD, Biesinger U, Bergkvist G, Goehl H, Weber H, Krauth E, Kulbe KD. Haemofilter efficiency as a result of membrane charge and wettability. In: Paul JP, Gaylor JDS, Courtney JM, Gilchrist T (eds) Biomaterials in artificial organs. Macmillan, London, 1984, p 238
241. Hill JD. Prolonged extracorporeal oxygenation for pulmonary insufficiency. In: Ionescu MI (ed) Techniques in extracorporeal circulation. 2nd edn. Butterworths, London, 1981, p 627
242. Neville WE, Kontaxis A, Gavin T, Clowes GHAJr. Postperfusion pulmonary vasculitis: its relationship to blood trauma. Arch Surg 1963;86:126
243. Signori EE, Penner JA, Kahn DR. Coagulation defects and bleeding in open-heart surgery. Ann Thorac Surg 1969;8:521
244. Salzman EW. Blood platelets and extracorporeal circulation. Transfusion 1963;3:274
245. McKenna R, Bachman F, Whittaker B, Gibson JR, Weinberger MJr. The hemostatic mechanism after open-heart surgery. II. Frequency of abnormal platelet functions during and after extracorporeal circulation. J Thorac Cardiovasc Surg 1975;70:298
246. Harker LA, Malpass TW, Branson HE, Hessel EA II, Slichter SJ. Mechanism of abnormal bleeding in patients undergoing cardiopulmonary bypass: acquired transient platelet dysfunction associated with selective α-granule release. Blood 1980;56:824
247. Davies GC, Sobel M, Salzman EW. Elevated plasma fibrinopeptide A and thromboxane B_2 levels during cardiopulmonary bypass. Circulation 1980;61:808

248. Addonizio VPJr, Smith JB Strauss JF III, Colman RW, Edmunds LHJr. Thromboxane synthesis and platelet secretion during cardiopulmonary bypass with a bubble oxygenator. J Thorac Cardiovasc Surg 1980;79:91

249. de Leval M, Hill JD, Mielke H, Bramson MI, Smith C, Gerbode F. Platelet kinetics during extracorporeal circulation. Trans Am Soc Artif Intern Organs 1972;18:355

250. Edmunds LHJr. Ellison N, Colman RW, Niewiarowski S, Rao AK, Addonizio VPJr, Stephenson LW, Edie RN. Platelet function during cardiac operation. Comparison of membrane and bubble oxygenators. J Thorac Cardiovasc Surg 1982;83:805

251. Hellem AJ. The adhesiveness of human blood platelets in vitro, Scand J Clin Lab Invest 12 (Suppl. 1) 1, 1960

252. Kowalski E, Kopec M, Wegrzynowicz Z. Influence of fibrinogen degradation products (FDP) on platelet aggregation, adhesiveness and viscous metamorphosis. Thromb Diath Haemorrh 1964;10:406

253. Mustard JF, Packham MA. Factors influencing platelet function: adhesion, release, and aggregation. Pharmacol Rev 1970;22:97

254. Adams T, Schutz L, Goldberg L. Platelet function abnormalities in the myeloproliferative disorders. Scand J Haematol 1974;13:215

255. Bick RL, Fekete LF. Cardiopulmonary bypass hemorrhage: aggravation of pre-op ingestion of antiplatelet agents. Vasc Surg 1979;13:277

256. Edmunds LHJr, Addonizio VPJr. Platelet physiology during cardiopulmonary bypass. In: Utley JR (ed) Pathophysiology and techniques of cardiopulmonary bypass. Williams & Wilkins, Baltimore, 1981, p 106

257. Hennessey VLJr, Hicks RE, Niewiarowski S, Edmunds LHJr, Colman RW. Function of human platelets during extracorporeal circulation. Am J Physiol 1977;232:H622

258. Beurling-Harbury C, Galvan CA. Acquired decrease in platelet secretory ADP associated with increased postoperative bleeding in post-cardiopulmonary bypass patients and in patients with severe valvular heart disease. Blood 1978;52:13

259. Addonizio VPJr, Macarak EJ, Nicolaou KC, Edmunds LHJr, Colman RW. Effects of prostacyclin and albumin on platelet loss during an in vitro simulation of extracorporeal circulation. Blood 1979;53:1033

260. Hicks RE, Dutton RC, Ries CA, Price DC, Edmunds LHJr. Production and fate of platelet aggregate emboli during venovenous perfusion. Surg Forum 1973;24:250

261. Hill JD, Aguilar MJ, Baranco A, Gerbode F. Neuropathological manifestations of cardiac surgery. Ann Thorac Surg 1969;7:409

262. de Vries SI, van Creveld S, Groen P, Müller E, Wettermark M. Studies on the coagulation of the blood in patients treated with extracorporeal circulation. Thromb Diath Haemorrh 1961;5:426

263. Müller N, Popov-Cenic S, Buttner W, Kladetzky RG, Egli H. Studies of fibrinolytic and coagulation factors during open heart surgery. II. Postoperative bleeding tendency and changes in the coagulation system. Thromb Res 1975;7:589

264. Bick R, Schmalhorst W, Crawford L, Holterman M, Arbegast N. The hemorrhagic diathesis created by cardiopulmonary bypass. Am J Clin Pathol 1975;63:588

265. Edmunds LHJr, Saxena NC, Hillyer P, Wilson TJ. Relationship between platelet count and cardiotomy suction return. Ann Thorac Surg 1978;25:306

266. ten Duis HT, de Jong JCF, van Asseldonk AGM, Smit Sibinga CTh, Wildevuur ChRH. Improved hemocompatibility in open heart surgery. Trans Am Soc Artif Intern Organs 1978;24:656

267. Liddicoat JE, Bekassy SM, Beall ACJr, Glaeser DH, DeBakey ME, Membrane vs bubble oxygenator: clinical comparison. Ann Surg 1975;181:747

268. Siderys H, Herod GT, Halbrook H, Pittman JN, Rubush JL, Kaselbaker V, Berry GRJr. A comparison of membrane and bubble oxygenation as used in cardiopulmonary bypass in patients. J Thorac Cardiovasc Surg 1975;69:708

269. Wright JS, Fisk GC, Torda TA, Stacey RB, Hicks RG. Some advantages of the membrane oxygenator for open-heart surgery. J Thorac Cardiovasc Surg 1975;69:884

270. Mortensen JD. Evaluation of tests for blood damage produced by oxygenators. Trans Am Soc Artif Intern Organs 1977;23:747

271. Clark RE, Beauchamp RA, Magrath RA, Brooks JD, Ferguson TB, Weldon CS. Comparison of bubble and membrane oxygenators in short and long perfusions. J Thorac Cardiovasc Surg 1979;78:655

272. de Jong JCF, Smit Sibinga CTh, Wildevuur ChRH. Platelet behaviour in extracorporeal circulation (ECC). Transfusion 1979;19:72
273. Peterson KA, Dewanjee MK, Kaye MP. Fate of indium III-labelled platelets during cardiopulmonary bypass performed with membrane and bubble oxygenators. J Thorac Cardiovasc Surg 1982;84:39
274. Peirce ECII. The membrane versus bubble controversy. Ann Thorac Surg 1980;29:497
275. Kendall AG, Lowenstein L. Alterations in blood coagulation and hemostasis during extracorporeal circulation. Can Med Assoc J 1962;87:786
276. Osada H, Ward CA, Duffin J, Nelems JM, Cooper JD. Microbubble elimination during priming improves biocompatibility of membrane oxygenators. Am J Physiol 1978;234:H646
277. Addonizio VPJr, Strauss JFIII, Colman RW. Edmunds LHJr. Effects of prostaglandin E_1 on platelet loss during in vivo and in vitro extracorporeal circulation with a bubble oxygenator. J Thorac Cardiovasc Surg 1979;77:119
278. Addonizio VPJr, Macarak EJ, Niewiarowski S, Colman RW, Edmunds LHJr. Preservation of human platelets with prostaglandin E_1 during in vitro simulation of cardiopulmonary bypass. Circ Res 1979;44:350
279. Pearson DT, McArdle B, Poslad SJ, Murray A. A clinical evaluation of the performance characteristics of one membrane and five bubble oxygenators: haemocompatibility studies. Perfusion 1986;1:81
280. Irvine L. Blood-biomaterial interactions: investigations into granulocyte elastase release and contact phase activation. PhD thesis, University of Strathclyde, Glasgow, 1989
281. Sundaram S. Investigation of contact phase activation during in vitro blood–biomaterial contact and cardiopulmonary bypass. MSc thesis, University of Strathclyde, Glasgow, 1989
282. Riegel W, Spillner G, Schlosser V, Hörl WH. Plasma levels of main granulocyte components during cardiopulmonary bypass. J Thorac Cardiovasc Surg 1988;95:1014
283. Schrader J, Gallimore MJ, Eisenhauer T, Isemer FE, Schoel G, Warneke G, Bruggeman M, Scheler F. Parameters of the kallikrein-kinin, coagulation and fibrinolytic systems as early indicators of kidney transplant rejection. Nephron 1988;48:183
284. Peskin GW, O'Brien K, Rabiner SF. Stroma-free hemoglobin solution: the "ideal" blood substitute? Surgery 1969;66:185
285. Bernstein EF, Blackshear PLJr, Keller KH. Factors influencing erythrocyte destruction in artificial organs. Am J Surg 1967;114:126
286. Blackshear PLJr. Summation: flow-related surface phenomena. Fed Proc 1971;30:1709
287. Indeglia R, Shea MA, Varco RL, Bernstein EF. Mechanical and biologic considerations in erythrocyte damage. Surgery 1967;62:47
288. Galletti PM. Laboratory experience with 24 hour partial heart-lung bypass. J Surg Res 1965;5:97
289. Kusserow BK, Clapp JF. Red blood cell survival after prolonged perfusion with a blood pump. Trans Am Soc Artif Intern Organs 1966;12:121
290. Indeglia RA, Dorman FD, Castaneda AR, Vacro RL, Bernstein EF. Use of GBH-coated Tygon tubing for experimental prolonged perfusions without systemic heparinization. Trans Am Soc Artif Intern Organs 1966;12:166
291. Bernstein EF, Indeglia RA, Shea MA, Varco RL. Sublethal damage to the red blood cell from pumping. Circulation 1967;35 [Suppl 1]:226
292. Solis RT. Blood filtration during cardiopulmonary bypass. J Extracorporeal Tech 1974;6:64
293. Chopra PS, Dufek JH, Kroncke GM, Dacumos GC, Celesia GG, Troner SP, Marshall JR, Jefferson JW, Loring LL, Kahn DR. Clinical comparison of the General Electric Peirce membrane lung and bubble oxygenator for prolonged cardiopulmonary bypass. Surgery 1973;74:874
294. Alon L, Turina M, Gattiker R. Membrane and bubble oxygenator;a clinical comparison in patients undergoing aortocoronary bypass procedures. Herz 1979;4:56
295. Kolobow T, Zapol WM, Sigman RL, Pierce J. Partial cardiopulmonary bypass lasting up to seven days in alert lambs with membrane lung blood oxygenation. J Thorac Cardiovasc Surg 1970;60:781
296. Hanson EL, Bartlett RH, Burns NE, Shults MC, La Cava EJ, Polet H, Drinker PA. Prolonged use of a membrane oxygenator in air-breathing and hypoxic lambs. 1. Venovenous bypass. Surgery 1973;73:284
297. Bartlett RH, Fong SW, Burns NE, Gazzaniga AB, Prolonged partial venoarterial bypass: physiologic, biochemical and hematologic responses. Ann Surg 1974;180:850

298. Hill JD, de Leval MR, Fallot RJ, Bramson ML, Eberhart RC, Schulte HD, Osborn JJ, Barber R, Gerbode F. Acute respiratory insufficiency: treatment with prolonged extracorporeal oxygenation. J Thorac Cardiovasc Surg 1972;64:551

299. Pranger RL, Mook PH, Elstrodt JM, Kessler M, Lubbers DW, Wildevuur ChRH. Improved tissue perfusion (PO$_2$ histograms) in extracorporeal circulation using membrane instead of bubble oxygenators. J Thorac Cardiovasc Surg 1980;79:513

300. Timmes JJ, Wilson JW. Microcirculatory considerations in extracorporeal oxygenation NY State J Med 1973;73:2337

301. Hohn DC, Meyers AJ, Gherini ST, Beckman A, Markison RE, Churg AM. Production of acute pulmonary injury by leukocytes and activated complement Surgery 1980;88:48

302. Del Maestro RF, Thaw HH, Bjork J, Planker M, Arfors KE. Free radicals as mediators of tissue injury. Acta Physiol Scand Suppl 1980;492:43

303. Westaby S, Fleming J, Royston D. Acute lung injury during cardiopulmonary bypass, the role of neutrophil sequestration and lipid peroxidation. Trans Am Soc Artif Intern Organs 1985;31:604

304. Royston D, Fleming JS, Westaby S, Desai J, Taylor K. Neutrophil kinetics and oxidative injury associated with cardiopulmonary bypass. Thorax 1985;40:240

305. Royston D, Fleming JS, Braude S, Nolop K, Taylor KM. Lung injury following cardiopulmonary bypass;the potential role of oxidant-free radicals. Life Support Systems 1986;4:151

306. Kusserow BK, Larrow R. Studies of leukocyte responses to prolonged blood pumping – effects upon phagocytic capabiligy and total white cell count. Trans Am Soc Artif Intern Organs 1968, 14:261

307. Silva JJr, Hoeksema H, Fekety FRJr. Transient defects in phagocytic functions during cardiopulmonary bypass. J Thorac Cardiovasc Surg 1974;67:175

308. Kirklin JK, Westaby S, Blackstone EH, Kirklin JW, Chenoweth DE, Pacifico AD. Complement and the damaging effects of cardiopulmonary bypass. J Thorac Cardiovasc Surg 1983;86:845

309. O'Neill JA, Ende N, Collins IS, Collins HA. A quantitative determination of perfusion fibrinolysis. J Thorac Cardiovasc Surg 1966;51:777

310. Kevy SV, Glickman RM, Bernhard WF, Diamond LK, Gross RE. The pathogenesis and control of the hemorrhagic defect in open heart surgey. Surg Gynec Obst 1966;123:313

311. Derman UM, Rand PW, Barker N. Fibrinolysis after cardiopulmonary bypass and its relationship to fibrinogen. J Thorac Cardiovasc Surg 1966;51:223

312. Gans H, Subramanian V, John S, Casteneda AR, Lillehei CW. Theoretical and practical (clinical) considerations concerning proteolytic enzymes and their inhibitors with particular reference to changes in the plasminogen-plasmin system observed during assisted circulation in man. Ann NY Acad Sci 1968;146:721

313. Tice DA, Worth MHJr. Recognition and treatment of postoperative bleeding associated with open-heart surgery. Ann NY Acad Sci 1968;146:745

314. Mammen EF. Natural proteinase inhibitors in extracorporeal circulation Ann NY Acad Sci 1968;146:754

315. Tsuji HK, Redington JV, Kay JH, Groesswald RK. The study of fibrinolytic and coagulation factors during open-heart surgery. Ann NY Acad Sci 1968;146:763

316. Porter JM, Silver D. Alterations in fibrinolysis and coagulation associated with cardiopulmonary bypass. J Thorac Cardiovasc Surg 1968;56:869

317. Gomes MR, McGoon D. Bleeding patterns after open-heart surgery. J Thorac Cardiovasc Surg 1970;60:87

318. Ekert H, Friedlander I, Hardisty RM. The role of platelets in fibrinolysis: studies on the plasminogen activator and anti-plasmin activity of platelets. Br J Haematol 1970;18:575

319. Ekert H, Montgomery D, Aberdeen E. Fibrinolysis during extracorporeal circulation: comparison of the effects of disc and membrane oxygenators. Circ Res 1971;28:512

320. Wildevuur ChRH, Oeveren WV. Artificial lung: current problems. Life Support Systems 1986;Suppl. 1:130

321. Rent R, Ertel N, Eisenstein R, Gewurz H. Complement activation by interaction of polyanions and polycations. 1. Heparin-protamine induced consumption of complement. J Immunol 1975;114:120

322. Kazatchkine MD. Alterations in host defence mechanism associated with cardiopulmonary bypass. Life Support Systems 1986;Suppl. 1:144

323. Craddock PR, Fehr J, Dalmasso AP, Brigham KL, Jacob HS. Hemodialysis leukopenia: pulmonary vascular leukostasis resulting from complement activation by dialyzer cellophane membranes. J Clin Invest 1977;59:879

324. Kaplow LS, Goffinet JA. Profound neutropenia during the early phase of hemodialysis. J Am Med Assoc 1968;203:1135

325. Craddock PR, Fehr J, Brigham KL, Kronenberg RS, Jacob HS. Complement and leukocyte-mediated pulmonary dysfunction in hemodialysis. N Engl J Med 1977;296:769

326. Wysocki H, Ponizynski A, Wierusz-Wysocka B, Braki Z, Czarnecki R. Cardiopulmonary bypass-induced complement activation. Evidence for C5a participation. Int J Artif Organs 1982;5:305

327. Wonders T, Huttemeier P, Berry D, Schuette A, Kong D, Watkins WD, Zapol WM. Complement depletion prevents pulmonary hypertension and leukopenia in sheep extra-corporeal membrane oxygenation. Trans Am Soc Artif Intern Organs 1983;29:210

328. Takahama T, Kanai F, Iizuka I, Hiraishi M, Yamazaki Z, Idezuki Y, Sudo K, Asano K, Morioka M Kazam M, Abe T, Sonoda T, Nishio S, Tanzawa H, Kawamura Y. Application of a new prostaglandin I_2 analogue (APS-306) on cardiopulmonary bypass. Trans Am Soc Artif Intern Organs 1984;30:44

329. Rådegran K, Arén C, Teger-Nilsson A-C. Prostacyclin infusion during extracorporeal circulation for coronary bypass. J Thorac Cardiovasc Surg 1982;83:205

330. Faichney A, Davidson KG, Wheatley DJ, Davidson JF, Walker JD. Prostacyclin in cardiopulmonary bypass operations. J Thorac Cardiovasc Surg 1982;84:601

331. Miyamoto H, Hirose H, Matsuda H, Nakano S, Ohtani M, Kaneko M, Nishigaki K, Nomura F, Kitamura H, Kawashima Y. Analysis of complement activation profile during cardiopulmonary bypass and its inhibition by FUT-175. Trans Am Soc Artif Intern Organs 1985; 31:508

332. Hagler HK, Powell WM, Eberle JW, Sugg WL, Platt MR, Watson JT. Five day partial bypass using a membrane oxygenator without systemic heparinization. Trans Am Soc Artif Intern Organs 1975;21:178

333. Roohk HV, Calabrese D, Sanematsu L, Castillo G, Cottonaro CN. Bound and circulating heparin in an ECMO system: thrombogenicity versus functionality. Trans Am Soc Artif Intern Organs 1984;30:639

334. Cottonaro CN, Roohk HV, Bartlett RH, Servas FM, Sperling DR. A new non-thrombogenic surface. Trans Am Soc Artif Intern Organs 1982;28:478

Chapter 3

Collagen in Cardiovascular Tissues

M.E. Nimni

Introduction

The structural and viscoelastic properties of the vascular tissues are determined to a large extent by the fibrous proteins collagen and elastin and to a much lesser degree by the contractile protein elements and the proteoglycans of the ground substance. Depending on the nature of the tissue (arteries, veins, heart valves) and on the anatomical area (intima, media or adventitia) endothelial cells, smooth muscle cells or fibroblasts are primarily reponsible for the biosynthesis of these macromolecules.

Collagen, the single most abundant protein in mammalian tissues, accounts for up to 30% of all proteins, but is not evenly distributed throughout the body [1]. In bone, collagen can account for over 90% of the organic matrix; the same holds true for ligaments and tendons. In elastic arteries, such as in the media of the human aorta, collagen accounts for approximately 25% of the dry fat-free and calcium-free weight and elastin for about 42%. These values do not change appreciably with age [2]. The muscular arteries contain approximately equal amounts of collagen and elastin, and veins about seven times more collagen than elastin. In human heart valves collagen represents 55% of the tissue on a dry weight basis while elastin is slightly over 10% [3]. Proteoglycans represent only a relatively small proportion of the extracellular matrix of the vascular tissues, usually around 1% of the dry weight [2]. The proportion of the individual components within this fraction can change significantly from tissue to tissue. In the human aorta, chondroitin sulphate is the major glycosaminoglycan, while hyaluronic acid constitutes one-seventh of the total, and decreases markedly with age. In heart valves, on the other hand, 65% of the glycosaminoglycans are made up by hyaluronic acid [4]. As will be discussed below, there is an interesting correlation between the nature of the macromolecules (charge, hydrophobicity, molecular size) and the way they organize (fibre diameter, orientation, relative distribution), and the function a particular tissue performs.

In higher animals there are nine types of collagen that have been well characterized, and many others are being studied. Whereas type I collagen is the most prevalent, and is the only collagen present in bone and almost exclusively present in tendons and ligaments, the vascular system, as well as embryonic and granulation tissues, contains large amounts of type III collagen.

Vascular tissues also contain significant proportions of basement membrane collagens (type IV) as well as other associated macromolecules such as laminin and fibronectin [1]. The aim of this chapter is to summarize some of the fundamental aspects of collagen structure, synthesis, assembly and degradation. These events play a major role during development, wound healing, and following implantation of devices that require some form of tissue ingrowth or generate a fibrotic response. In addition, collagen as a biomaterial, its application to the cardiovascular system, and some of the problems which follow the implantation of such devices will be discussed. For further details on the metabolic aspects of collagen and its relationship to fibrosis, the reader is referred to a recent review [1].

Collagen in Health and Disease

Collagen molecules, after being secreted by the cells, assemble into characteristic fibres responsible for the functional integrity of tissues such as bone, cartilage, skin and tendon (Fig. 3.1). Collagen contributes a structural framework to other tissues such as blood vessels and most organs. Cross-links between adjacent molecules are a prerequisite for the collagen fibres to withstand the physical stresses to which they are exposed. Significant progress has been made towards understanding the functional groups on the molecule that are involved in the formation of such cross-links, and their nature and location. A variety of human conditions, both normal and pathological, involve the ability of tissues to repair and regenerate their collagenous framework. Some of these conditions are characterized by excessive deposition of collagen (e.g.

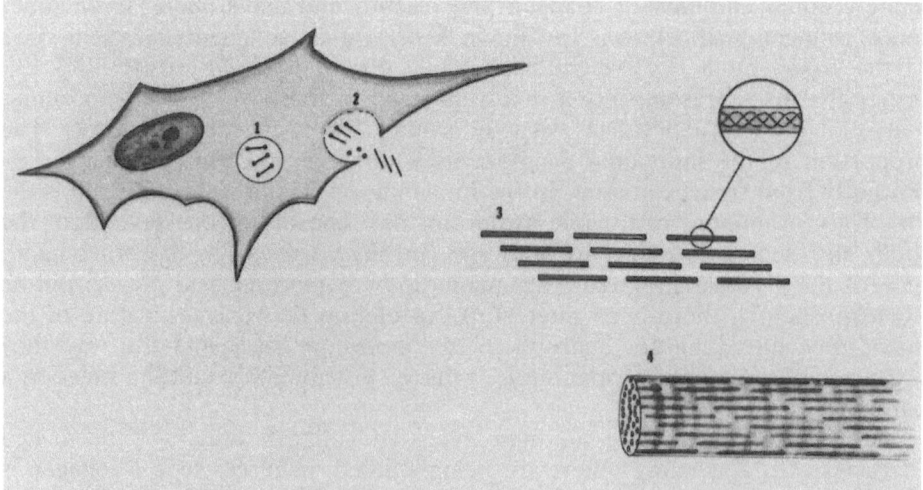

Fig. 3.1. Diagram showing a cell synthesizing collagen: (1) synthesis and inclusion, (2) extrusion, (3) self assembly, (4) fibril.

cirrhosis, scleroderma, keloid, pulmonary fibrosis, diabetes). After trauma or surgery, abnormal deposition of collagen may impair function (adhesions following repair of long tendons, scar formation during healing, etc.). In addition, many disabling conditions result from changes in the nature and organization of collagen (heart valve lesions, osteoarthritis, rheumatoid arthritis, and congenital collagen diseases such as Marfan's and Ehlers–Danlos syndromes, osteogenesis imperfecta, etc.).

In human tissues there are nine different collagen types that have been very well characterized. Collagen molecules in cartilage differ from those in cornea, tendon, bone matrix, dermis, the parenchyma of organs, periodontal ligaments, and many other locations within the organism. Why is cornea transparent, tendon tough and inelastic and able to sustain significant stresses, and cartilage resilient and viscoelastic? What is unique in the chemical structure of collagen that enables these tissues to perform such diverse biological functions? What regulates fibre diameter, orientation, concentration of fibres in a particular volume of tissue, and packing of the fibres into larger bundles? How can we understand the problem of ageing of connective tissues and changes related to pathology? It now seems as if cells that have acquired the ability to make a particular type of collagen can be influenced by environmental factors to change the rate and nature of the collagen molecules that they synthesize, and that in some instances these changes are reversible.

In order to understand the functional and structural relationships that operate in normal tissues and how an imbalance can lead to disease, an understanding of the genesis of the collagen fibril is necessary.

The Collagen Molecule

The arrangement of amino acids in the collagen molecule is shown schematically in Fig. 3.2. Every third residue is glycine. Proline and hydroxyproline follow each other relatively frequently, and the gly–pro–hyp sequence makes up about 10% of the molecule. This triple helical structure generates a symmetrical pattern of three left-handed helical chains that are, in turn, slightly displaced to the right, superimposing an additional "supercoil" with a pitch of approximately 86 Å units. The amino acids within each chain are displaced by a distance $h = 2.91$ Å with a relative twist of $-110°$, making the number of residues per turn 3.27 and the distance between each third glycine 8.7 Å. The individual residues are nearly fully extended in the collagen structure, since the maximum displacement within a fully-stretched chain would be approximately 3.6 Å. This separation is nevertheless such that it will not allow intrachain bonds to form (as does occur in the α-helix), and only interchain hydrogen bonds are possible [5]. The exact number of hydrogen bonds that stabilize the triple helical structure has not been determined. The model that Ramachandran [5] describes has two hydrogen bonds for every three amino acids, whereas the Rich and Crick [6] version assumes one hydrogen bond for every three residues.

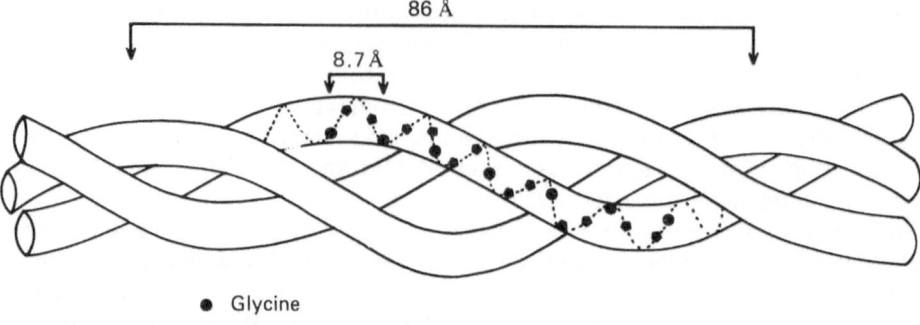

● Glycine

● Predominantly imino acids

Fig. 3.2. Schematic drawing showing the collagen triple helix. The individual a chains are left-handed helices with approximately three residues per turn. The chains are in turn coiled around each other following a right-handed twist. The hydrogen bonds which stabilize the triple helix (not shown) form between opposing residues in different chains (interpeptide hydrogen bonding), and are therefore quite different from α-helices which occur between amino acids located within the same polypeptide.

In addition to these intramolecular conformational patterns, there seems to exist a supermolecular coiling. Microfibrils, possibly representing intermediate stages of packing, may be present; such possibilities will be discussed below.

Figure 3.3 shows a native collagen fibre with its repeating 680 Å (68 nm) periodicity alongside a schematic drawing of a collagen molecule (3000 Å length). The relationship between the length of the molecule and the periodicity that prompted the quarter-staggered theory of packing [7] can be clearly seen. The stacking of collagen molecules to give rise to SLS (segment long spacing) crystallites (Fig. 3.4) has provided a very useful tool for understand-

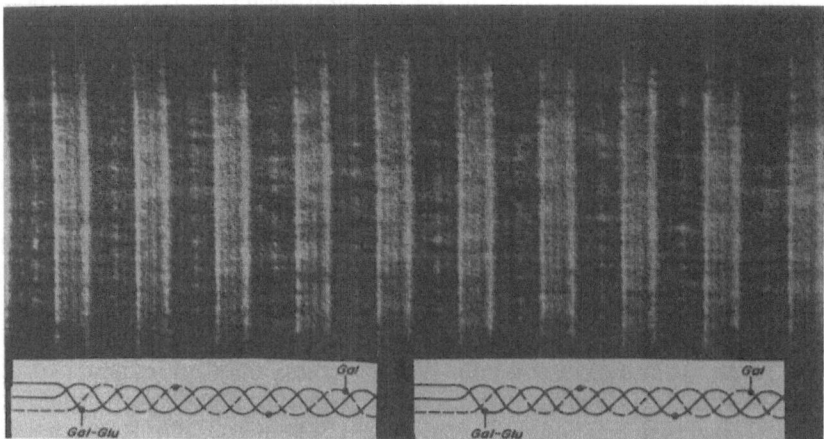

Fig. 3.3. Native collagen fibre stained with phosphotungstic acid showing the 68 nm periodicity and a schematic representation of collagen molecules measuring approximately 300 nm. (Courtesy of Dr J. Petruska.)

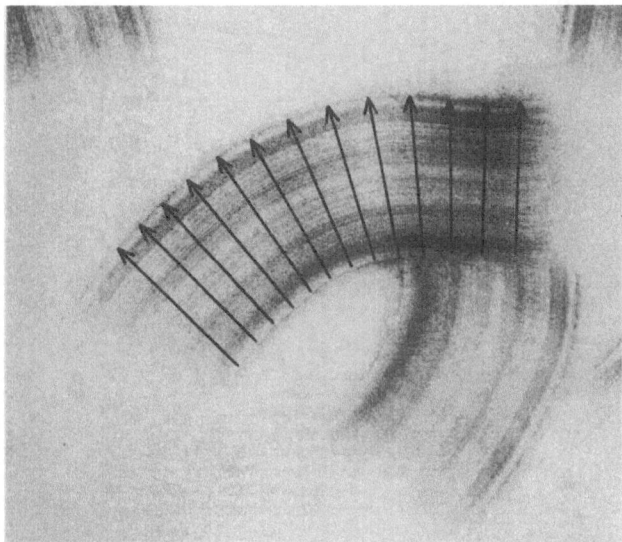

Fig. 3.4. Segment-long-spacing (SLS) form when ATP is added to a solution of collagen. The negatively charged ATP, by altering the charge density around the molecules, causes them to aggregate side by side in register in such a way that the individual molecules can now be visualized. The arrows indicate the positions of the molecules in the crystallite and represent their orientation. It is of interest that structures similar to these have been observed within intracellular vesicles which transport procollagen to the cell surface.

ing the dimensions of the molecule, to order the peptides originating after cyanogen bromide (CNBr) cleavage of the molecule, and to identify and characterize the various collagen types. This form of packing, which does not lead to normal fibre formation, will also be discussed in connection with the intracellular translocation of procollagen.

The process of self-assembly that causes the collagen molecules to organize into fibres is shown schematically in Fig. 3.5. The thermodynamics of such a system involve changes in the state of the water molecules associated with the non-polar regions of the collagen molecule. Also illustrated is the role of the polar groups on the surface of collagen, which we now know are distributed so as to effectively aid in the quarter-staggered packing that leads to the native fibrillar banded structure [8–10].

Biosynthesis

The Procollagen Molecule

In order for the organism to develop an extracellular network of collagen fibres, the cells involved in the biosynthetic process must first synthesize a precursor known as procollagen. This molecule is later enzymatically trimmed

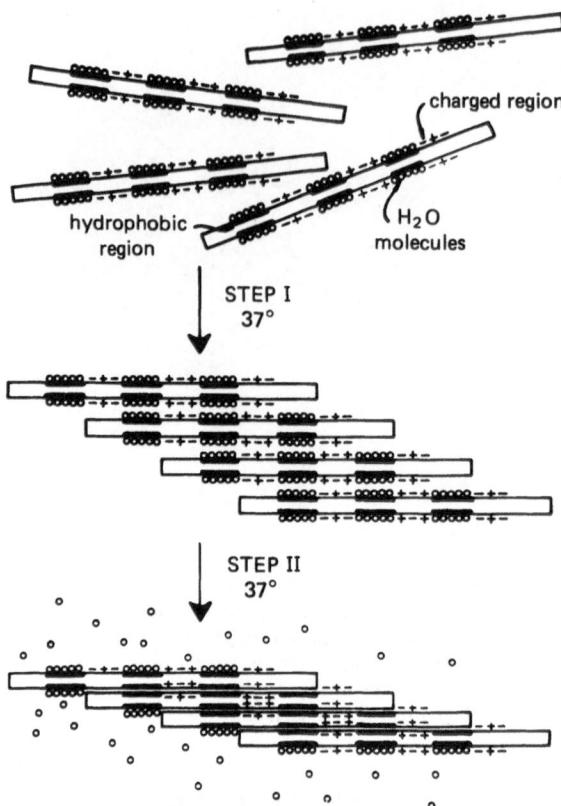

Fig. 3.5. Soluble collagen can be extracted from most tissues by cold neutral salt solutions. If these solutions are warmed to 37°C the collagen molecules re-assemble into native fibres. The upper part of the drawing represents molecules that have begun to align in a quarter-staggered overlap. The alignment is primarily due to interactions of opposing electrostatic charges as depicted by the + and − signs. As the temperature approaches 37 °C the hydrogen-bonded water molecules (open circles), clustered around the hydrophobic regions of collagen, "melt" and expose these non-polar surfaces. Exclusion of water allows these surfaces to interact with each other, giving rise to hydrophobic bonds that greatly enhance the stability of the fibre. The driving force results from an increase of entropy of the system since the release of "organized" water from initial sites and its transformation into "random" water increases the state of disorder of the system. Part of the ageing process which leads to a gradual insolubilization of collagen may be associated with this phenomenon which continues to operate through the lifespan of the individual.

of its non-helical ends, giving rise to a collagen molecule that spontaneously assembles into fibres in the extracellular space. Procollagen molecules have been identified as precursors of the three interstitial collagens (types I, II and III). Several of the N- and C-terminal peptides (propeptides) have been characterized and, in some instances, the primary sequence determined [11]. The N-terminal propeptides for both proα1(I) and proα1(III) chains have a terminal globular domain of 77–86 amino acids, followed by a collagen-like domain of about 40 amino acids. The collagen-like domain is joined to the chain by a short non-collagen sequence of two to eight amino acids. The N-terminal propeptide of proα2(I) has not been as well characterized and in some species may lack the N-terminal non-globular domain [12]. Type II procollagen isolated from chick embryos seems to contain a similar amino-propeptide but with a smaller N-terminal globular domain [13]. The N-terminal propeptide of type I collagen contains one residue of N-acetylglucosamine [14] and intrachain but no interchain disulphide links. On the other hand, interchain disulphide links seem to be present in the N-terminal propeptides of type III procollagen [15,16].

The carboxyterminal propeptides of both proα1 and and proα2 chains have molecular weights of 30000 to 35000 daltons and globular conformations without any collagen-like domain [17]. These peptides contain asparagine-linked oligosaccharide units composed of N-acetylglucosamine and mannose [18,19]. This carbohydrate side-chain is located in the carboxy-terminal half of the carboxyl propeptide in a region containing the sequence Asn−X−Thr [20], which is compatible with the structural requirement for glycosylation of asparaginyl residues by oligosaccharide transferases [21]. The functional importance of the carbohydrate in the carboxy-end of procollagen is unknown but may be part of a recognition mechanism for alignment, secretion or assembly into microfibrils. A diagram summarizing the major characteristics of procollagen type I is shown in Fig. 3.6. The central segment of the molecule is arranged in a triple helical conformation characteristic of collagen, and the globular extensions can be seen at both ends. Also shown in the diagram (indicated by arrows) are the sites of cleavage by specific procollagen peptidases.

The extensions play a key role in the assembly of the tri-helical collagen molecule and their possible functions in this connection will be discussed later in this section. Once the molecule is completed and translocated to the cell surface the extensions are enzymatically removed (in the case of types I, II and III collagens) and fibrillogenesis occurs. Enzymes that selectively remove these extensions can be found in a variety of connective tissues and in the culture media derived from collagen-secreting cells [19].

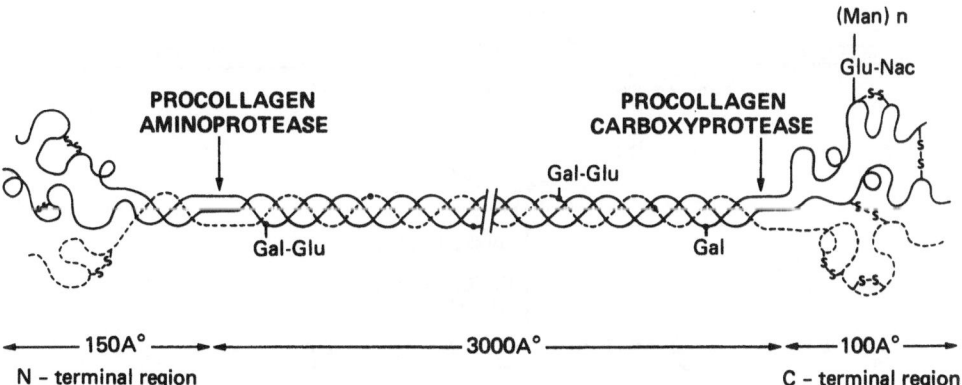

Fig. 3.6. Procollagen molecule showing the non-helical terminal extensions. The N-terminal end contains a small helical domain and the C-terminal end is stabilized by interchain disulfide bonds. The sites of cleavage by procollagen peptidases are indicated by arrows.

Intracellular Events Leading to the Synthesis of Procollagen

Since the discovery, about 12 years ago, of a distinct form of collagen in cartilage, labelled type II collagen, more than a dozen collagen types have been characterized in different tissues of the same animal species. The best defined (types I to V) clearly represent unique amino acid sequences coded by different genes. Cell hybridization has shown that human chromosome number 17 contains the coding information for the α1 and α2 chains of type I collagen [22,23]. Type III collagen seems to be encoded in another chromosome. Recent advances in recombinant DNA technology have opened the way for study of the structure and regulation of the collagen gene. In part this interest is generated by the fact that collagens constitute a family of closely-related proteins, and are synthesized by specialized cells that can be experimentally manipulated to synthesize different collagen types.

The collagen gene is quite large, about ten times the size of the functional mRNA [24]. These mRNAs have a unique sequence of codons, signal codons, to the right of the initiation codon. These are translated on a free ribosome to a unique sequence of about 15–30 amino acid residues (signal sequence) on the amino terminal of the nascent chain. In the case of collagen, the 2(I) collagen gene from chick is 38 kilobases(kb) in length and contains at least 52 coding sequences (exons). Many of these exons are 54 base pairs(bp) in length and are separated from each other by large intervening sequences (introns) that range in size from about 80 to 2000 [25]. The gene itself contains 38 000 base pairs and is the most complex gene so far isolated [26]. It was quite surprising to find that a molecule as uniform and regular as collagen should be coded by a gene of such complexity and divided into so many domains. In particular, the finding that most exons of the gene for the 2 chain have identical lengths may have important implications in the understanding of evolution, since it suggests that the ancestral gene for collagen was assembled by multiple duplications of single

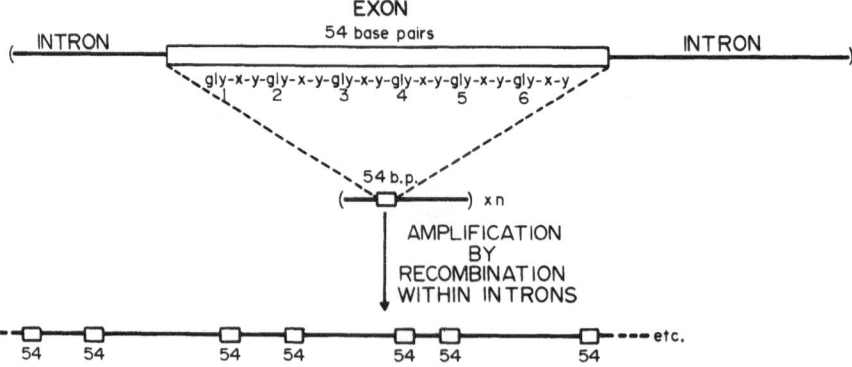

Fig. 3.7. The collagen gene is made up of multiple units containing 54 base pairs, each of which corresponds to sequences of 18 amino acids. The conservation of this minimum sequence, and the fact that it is repeated in such an exacting fashion, provides valuable information to investigators interested in the process of evolution of proteins [21].

genetic units containing an exon of 54 bp (Fig. 3.7). It is quite likely that a primordial exon this size could have encoded for a gly–pro–pro tripeptide repeated six times (3 × 3 × 6). Such a polypeptide of 18 amino acids probably had the minimal length needed to form a stable triple helical structure. The 54 bp exon structure may be common to all collagen genes. These observations generate interesting possibilities, and may allow us to better understand the nature of defects associated with some of the heritable collagen diseases.

Translational, Co-translational and Early Post-translational Events

After the gene is transcribed it is spliced to yield a functional mRNA that contains about 3000 bases. Specific mRNAs for each chain and collagen type are translocated to the cytoplasm and translated in the rough endoplasmic reticulum (RER) on membrane-bound polysomes (Fig. 3.8). A pre-pro chain that contains an unusually large N-terminal hydrophobic signal or πleaderπ sequence is the final translational product. The signal portion facilitates transfer of the chain into the lumen of the RER and is probably removed by an intramembranous endopeptidase after it has served its function of orienting compatible proS chains in apposition. As the collagen polypeptide is synthesized in the RER, important co-translational events accompany this process. It is a well known observation, extensively documented in the literature, that neither hydroxyproline nor hydroxylysine can be directly incorporated into proteins [27]; it is only after peptide bond formation that hydroxylation of proline and lysine can occur, mediated by two enzymes, prolyl and lysyl hydroxylases. These enzymes are quite specific and require for their activity ferrous iron, ascorbate and α-ketoglutarate. They seem to recognize sequences surrounding the target imino or amino acids with differing affinities and thus selectively modify randomly alternating proline and lysine residues. The degree of hydroxylation differs from tissue to tissue and probably with availability of substrate, rates of synthesis and turnover as well as the time that the molecule remains in the presence of the hydroxylating enzymes. As we shall see later, these factors may also affect the position of the carbon atom in the peptide bound proline that is hydroxylated (e.g. the 3- or 4-carbon).

The time required for the synthesis of a complete pro chain is about 6.7 min [28]. The radioactive label, however, appears in fully aligned triple helical chains after a further delay, a fact that may have significant physiological implications as the time lapse between polypeptide synthesis and folding may affect the nature and extent of hydroxylation and glycosylation, another important post-translational event.

The enzyme prolyl hydroxylase (4-hydroxylase) has been isolated from several sources and extensively characterized [19,29,30]. The active enzyme is a tetramer with a molecular weight of 240 000 daltons, and consists of two different types of monomers with molecular weights of about 64 000 and 60 000 daltons. Lysyl hydroxylase has been extensively purified and is apparently a dimer with two subunits, each having a molecular weight of about 90 000 daltons [31]. Prolyl 3-hydroxylase has been only partially purified and characterized [32]. These three enzymes are quite specific and act only on chains in

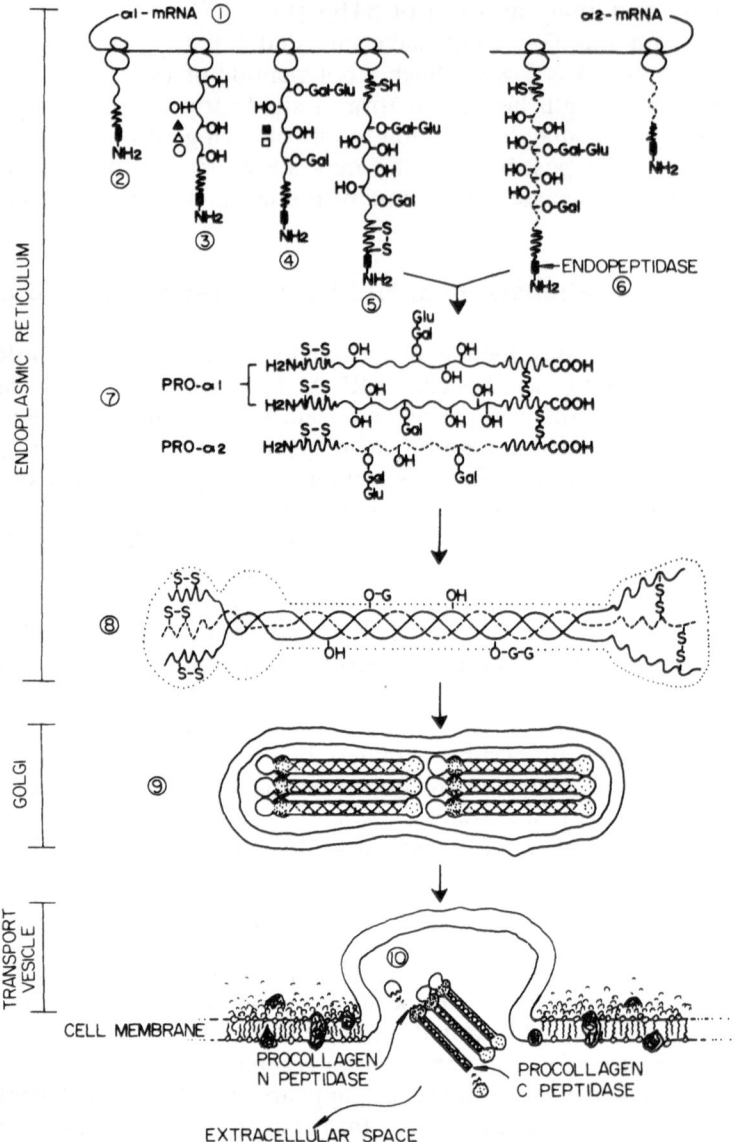

Fig. 3.8. Sequence of events in the biosynthesis of collagen: (1) Synthesis of specific mRNAs for the different procollagen chains. (2) Translation of the message on polysomes of the rough E.R. (3) Hydroxylation of specific proline residues by 3-proline hydroxylase (△) and 4-proline hydroxylase (▲) and of lysine by lysyl hydroxylase (○). (4) Glycosylation of hydroxylysine by galactosyl-transferase (■) and addition of glucose by a glucosyltransferase (□). (5) Removal of the N-terminal signal peptide. (6) Release of completed α-chains from ribosomes. (7) Recognition of three α-chains through the C-terminal propeptide end and formation of disulphide crosslinks. (8) Folding of the molecule and formation of a triple helix. (9) Intracellular translocation of the procollagen molecules and packaging into vesicles. (10) Fusion of vesicles with the cell membrane and extrusion of the molecule accompanied by the removal of the C-terminal non-helical extensions and part of the N-terminal non-helical extensions by specific peptidases.

the non-helical conformation, a reason why the time elapsed between peptide synthesis and folding may be so important. This time varies considerably, being approximately 10 min in cells synthesizing type I procollagen [33], 20 min in cells synthesizing type II procollagen [34], and 60 min in cells synthesizing basement membrane collagen [35]. After folding of the procollagen poly-peptides, there is an additional time interval before the collagen molecule is secreted: this varies between 18 min for tendon cells [36], 36 min for cartilage cells [37], and 60 min in parietal yolk sac tissue [38].

Proline analogues, such as cis-hydroxyproline and azetidine 2-carboxylic acid, are known to be incorporated into collagen in the proline position and to inhibit triple helix formation within the cell. Using such an experimental tool it was shown that the glycosylation of hydroxylysine [39] and the hydroxylation of proline at the 3 position [32] are increased approximately twofold by inhibiting helix formation. These observations, coupled with the time factors noted above, may be linked to the increased hydroxylation of proline in the 3 position, the increased content of hydroxylysine and the greater degree of glycosylation seen in basement membrane collagen, and may explain dif-ferences in hydroxylation seen in pathological connective tissues.

As lysyl residues in the newly synthesized pro-α-chains are hydroxylated, sugar residues are added to the resulting hydroxylysyl groups. Glycosylations are catalyzed by two specific enzymes, a galactosyltransferase and a glucosyl-transferase [40]. The first of these enzymes adds galactose to the hydroxylysyl residues, and the second adds glucose to the galactosylhydroxylysine that is formed. The galactosyltransferase from chick embryo has been purified about 1000-fold and the glucosyltransferase has been isolated as a homogeneous protein. Both enzymes are glycoproteins and their activity requires the pre-sence of sulphydryl groups. The activity of partially purified galactosyl-transferase is separated by gel filtration into three species with apparent molecular weights of 450 000, 200 000 and 50 000 daltons. The purified glucosyl-transferase has a molecular weight of 70 000 daltons. Both these transferases use sugar in a form of a uridine diphosphate glycoside, and require the pre-sence of bivalent cations, preferably manganese [41]. These enzymes, like the hydroxylases, require that the pro α-chains be in a non-helical conformation. In intact cells, glycosylation is initiated while the polypeptides are still being assembled on the ribosomes, but probably continues after the release of com-plete pro α-chains in the cisternae of the RER; activity ceases when the chains acquire a triple helical conformation. The oligosaccharides present in the extension peptides associated with the C-terminal region of collagen resemble those present in most other glycoproteins; they contain N-acetylglucosamine and mannose, and are attached to asparagine residues [42,43]. Their com-position suggests that they are added as intermediates via the dolichol phos-phate pathway, and that final remodelling occurs in the Golgi bodies after the helix has been formed [44]. Once the translation, modifications and additions are completed it is essential that the individual pro α-chains become properly aligned for the triple helix to form. It is not known if this alignment occurs while the polypeptides are still attached to the ribosome or if they have to detach, or if the N-terminal "signal" peptide plays a role in this connection. In any case, proper alignment should juxtapose the appropriate cysteine residues as a prerequisite for formation of the disulphide bridges that link the individual pro α-chains at the C-terminal end. Earlier studies involving subcellular fractionation suggested that the disulphide bridges could appear during translocation of procollagen from the ribosome to the smooth endoplasmic reticulum, probably in the cisternae [45]. More recently it has been proposed that disulphide bond formation occurs while the propeptides are still attached to the ribosome [46]. In any case, it seems clear that for assembly and secretion the C-terminal extensions must be present [47–49].

Although helix formation seems to be a spontaneous, entropy-driven process, the possibility that an enzymatic system, similar to that which regulates the coiling of DNA and shifts it from one topological form to another involving DNA girases and topoisomerases [50], could be associated with the RER, and controls and monitors this step cannot be discounted. The kinetics of triple helix formation of type I procollagen within fibroblasts have been measured in pulse-chase experiments followed by proteolytic digestion [49]. Production of triple helical molecules requires 8–9 min after completion of pro α-chains [51]. Disulphide bond formation precedes triple helix formation and seems to serve as a catalyst for it to occur. Similar observations and conclusions have been derived from studies on the biosynthesis of type III procollagen by chick embryo blood vessels [48,52]. In this case further stability may be added by interchain disulphide bond formation in the helical region as well as in the N-terminal non-helical region, but the exact timing of these subsequent events remains difficult to ascertain.

Intracellular Translocation of Procollagen and Extrusion into the Extracellular Space

As discussed previously, the synthesis of procollagen chains involves the translation of a specific mRNA on membrane-bound ribosomes similarly to secretory proteins in general [53] and core protein of proteoglycans [54]. The signal sequence, an unusually large one in the case of collagen [55], may trigger the attachment of the ribosome that generated it to a specific binding site on the membrane. In most instances the signal sequence is removed from the nascent polypeptide chain by a specific endopeptidase before chain completion [56,57]. It is not clear whether this is the case with collagen since before movement along the secretory pathways begins three separate specific chains have to register to form the triple helical structure. It is quite likely that the signal peptide, due to its hydrophobic character, guides the nascent chain to the interior of the rough membrane intracisternal space where the translational and post-translational events occur. Once the procollagen molecule is assembled (devoid of the signal peptide) the secretory pathway seems to be similar to that followed by other glycoproteins. These experimental findings have been recently reviewed [58]. Essentially the procollagen molecules, now detached from the ribosome, emerge from the endoplasmic reticulum and move towards the Golgi apparatus through the microsomal lumen (Fig. 3.9). In the Golgi its C-terminal mannose-rich carbohydrate extension is probably remodelled and the completed procollagen molecules packaged in Golgi-derived vesicles and

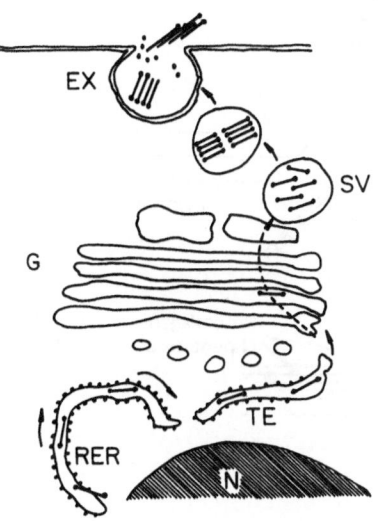

Fig. 3.9. Movement of procollagen through the cisternae of the rough endoplasmic reticulum (RER) and through a transitional endoplasm (TE) to the Golgi (G) where it is packaged into secretory vesicle (SV) prior to extrusion (EX) by exocytosis.

carried towards the cellular membrane by cytoskeletal movements. During transit they seem to sit side by side to form structures that can sometimes be identified with the electron microscope as SLS crystallites (see fibrillogenesis). The small aggregates of oriented procollagen molecules are probably trimmed of their non-helical amino and carboxyl extensions by specific peptidases when they reach the extracellular space. In the case of type I collagen, the first peptidase to act seems to be the amino protease; this is followed by a carboxyprotease. In type III collagen the sequence of removal may be reversed [58,59]. Recent immunoelectron microscopical studies have shown that the thinner collagen fibres (200–400 Å) contain procollagen molecules that still retain their NH_2-terminal extensions [60]; this is not the case for larger collagen fibres. Thus, certain fibres in normal human skin still possess, at least on their outer surface, procollagen or pN-collagen molecules. The latter possibility is most likely in view of earlier work [61] and because antibody reactivity could be eliminated by treating the tissues with procollagen NH_2-terminal protease. These findings support suggestions that removal of extension aminopropeptides could be involved in the control of fibre growth. It is possible that selective removal of portions of the extensions may occur at the cell surface thus allowing for formation of 4-D staggered microfibrils, and that final removal of these propeptides occurs in the extracellular space. This process would allow for modulation of fibre growth by apposition and elongation as well as for fusion of thin fibres (20–40 nm) into larger diameter fibres (Fig. 3.10).

Lysyl Oxidase

Somewhere in the process of extrusion, recently formed microfibrils must be recognized by the enzyme lysyl oxidase, which converts certain peptide-bound lysines and hydroxylysines to aldehydes. This enzyme initiates the biosynthesis of cross-links in collagen. A recent review summarized most of the current

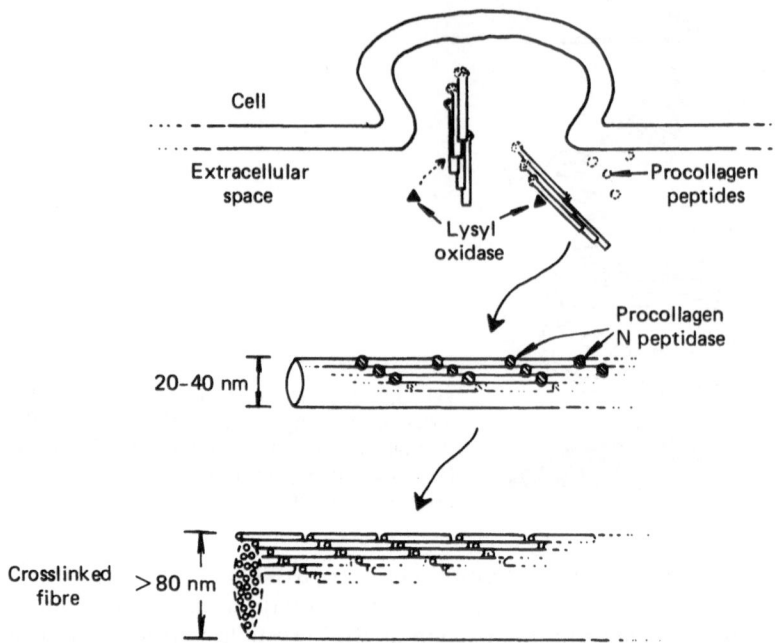

Cell

Extracellular
space

Lysyl
oxidase

Procollagen
peptides

Procollagen
N peptidase

20–40 nm

Crosslinked
fibre

> 80 nm

Fig. 3.10. Fibrillogenesis: Microfibrils in a quarter-staggered configuration have lost their C-terminal non-helical extensions and part of their N-terminal extensions. In this form they seem to organize readily into small diameter fibres which retain part of the N-terminal non-helical extensions. After being relieved of these peptides by a procollagen peptidase, fibres are able to grow in diameter by apposition of microfibrils or by merger with other small diameter fibres.

knowledge in this field [62]. This enzyme, first described by Pinnell and Martin [63], catalyses the oxidative deamination of lysine and hydroxylysine, as summarized in Fig. 3.11. The enzyme is an extracellular amine oxidase, and has been purified from a variety of connective tissues. The molecular weight in most species is 30 000 daltons, or a multiple thereof. It requires Cu^{22+} and probably pyridoxal as cofactors, and molecular oxygen seems to be the cosubstrate and hydrogen acceptor. It is irreversibly inhibited by the lathyrogen

$$
\begin{array}{ccc}
\begin{array}{c}
R \\
| \\
C = O \\
| \\
C - (CH_2)_4 - NH_2 \\
| \\
NH \\
| \\
R
\end{array}
&
\xrightarrow{\text{Lysyl oxidase}}
&
\begin{array}{c}
R \\
| \\
C = O \\
| \\
C - (CH_2)_3 - C = O \\
| \qquad\qquad\ \ H \\
NH \\
| \\
R
\end{array}
\end{array}
$$

Peptide bound lysine   α-aminoadipic δ-semialdehyde

Fig. 3.11. The oxidative deamination of peptide-bound lysine by the enzyme lysyl oxidase generates the aldehydes associated with the collagen molecule.

BAPN. This enzyme exhibits maximal activity when acting on reconstituted collagen fibres rather than upon monomeric collagen. Because of this it is felt that the enzyme is most likely to act upon microfibrillar aggregates of collagen molecules at the time of extrusion. It would be difficult to conceive how it could act otherwise on collagen, since once assembled into the quarter-staggered array and compacted into fibres, it would be difficult for the enzyme to gain access to the interior of the fibre.

Fibrillogenesis

During the preceding discussion the tendency of collagen molecules to form macromolecular aggregates has been constantly emphasized. This tendency is common with most fibrous proteins that form filaments with helical symmetry and which occupy equivalent or quasiequivalent positions. Both electron micrographic and X-ray diffraction data support the view that within collagen fibres there is a regular arrangement of molecules that could result from such an ordered assembly [64–66].

A five-stranded microfibril was first suggested to account for such a sub-structure, one that would satisfy the condition that adjacent molecules were equivalently related by a quarter-stagger, as suggested by Hodge and Petruska [7]. The exact mode of organization, that is the mode in which the collagen molecules pack in the microfibril, their exact number, and the nature and location of cross-links within and between microfibrils still remains a subject for speculation (Fig. 3.12). The five subunit assembly proposed earlier by Smith [67] seems to be the most widely accepted basic unit. For detailed discussion the reader is referred to the reviews mentioned earlier, as well as to recent

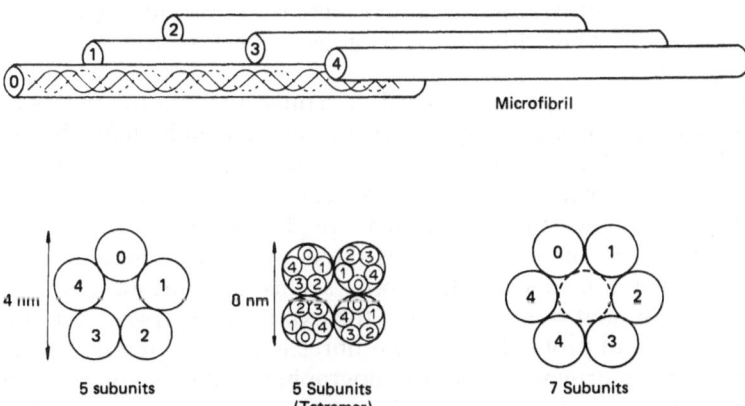

Fig. 3.12. Microfibrils represent early forms of organization of collagen on its way to becoming a fibre. The most widely accepted form of microfibril is that which involves five collagen molecules. The cross-sectional view indicates the degree of displacement measured in D values (0–4). Also shown is a higher degree of organization where four five-stranded microfibrils are packed in a unit cell 8 nm in width as well as an alternate way of packing which would accommodate seven collagen molecules allowing for some molecules to sit side-by-side without lateral displacement.

detailed publications [68–73]. The earliest form of intracellular interaction is documented by the appearance of what seem like side-to-side non-staggered arrangements of collagen molecules resembling SLS and end-overlapped SLS crystallites. These formations have been found in vacuoles within odontoblasts, epithelial cells and fibroblasts [74–78]. SLS crystallites normally do not form under physiological conditions of pH and ionic strength but occur if negatively charged counterions (such as ATP) are added to the solution to mask and interfere with ionic interactions that normally cause collagen molecules to form quarter-staggered arrays (Fig. 3.4). What causes such associations to occur early within the cell is not known, but they could be due to the presence of the C- and N-terminal extensions of procollagen or to the existence of ionic species within the vacuoles that may favour lateral stacking. In any case, such a conformation may prove to be of advantage at the time of intracellular transport since it would inhibit normal fibrillogenesis and probably position the procollagen molecules favourably for the procollagen proteases to exert their enzymatic activities during the process of extrusion. After removal of the non-helical extensions, the newly formed collagen molecules could then be free to organize into quarter-staggered microfibrils and proceed to form native fibres. Under pathological conditions, cells that are actively synthesizing collagen and that have accumulated large concentrations of proteoglycans have been shown to exhibit intracellular deposits of collagen fibrils within cytoplasmic inclusions [78].

The process of in vivo fibrillogenesis has been equated for a long time with the ability of monomeric collagen to form fibres in vitro (Figs. 3.5 and 3.13). When monomeric collagen is heated to 37 °C it progressively polymerizes, generating a turbidity curve that reflects the presence of intermediate aggregates. This phenomenon has been the focus of intensive investigation, and it has also led to the assumption that analogies exist between in vitro and in vivo situations. The lag phase (monomers), the nucleation and appearance of turbidity (microfibrils), and the rapid increase in turbidity (fibre formation) have been equated while attempting to understand how the cell handles these processes [79–82].

The experimental approaches used to study the nature and size of the aggregates formed during early stages of self assembly have been recently reviewed [83,84]. The reverse process, the disassembly of recently synthesized rat tail tendon collagen fibres by 0.1 M acetic acid, has also led to the conclusion that dimers and higher molecular weight aggregates can be recognized, since, as long as stable covalent cross-links are not formed, the process is reversible. Current evidence, therefore, seems to indicate that monomeric collagen does not float freely around in the extracellular space, but polymerizes into microfibrils and probably even into fibres before leaving the surface of the cell from which it originates. Autoradiographic studies show that the site of matrix deposition is very near the cell surface [74,85,86]. Similar observations have been made for other tissues such as the developing chick embryo, tendon, cornea and basement lamella of fish, all of which provide good models for fibre growth and elongation [76,83,87].

Although we are still not able to completely understand the detailed nature of the microfilaments nor the mechanism by which collagen fibres are deposited

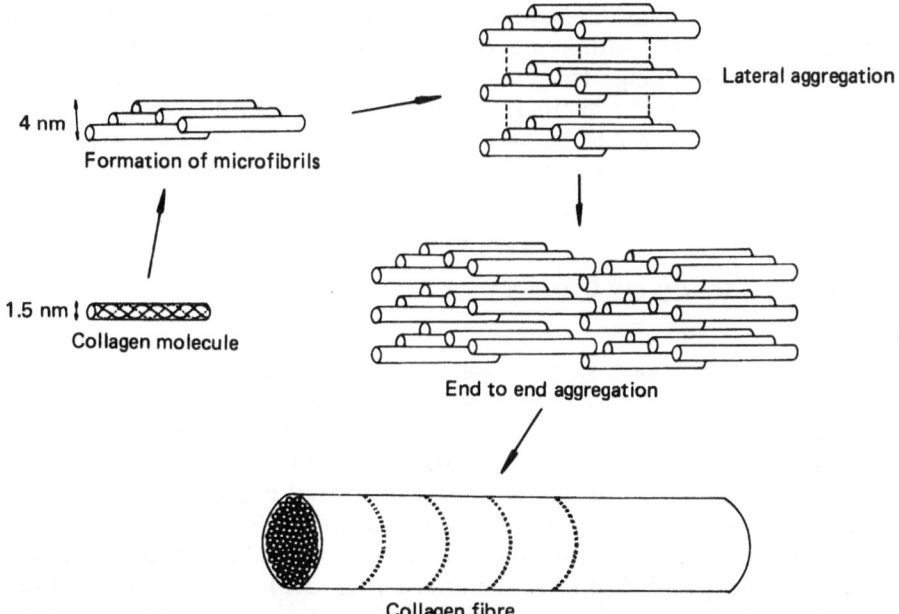

Fig. 3.13. Formation of the five-membered microfibril and its potential for lateral and end-to-end aggregation to form fibres.

in the connective tissues in an ordered and specific manner, the overall picture is becoming more clear. From the folding of the procollagen molecule, to its transport through the cisternae of the endoplasmic reticulum, its packaging into vacuoles in the Golgi to extrusion and filament elongation at the cell surface, the sequence seems logical and amenable to further investigation.

Collagen Metabolism

Collagen is the most abundant of all body proteins. It therefore has to be synthesized and accumulated in large amounts during periods of growth and at sites of injury or tissue repair. Its rate of turnover is also rapid at these times and locations. Tissues such as bone, which are involved in active remodelling, are responsible for the major turnover, while other less dynamic tissues in the fully-grown individual, such as skin and tendons, may exhibit very slow and almost negligible turnover. Although some specific cellular metabolic products have been implicated in stimulating or inhibiting collagen synthesis [88], the mechanisms involved are not understood. Under normal circumstances of growth and activity, mechanical stress, piezoelectric phenomena, cell density, and cell—cell interactions are likely to affect cell membranes and modulate the synthesis and secretion of collagen. This area of research is difficult to investigate and, therefore, has not received much attention and our knowledge is very scanty. Some aspects of these events will be discussed when we review the synthesis of collagen by cultured cells and the effects of specific drugs and inhibitors on such systems. Control could be exerted at both the transcriptional and translational levels within the cells, as well as during the extracellular assembly and crosslinking. In general the activity of cells and tissues with regard to their ability to synthesize collagen are assessed by their ability to synthesize hydroxyproline or by measurement of the activities of specific enzymes, the proline and lysyl hydroxylases being the most commonly assayed.

Different Types of Collagen

Fifteen years have passed since it was first realized that all collagen fibres within a particular organism are not made up of identical molecules. Since 1970 a great deal of experimental work has been devoted to understanding these various collagen types, their molecular structure, biosynthesis, cells of origin, distribution and turnover. In spite of great advances it is still not clear how the structure of these molecules relates to their function. The different collagen types have been identified using Roman numerals, which have been assigned to them as they are purified and characterized (Fig. 3.14). In addition to these major types (I to V), many lesser, albeit well characterized collagens have been described (Table 3.1). These have been identified using a variety of capital letters and Greek symbols. We shall describe in detail the major characteristics of types I, III, IV, V and other basement membrane components since they are most important in the function of the cardiovascular tissues.

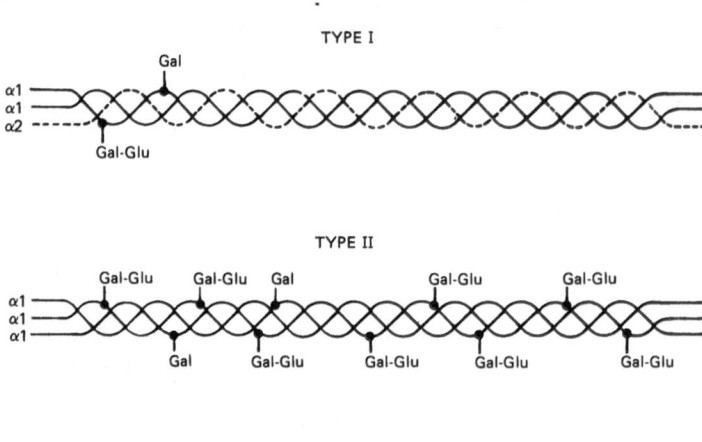

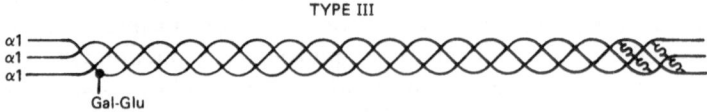

Fig. 3.14. Diagram of the three interstitial types of collagen. Type I is present in skin, bone, tendon, etc, type II in cartilage, and type III in blood vessels, developing tissues and as a minor component in skin and other tissues. There are differences in chain composition and degrees of glycosylation. Disulphide cross-links are only seen in type III collagen.

Table 3.1. The different types of collagen so far characterized

Type	Disulphide crosslinked	Tissue distribution	Chain composition	Mol. wt of each chain	References
I	–	Skin, bone, blood vessels and most organs	$\alpha1(I)_2 \alpha2(I)$	100 000	Nimni (1983)
I-trimer	–	Cell culture, tumors	$\alpha1(I)_3$	100 000	Nimni (1983)
II	–	Cartilage	$[\alpha1(II)]_3$	100 000	Nimni (1983)
III	+	Blood vessels, granulation tissue, skin	$[\alpha1(II)]_3$	100 000	Nimni (1983)
IV	+	Basement membrane	$[\alpha1(IV)]_3$	175 000–185 000	Kefalides et al. (1979) Timpl & Martin (1982) Kav et al. (1982)
V	–	Most tissues except hyaline cartilage, usually pericellular.	$[\alpha1(V)]_2 \alpha2(V)$	Unknown Globular and helical domains?	Linsenmayer et al. (1983)
VI	+	Uterus, placenta and skin		Short triple helical domains 40 000– 70 000	Furthmayr et al. (1983)
VII	+	Epithelial basement membrane	$[\alpha1(VII)]_3$	Seems larger than any known collagen (~170 000)	Bentz et al. (1983)
VIII	–	Aortic endothelial cells, corneal endo cells	$[\alpha1(VIII)]_3$	180 000	Sage et al. (1980) Benva (1980)
IX	+	Cartilage	$\alpha1(IX)\alpha2(IX)\alpha3(IX)$[a]	69 000–85 000	Yasui et al. (1984) Vander Rest (1985)
X	–	Hypertrophic cartilage	$[\alpha1(X)]_3$	59 000	Schmit (1983) Gibson (1983)

[a] 1α, 2α and 3α may be the type V equivalent for hyaline cartilage.

Type I Collagen

Before 1969 this was the only mammalian collagen known. The basic molecule was called "tropocollagen" or "collagen molecule"; the latter term has survived. It is composed of three chains, two identical, termed α1 chains, and one different from the other two, called α2. Using the new terminology we now call the chains α1 type I or α1(I) and α2 type I or α2(I) or simply α2, since there is no α2 chain among the other collagen types. This molecule has been almost completely characterized both physically and chemically (amino acid sequence, sedimentation, molecular dimensions, carbohydrate attachments, viscosity, crosslinking, etc.) [89]. Type I collagen is most abundant in skin, tendon, ligament, bone, cornea, etc. where it comprises between 80 and 99% of the total collagen. Bone matrix is almost exclusively type I collagen. As discussed below, the proportion of type I collagen in a particular tissue can vary at different sites, during development, with age and pathology. The most common technique used to isolate this molecule, and distinguish it both qualitatively and quantitatively from the other collagens, involves the use of solvents of different ionic strength and pH followed by differential salting out [90]. This fractionation is usually followed by identification of the intact chains and CNBr-derived peptides using polyacrylamide gel electrophoresis [1,91].

Type III Collagen

When the residue of human skin remaining after prolonged extraction with neutral salt and dilute acetic acid solutions is subjected to digestion with CNBr, a series of peptides appear that do not correspond to any of the known peptides derived from types I or II collagens [92,93]. Because of the similarities of two of these peptides to well characterized regions of the α1(I) and α1(II) chains it seemed related to the α1 family of chains and was therefore designated α1(III).

When human dermis was digested with pepsin under conditions that allowed the collagen molecules to maintain their helical conformation, it was found that type I molecules could be separated from type II by differential salt precipitation at pH 7.5 [94]. The type III molecules were composed of three identical chains, α1(III), which eluted on carboxymethylcellulose in a position intermediate between α1(I) and α2. The pepsin resistant portion of the new chains is similar in size to the previously isolated collagen chains and can migrate with α1(I) and α1(II) on conventional SDS-polyacrylamide gels during electrophoresis, although in some systems it can be seen to migrate slightly slower [95]. A characteristic of this collagen is the relatively high degree of hydroxylation of proline, its higher glycine content (more than 33% of the residues) and above all the presence of intramolecular disulphide bonds involving two cysteine residues very close to the C-terminal region of the triple helix. Because the ratio of type I to type III collagen changes with age, type III being predominant in fetal skin, this type of collagen is often referred to as fetal or embryonic collagen. Some interesting conclusions can be derived from observing Epstein's data on the ratio of type I to type III collagen present in the dermis of people of various ages, as well as in the insoluble residue remaining after the soluble collagen has been removed. In early fetal life (16 weeks) type III collagen is more abundant than type I. This coincides with the rapid rate of synthesis seen in the developing fetus [96]. At time of birth the ratio of I to III is 2.6 in the total dermis but around 1.7 in the insoluble dermis. In fetal life type III collagen seems to enhance significantly the strength of the dermis, since insolubility and cross-links go hand in hand. The possibility that type III collagen can become instantly crosslinked through intermolecular disulphide bridge formation is supported by the recent findings of Cheung et al. [97]. The ability of this collagen to rapidly crosslink through this mechanism could be of great advantage during early development and wound healing, where collagen is layed down at a rapid rate in an area where no previous connective tissue existed.

The distribution of types I and III collagen in human skin has been assayed by biochemical and immunohistochemical techniques [98–101]. Whereas biochemical determinations of collagens failed to show relative changes in dermis cut with a dermatome, immunohistochemical studies seemed to indicate that type III collagen is present primarily in the papillary dermis, just beneath the epidermis and around dermal blood vessels and appendages. The reasons for these discrepancies are not clear but age-related changes in solubility or preferential masking of the antigenic determinants could be responsible. Type III collagen, when reconstituted in vitro, gives rise to thinner fibres than type II collagen [102]. The physiological significance of these findings is not yet clear.

Although the denaturation temperatures of type III and type I collagen molecules do not differ, renaturation is more rapid and complete with the type III preparations, due to the presence of interchain disulphide bonds [103]. This property has been used to further purify type III collagen which still retains type I collagen as a contaminant [104]. Separation and quantitation of types I and III α1 chains has most recently been accomplished using HPLC and HEMA 1000 Glc (a copolymer of 2-hydroxyethyl methacrylate and ethylene dimethacrylate covalently coated with glucose) [105].

Conversion of type I procollagen to collagen is more efficient than that of type III procollagen [91,106,107]. These findings are consistent with the greater yields of type III procollagens extracted by neutral salt solutions from tissues and cell cultures, and with the estimated half-lives determined in growing rabbit skin: 26 min for type I procollagen and 3.9 h for type III [108]. The amino acid sequence of the α1(III) chain, consisting of 1028 residues, was determined by Fietzek and coworkers [109].

Following the demonstration that type III collagen was a normal constituent of skin (10–20% of the total collagen), it has been found in many other connective tissues [110]. Normal bone matrix may be the only tissue containing type I collagen that lacks type III. It is present in variable amounts associated with type I collagen in lung, heart muscle, heart valves, uterus, nerves, liver, placenta, umbilical cord, blood vessels, spleen, gingiva, kidney, lymph nodes, sclera and other eye structures. Blood vessels are particularly rich in type III collagen. The actual amounts determined vary with the method of assay, but 20–30% of the total collagen in human aorta seems to be type III [111, 112].

The media seems to contain the highest proportion of type III collagen and the atherosclerotic plaque the least.

Contrary to what had been observed in earlier studies [113], where atherosclerotic plaque was found to have more type I than type III collagen, more recent work [114] has failed to substantiate such a dramatic reversal, even though a small shift in favour of type I collagen was observed. In the latter studies, CNBr treatment solubilized around 80% of the total collagen in the intima and plaque and around 65% of that in the media. Solubilization with pepsin was very much less, generally under 20%. In vitro biosynthetic studies with arterial tissues have also yielded conflicting data since both an increase and a decrease in the relative proportions of types I and III have been reported in diseased tissue [115]. It is conceivable that, as in dermal wound repair, there is in the early stages of plaque formation a preponderance of type III and later a reversion in the III:I ratio towards normal. It is of significant interest in connection with this type of collagen that cells in fibrous joints, such as those present in the sagittal sutures in young rabbit calvaria (which normally synthesize only type I collagen), can be stimulated to synthesize significant quantities of type III collagen when tensile mechanical stresses are applied to this structure [116]. Further studies are required to elucidate the sequence of events and the implications of these findings.

Type IV Collagen and Other Basement Membrane-Associated Macromolecules

Type IV collagen is the major component of basement membranes and is generally regarded as the most characteristic of a large number of macromolecules that comprise these structures. Basement membranes are specialized connective tissue structures that underlie epithelia and endothelia and perform a multiplicity of structural and functional roles. For instance, they are involved in cell differentiation and orientation, membrane polarization, selective permeability to macromolecules, and are a target for a large number of diseases. The thickening of glomerular basement membrane in diabetics and the deposition of antibodies and complement in bullous pemphigoid, Goodpastures syndrome and dermatitis herpetiformis are some of the associated pathological processes.

The literature on basement membrane is very extensive and the reader is referred to recent reviews on the subject [117–121]. In addition to collagen, a large number of other macromolecules, which include glycoproteins such as laminin, fibronectin, proteoglycans and other less well-defined structures, participate in the formation of basement membranes. This discussion will focus on some of the better documented aspects of basement membrane research: it will discuss individually the most relevant characteristics of the macromolecules that have been isolated from basement membranes while trying to provide the reader with an overview of the molecular structure and organization of this vital connective tissue matrix. For a more detailed discussion of the macromolecules involved, the review by Timpl and Martin is suggested [117].

Kidney glomeruli and lens capsules have been frequently used as a source of basement membranes since they can be readily isolated free from other tissue elements [122]. By treating these tissues with pepsin, Kefalides [123] was able to solubilize and characterize a collagenous protein, now called type IV, that contains a single type of chain, the α1(IV) chain. It was suggested that basement membranes were composed of type IV collagen linked to non-collagenous glycoproteins by disulphide bonds [121,124].

Spiro and his collaborators [125–127], using denaturing solvents and reducing agents, were able to extract collagenous proteins ranging in size from 20 000 to over 200 000 daltons, from isolated glomeruli. These investigators proposed that glomerular basement membrane was composed of a number of dissimilar peptide subunits with collagenous and non-collagenous sequences of variable length.

Type IV collagen differs from interstitial collagens in its amino acid composition (Table 3.1). In comparison to the interstitial collagens, it contains higher amounts of hydroxylated amino acids (including 3-hydroxyproline) and a lower content of alanine and arginine. The glycine content is less than one-third, indicating the presence of non-collagenous segments. Most of the hydroxylysine residues are substituted by glucosyl-α(1–2)-galactosyl-7 groups linked to the hydroxyl group. Heteropolysaccharide side chains consisting of glucosamine, mannose, galactose, fucose, and sialic acid have also been identified as part of the type IV collagen molecules [128,129]. Carbohydrate accounts for some 10% of the mass of type IV collagen, a higher level than that found in most other collagens. A schematic diagram of type IV is shown in Fig. 3.15. It consists of a large triple helical domain and non-collagenous extensions that make it resemble procollagen. There are frequent interruptions of the triplet sequence Gly–X–Y within the triple helical domain with glycine replaced by other amino acids [130].

Soluble forms of type IV collagen can be extracted with acidic solvents (usually dilute acetic acid) from the matrix of EHS tumour [131] and from bovine lens capsule [132,133]. When electrophoresed, the reduced tumour collagen migrates as two chains α1(IV) and α2(IV), with apparent molecular

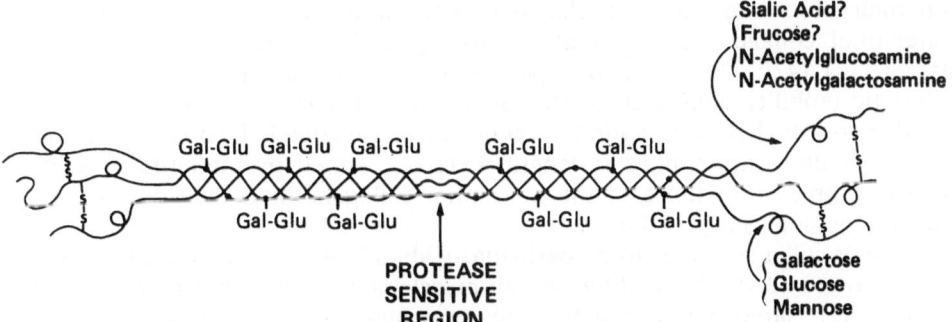

Fig. 3.15. Basement membrane collagen: Type IV collagen is a major component of basement membrane. It characteristically contains significant amounts of 3-hydroxyproline and sugar residues and seems to retain most of its non-helical extensions in the extracellular environment. A protease-sensitive area is located within the helical region which complicates the problem of isolation from insoluble matrices.

weights of about 160 000 and 140 000 [133,134]. The chains are not separated by molecular sieve chromatography and their resolution on electrophoresis may be due to compositional differences more than to differences in molecular weight. Evidence exists for a third constituent polypeptide chain. Ultra-structural studies suggested that the pepsin-solubilized collagens contain globular structures at each end of the molecule [135,136].

Pepsin and other proteases are used to dissolve otherwise insoluble collagen. Considerable heterogeneity is observed in the type IV collagen solubilized by pepsin from various tissues such as glomeruli or kidney cortices, lens capsule, placenta, muscle and the EHS tumour, with polypeptides ranging from 15 000 to 140 000 daltons [117]. As mentioned above, type IV collagen contains non-helical regions interrupting the helical domain which are sensitive to various proteases, resembling that found in the triple helical domain, of the comple-ment component Clq where it is associated with a bend in the triple helical strands [137]. These breaks in the helix of type IV collagen may impart a similar flexibility to these molecules.

The chains in the triple stranded molecules of type IV collagen are con-nected by disulphide bonds. In the $\alpha 1(IV)$ chain, the disulphides are located at the N-terminal end of the triple helical domain [138].

Type V Collagen

Type V collagen was discovered in pepsin digests of placental membranes [138–140] and other tissues. Type V collagen is more soluble than other collagens, particularly at high concentrations of NaCl (3–3.5 M) and at neutral pH, conditions that readily precipitate the interstitial collagens. Its amino acid composition in large part resembles interstitial collagens, except for a high ratio of hydroxylysine to lysine and a low alanine content. Similar to interstitial collagens, the hydroxylysines are only partially glycosylated with glucosylgalactose or galactosyl groups.

So far three chains $\alpha 1(V)$, $\alpha 2(V)$, and $\alpha 3(V)$ (formerly named B, A and C) [138] have been obtained from type IV collagen. They are similar in size, based on their behaviour on molecular sieve chromatography, to the α chains of interstitial collagens except that the $\alpha 1(V)$ chains appear to be somewhat larger [141,142]. The chains of type V collagen show a slightly lower electro-phoretic mobility compared to the chains of type I [139,143–146]. This may be due to a higher carbohydrate content or anomalous behaviour, since their SLS crystallites are similar in length to those formed by interstitial collagen and resemble more those of the interstitial collagens than they do basement membrane collagen [143,146].

Type V collagen seems to be particularly abundant in vascular tissues, where it appears to be synthesized by smooth muscle cells, although it is also present in relatively large amounts within the avascular corneal stroma [147]. Anti-bodies specific for type V collagen appear to be closely associated with cell surfaces. In muscle it surrounds the individual myotubules functioning as a boundary not only between cells but between cells and connective tissue elements of the peri- and epimysium [148]. In differentiated cartilage, antibodies to type V collagen localize around the pericellular matrix within the chondrocyte lacunae [149]. Electron immunohistochemical localization of type V collagen in rat kidney shows that it is present in the renal interstitium as individual fibres in close apposition to interstitial collagens and vascular basement membranes [150]. These observations suggest that type V collagen may be a unique form of collagen that contributes to cell shape by localizing on the surface of the cells and to the formation of an exocytoskeleton, as well as to binding to other connective tissue components.

Non-collagenous Proteins Associated with Basement Membranes

Basement membranes also contain significant amounts of non-collagenous glycoproteins that presumably account for their positive periodate-Schiff reaction [151].

Laminin

Laminin comprises almost half of the matrix proteins of EHS tumour, most of which can be extracted in neutral buffers of moderate ionic strength [152]. It has also been isolated from cultured endodermal and teratocarcinoma cells, in some instances in native form after collagenase treatment [117]. Immunohistochemical localization of laminin indicates that it is abundant in all basement membranes [153].

The amino acid composition of laminin distinguishes it from fibronectin [154]. It contains about 12–15% carbohydrate [155]. While the native protein migrates in electrophoresis as a narrow band, reduction of disulphide bonds produces two broad, faster migrating bands with molecular weights 200 000–220 000 and 400 000–440 000 daltons. Ultracentrifugal analyses indicate that laminin has a molecular weight in the range 800 000–1 000 000 daltons both in neutral buffer and under dissociating conditions (6 M guanidine). Laminin interacts with heparin, heparan sulfate [155] and type IV collagen, and seems to link endothelial cells to basement membranes [156].

Fibronectin

Fibronectin is a major biosynthetic product of cultured fibroblasts [157]. It is similar to the cold-unsoluble globulin of human plasma described earlier [158,159]. It is also produced by a variety of cells [160], including endothelial and smooth muscle cells and some epithelial cells. Immunohistology studies have shown that fibronectin is produced early in development and is associated with most embryonic basement membranes, but is not always detectable in fully developed basement membranes [161,162].

Fibronectin binds to a variety of macromolecules, including several types of collagens and denatured collagen [163–165]. One of the major binding sites for fibronectin on the collagen molecule has a hydrophobic nature and resides in CNBr peptide $\alpha 1$(I)-CB7, close to or including the cleavage site for animal collagenase [164–166]. Denatured collagen competes with native collagen in binding fibronectin [167] and, since fibronectin inhibits fibrillogenesis, it may play a role in regulating this process as well as fibre size and distribution.

The region of fibronectin responsible for its collagen-binding activity is located in the NH_2-terminal third of each chain [168] and since there are two such sites, it may enable the molecule to interact with collagen to form extended polymers. The collagen-like region of Clq, a subcomponent of the first complement component, can also bind to this region and coexist as complexes [169].

Proteoglycans

Glycosaminoglycans were first detected in basement membranes of embryonic tissues [170,171]. Polyanionic sites in native basement membranes observed by staining the glomerulus with ruthenium red were shown to disappear after treatment with heparitinase or heparinase [171,172], as did the permeability of the kidney and the basement membrane of the glomerulus [172,173]. Heparan sulfate and hyaluronic acid were isolated after proteolytic digestion from purified glomerular basement membranes, where they accounted for about 1% of the dry weight of the material [174].

A heparan sulfate containing proteoglycan, BM-1 proteoglycan (molecular weight 500 000–1 000 000 daltons) containing equal amounts of protein and heparan sulfate has been extracted from the EHS tumour matrix [175]. Antibodies prepared against these proteoglycans react mainly with the protein core and localize in various basement membranes.

In addition to the glycoproteins discussed above, a variety of other macromolecules have been detected in basement membranes, these are discussed in the reviews cited.

A Continuum Between Cytoplasm and Extracellular Matrix

The role of the extracellular matrix in determining cell shape, orientation, movement and metabolic activity has generated considerable interest [176]. Corneal fibroblasts, which have the capacity to migrate through extracellular matrices, can provide a good model to understand this phenomenon [177]. The migrating corneal fibroblast is an elongate, bipolar cell, possessing a leading pseudopodium and a trailing cell process that, by successive attachments and retractions, seems able to change shape and location. Using antibodies to various fibrillar proteins, it was observed that fibroblasts grown in collagen gels exhibit significant ultrastructural differences from those attached to glass surfaces [177]. The fibroblasts grown on glass exhibit a network of well-defined fibres, "stress fibres" that stain for actin, α-actinin and mysosin. These fibres seem to traverse the cell in all directions radiating from the cell surface along lines of stress. In contrast, the cells grown in collagen gels fail to show such patterns but, rather, show diffuse cytoplasmic staining, and actin and α-actinin but not mysosin, and seem to concentrate in the cell cortex and in filipodia.

It would seem reasonable to visualize how developing and adult living tissues could possess both of these characteristics at different times, and in different regions of the cell depending on their degree of activity. Even though such stress fibres have not been detected in vivo [178], it is conceivable that such structures could be found in areas of cell attachment. In many ways the phenomenon described resembles the organization of microfilaments in smooth muscle cells at the time of contraction. The association of myosin to actin and α-actinin in the stress filaments, and the absence of myosin in the cortical microfilaments of the "non-stressed" cell supports this analogy (Fig. 3.16).

The possible penetration of fibronectin into the cell membrane, its affinity for actin, its general characteristics and distribution, and the fact that the chemotaxis of the fibroblast requires a cytoskeletal organization that seems to be associated with the presence of fibronectin [179] suggests that a network must exist which connects the extracellular matrix with the cell cytoplasm (and

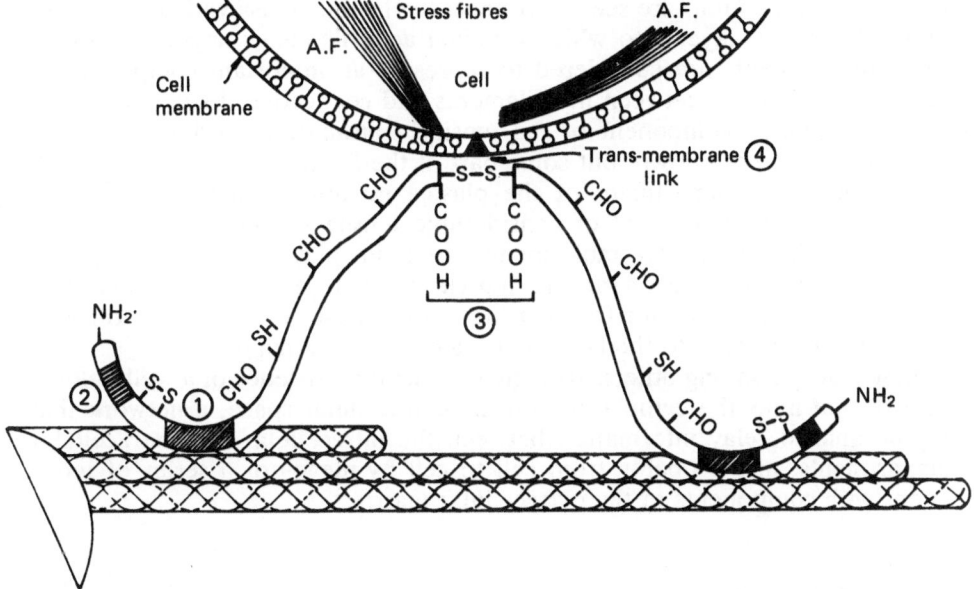

Fig. 3.16. A fibronectin molecule is shown attaching a cell to the surface of a collagen fibre. Fibronectin, a dimeric molecule composed of two subunits linked via disulphide bonds located near the C-terminal ends, is attached to collagen molecules placed in a quarter-staggered arrangement and separated by a 68 nm period. The attachment involves a specific binding site on fibronectin and a site on collagen located close to the collagenase cleavage area (1). Fibronectin contains in addition a fibrin binding site (2) and a sulphated glycosaminoglycan binding site (3) which is close to the cell attachment site. Shown in this diagram is a "trans-membrane link" (4) which has not been clearly identified and which may allow fibronectin to attach to actin filaments (AF) present in different forms of organization within the cell (stress fibres or tangentially oriented microfilaments).

probably the cell nucleus). This network could link the collagen–proteoglycan extracellular matrix via fibronectin, laminin, or chondronectin (or combinations of these molecules with other basement membrane components discussed earlier) to the actin-binding protein and the microfilamentous network within the cell. The transmembrane mode of communication is not known, but transmethylation reactions involved in chemotaxis of fibroblasts supports membrane involvement [179].

Epithelial cells may also be part of such a communication network, but less information is available. Evidence exists for the presence of a receptor for type I collagen on the cell surface of fibroblasts, but not on the apical surface of epithelial cells grown in culture [180]. Epithelial cells do not bind directly to collagen but seem to do so through laminin [156]. On the other hand, the basal cell surface of corneal epithelial cells seems to respond directly to collagen molecules added to the medium, without the presence of intermediates, suggesting that this surface may contain a collagen receptor that interacts across the plasmalemma with the actin-rich cortical cytoskeleton [181].

This modality of interaction seems also to hold true at a more macro-structural level. The electron microscopic analysis of the extracted muscle–tendon junctions reveals that the relationship between the terminal myofilaments and the lamina densa of the basal lamina is retained, despite the extensive extraction of the plasma membrane by non-ionic detergents [182]. Fine filaments (2–7 nm) are seen to connect the lamina densa with an electron-dense intracellular layer into which terminal actin filaments appear to insert. These fine filaments are considered to represent an important component of the structural linkage between myofilaments and connective tissue, and hence to be a significant component of the tension transmitting mechanism. Their precise nature is not known, but some part of the filaments must pass through the hydrophobic compartment of the plasma membrane and thus must be a transmembrane component of considerable tensile strength. These studies suggest that detergent-extractable membrane lipids play no significant role in the transmission of tension at the muscle–tendon junction, and that fine filaments are responsible for transmitting tension from myofilaments, through the plasma membrane, to the lamina densa of the basal lamina.

These studies, among others, strongly support the existence of a well-defined network that links the cytoplasm with the extracellular space, a network that may be able to relay information between the intracellular and extracellular compartments, and probably from cell to cell by means of a series of interactions with components of the extracellular matrix.

Wound Healing

There is an inherent tendency of tissues to repair after they have been damaged, with the nature of the repair process varying with the site and mode of injury. Connective tissues repair by regeneration of their extracellular matrices. Therefore, a major part of the process involves the deposition of newly-synthesized collagen and proteoglycans. Healing of experimentally-induced skin lesions has been studied extensively in animal models. In general, the cellular population of healing wounds changes from one associated with the initial inflammatory response (i.e. granulocytes and macrophages) to that associated with a proliferative and anabolic response (fibroblasts). Immediately after wounding, no obvious fibroblasts are present. Before recognizable fibroblasts enter the wound, cells that resemble immature fibroblasts are seen in the perivascular connective tissue. The development of these cells into mature fibroblasts has been followed through the different stages of wound repair [183]. Collagen synthesis has been reported to increase significantly by 24 h in open skin wounds of the rat [184]. A high proportion of type III collagen is produced in response to turpentine injection or to sponge implantation [185], and in the initial phase of wound repair in humans [186]. More quantitative studies on the nature of the collagen synthesized during the early phase of wound healing [187] show an increase in synthesis of type III collagen 10 h after infliction of the wound; by 24 h the percentage of type III collagen synthesized returned to a normal value.

The early increase in type III collagen observed by these investigators is probably derived from local fibroblasts that are activated by the wounding process, and the early type III collagen deposited may be important in establishing the initial wound structure and in providing a basic lattice for subsequent healing events. The ability of type III collagen to crosslink via disulphide bonds may greatly assist in this connection [97]. However, it is unlikely that type III collagen contributes significantly to wound tensile strength as the greatest increase in tensile strength is not observed until later phases of wound repair. In young guinea pigs the rate of collagen synthesis in dermal scars is initially high, but gradually approaches that of the surrounding dermis after a period of about 6 months [188]. Concomitant with the increased rate of collagen synthesis, the extent of hydroxylation of lysine in the early wound is significantly elevated, but declines to approach normal values about 3 weeks after wounding.

Dihidroxylysinonorleucine, derived from two residues of hydroxylysine, is the major reducible cross-link detectable in the early wounded tissue [189], but this is subsequently replaced by hydroxylysinonorleucine [190]. In addition to this increase in hydroxylation of lysine and hydroxylysine-derived cross-links, the amount of type III collagen is also increased in guinea pig dermal scars compared to uninvolved normal skin. It is noteworthy that the sequence described resembles very much that seen during early phases of growth and development. Further studies on the quantitative and qualitative distribution of collagen types in a variety of normal and injured tissues might thus provide further insight into the specific role that the different collagen types play in relationship to the normal structure and function of the connective tissues.

Fibrosis

Accumulation of collagen in excessive amounts is a major pathological event that underlies several clinical conditions, including pulmonary fibrosis, liver cirrhosis, retrocorneal fibrous membrane formation, as well as various forms of dermal fibrosis, such as scleroderma, keloids, hypertrophic scars and familial cutaneous collagenoma. Although in many of these diseases the terminal fibrotic lesion is considered to be the sequela of cellular injury, the cell populations injured and the endogenous mediators responsible for the post-injury fibrotic response vary from organ to organ. In many instances we seem to be dealing with an uncontrolled repair mechanism, where less organized and less specific connective tissue replaces a previously functional and carefully constructed matrix. In other instances we see an imbalance in the homeostasis of the extracellular matrix, where synthesis of macromolecules exceeds break-down, the end result being an excessive accumulation of collagen.

Fibrotic Response to Implantation of Foreign Materials

Most biomaterials cause a host tissue inflammatory response resulting in collagen synthesis and deposition around the implanted material. In some instances, marked inflammation and collagen synthesis is desired in order to produce a firm fibrous capsule of collagen, as around the sewing ring of a valve implant to secure it in place. Similarly, a mandibular defect is best repaired with a biomaterial which not only fills the defect, but also stimulates collagen production to allow a strong fibrous connection between bone and the bio-material. In other instances, however, minimal collagen deposition is desirable. For example, breast augmentation requires a material with minimal collagen response, thereby producing a soft, natural breast.

The granulomatous response that results from the implantation of clay cor-relates well with the significantly increased relative rates of collagen synthesis. Sand, on the other hand, which causes minimal histological reactivity, does not increase the relative rate of collagen synthesis compared to control wounds [191].

Implantation of soft silicone rubber prostheses is followed by growth of an enclosing connective tissue capsule that may undergo a process of contracture that results in pain, tissue deformity, and extrusion of the prosthesis [192,193]. Capsules developing in animals are histologically and ultrastructurally similar to those seen in human, and also show contracture [194,195]. The total collagen content of experimental capsules implanted in rats reaches a plateau with little change after 60 days [196].

When fibrous tissue capsules around silicone gel and saline-filled breast implants were examined by light, transmission, and scanning electron micro-scopy, regularly-arranged dense, connective tissue capsules were seen [195]. This tissue contains bundles of collagenous fibres that are densely packed and lie parallel to each other, forming structures of great tensile strength.

The outer surface of the connective tissue capsule contains reticulum fibres, small in diameter, that branch to form a net-like framework which supports the collagenous material. At the inner surface, fibrocytes and histiocytes are present in single layers and form an epithelial-like structure. The connective tissue of the capsules also contains capillaries and fibrocytes, which are usually deployed along bundles of collagen fibres and appear as fusiform elements with long processes. Contractile fibroblasts (myofibroblasts) are also found in these fibrous capsules. However, deformation of the augmented breast does not seem to be caused by the action of the myofibroblasts, because their number is too small. Rather it is more likely caused by the inelastic arrangement of large amounts of collagenous material layered around the capsule. Contracting capsules seem to present elevated levels of total glycosaminoglycans and chondroitin-4-sulphate compared to non-contracted capsules [196].

There is evidence that the ultrastructure of contracted capsules is similar to that of hypertrophic scars [193,195–197]. The kinetics of collagen deposition and of proteoglycan accumulation in fibrous capsules surrounding implants are similar to those of normal wound healing.

Collagen Degradation

The changing patterns of the connective tissue matrix during growth, development, and repair following injury, require a delicate balance between synthesis and degradation of collagen and proteoglycans. Under normal circumstances this balance is maintained, while in many diseased states it is altered, leading to an excessive deposition of collagen or to a loss of functional tissue. The first animal enzyme capable of degrading collagen at neutral pH was isolated from the culture fluid of tadpole tissue [198]. This was shown to cleave the native molecule into two fragments in a highly specific fashion at a temperature below that of denaturation of the substrate [199]. These fragments were characterized by electron microscopy and shown to reflect the cleavage of a native collagen molecule at a specific site closer to the C-terminal end of the molecule, yielding segments of one-quarter and three-quarters the length of the native collagen molecule. The larger fragment was termed TC_A and the smaller fragment TC_B.

Collagenolytic enzymes have been obtained following cell and organ culture from a wide range of tissues from animal species in which collagen is present [200–205]. In general, these enzymes have a number of fundamental properties in common: they all have neutral pH optima, they are not stored within the cell but, rather, appear to be secreted either in an inactive form or bound to inhibitors. Figure 3.17 summarizes schematically the fundamental aspects of this enzyme and its mode of action.

A factor that seems to slow down the breakdown of collagen is the presence of cross-links. The introduction of artificial methylene bridges with formaldehyde [206], or of native cross-links by the use of purified lysyl oxidase [207], increases the resistance of collagen to collagenase degradation. Native collagen fibres crosslinked by glutaraldehyde cannot be digested even by bacterial collagenase [208]. Collagen from individuals of increasing age becomes more resistant to enzymatic digestion, suggesting that an age-related accumulation of cross-links may be responsible [209]. It is therefore possible that crosslinking of collagen plays a role not only in generating mechanical stability to the fibres but also in the regulation of collagen turnover in vivo.

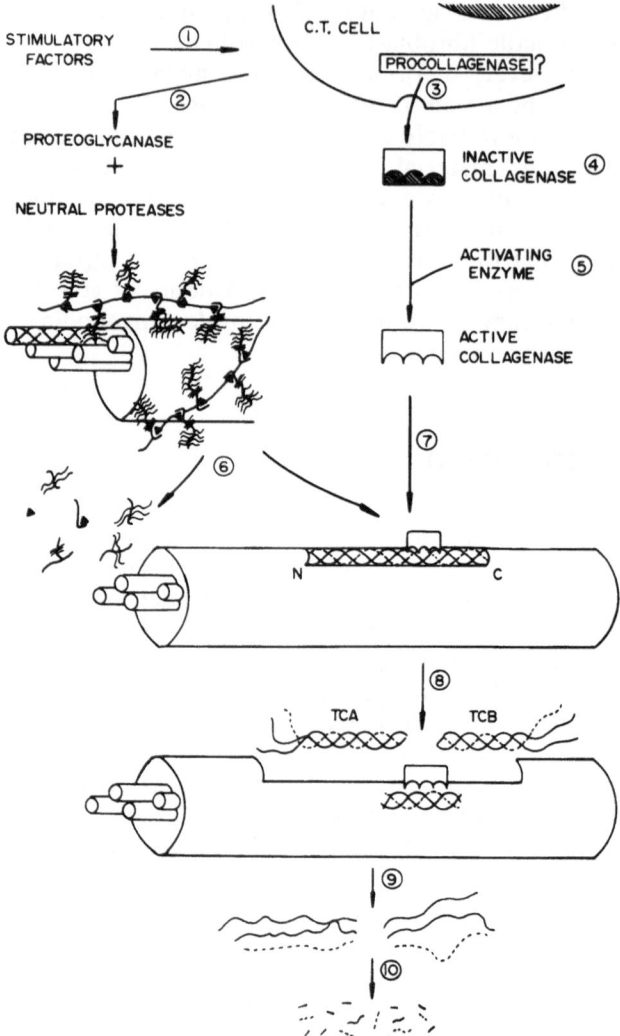

Fig. 3.17. Sequence of events leading to the degradation of collagen fibres by the enzyme collagenase. (1) A variety of factors have been described which stimulate connective tissue cells to synthesize collagenase, glycosidases and neutral proteases. (2) The proteoglycan degrading enzymes remove the mucopolysaccharides which surround collagen fibres and expose it to collagenase. (3) Inactive collagenase is secreted. (4) The enzyme is usually found in the extracellular space bound to an inhibitor. (5) An activating enzyme removes the inhibitor. (6) Glycosidases complete the degradation of the proteoglycans. (7) The active collagenase binds to fibrillar collagen. (8) Collagenase splits the first collagen molecule into two fragments (TC_A and TC_B) which denature and begin to unfold at body temperature. The enzyme now moves on to an adjacent molecule. (9) The denatured collagen fragments are now susceptible to other proteases. (10) Non-specific neutral proteases degrade the collagen polypeptides.

Crosslinking

Crosslinking renders the collagen fibres stable, and provides them with an adequate degree of tensile strength and viscoelasticity to perform their structural role. The degree of crosslinking, the number and density of the fibres in a particular tissue, as well as their orientation and diameter, combine to provide this function. Crosslinking begins with the conversion to peptide-bound aldehydes of specific lysine and hydroxylysine residues in collagen, a reaction that was illustrated earlier (Fig. 3.11). It involves the oxidative deamination of the ξ-carbon of lysine or hydroxylysine to yield the corresponding semialdehydes (allysine or hydroxyallisine) and is mediated by lysyloxidase [210–213]. Since this enzyme remains tightly bound to collagen, purified by conventional precipitative methods, incubation of such collagen at 37°C, neutral pH and physiological ionic strength, will cause additional aldehydes to form on the molecule [213]. This effect can be enhanced by tissue extracts that possess lysyl oxidase activity or by the purified enzyme. This strong affinity of lysyl oxidase for collagen has been used for purifying the enzyme by affinity adsorption [214]. Enzymatic activity is inhibited by β-aminopropionitrile, chelating agents such as EDTA and D-penicillamine, and isonicotinic acid hydrazide and other carbonyl reagents. Lysyl oxidase exhibits particular affinity for the lysines and hydroxylysines present in the non-helical extensions of collagen, but can, at a slower pace, also alter residues located in the helical region of the molecule [215]. It has been proposed that it binds initially to the carboxyl terminal non-helical end of the fibrillar collagen since it has been observed that the ξ-NH_2 groups in this region are the first to be converted to aldehydes [216].

Intramolecular and Intermolecular Cross-Links

Inhibitors of crosslinking, such as BAPN and D-penicillamine, made it clear that aldehydic groups were essential for formation of cross-links (Fig. 3.18). Additional progress was made when it was discovered that agents that can add across double bonds or stabilize Schiff bases, such as CN^-, and $NaBH_4$, could decrease the solubility of collagen and increase its mechanical strength [217–220]. In particular, the use of tritiated $NaBH_4$ became very useful in the identification and characterization of reducible cross-links [219]. Analysis of the radioactive compounds revealed the presence of aldehydes that have been converted to the parent alcohols (e.g. hydroxynorleucine) and reduced Schiff bases (lysinonorleucine, hydroxylysinonorleucine and dihydroxylysinonorleucine) [221]. These fundamental chemical reactions are summarized in Fig. 3.18. Alkaline hydrolysis of the reduced collagen yielded the reduced form of the aldol condensation product that generates intramolecular cross-links. Although these experiments provided basic information on the crosslinking precursors and their early reaction products, they did not allow all of the intricacies of the crosslinking process to unfold. Simple Schiff bases are acid labile, which means that dilute organic acids, such as acetic acid,

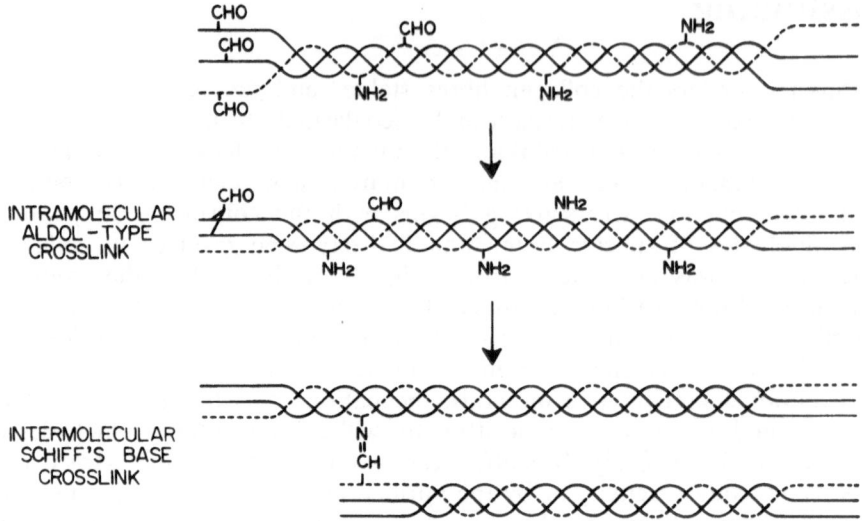

Fig. 3.18. Formation of intramolecular and intermolecular crosslinks in type I collagen. Intramolecular cross-links occur in the non-helical regions and involve an aldol condensation reaction between lysine or hydroxylysine derived aldehydes within a single molecule. Intermolecular cross-links on the other hand involve aldehydes and ε-amino groups of lysine present in different molecules.

should be able to cleave them. Yet we know that a significant amount of collagen is insoluble in this reagent, particularly when the tissue originates from older individuals. In recent years the details of the cross-linking of collagen have become much clearer, several unique crosslinking entities have been characterized and their exact location on adjacent molecules established. Detailed information is provided in a recent review by Nimni [1].

Collagen Composition of the Normal and Diseased Blood Vessel Wall

Blood vessels contain types I and III collagen as major components and lesser amounts of basement membrane collagen type IV, type V and a newly described endothelial cell type collagen labelled type VIII. Estimation of collagen types I and III in pepsin digests and by analysis of specific CNBr derived peptides has revealed that both the normal aorta as well as the atherosclerotic plaque of the diseased intima contain more type I than type III collagen [222]. There seems to be only a relatively small shift in composition in favour of type I collagen in the diseased tissue, in contrast to earlier studies which suggested a larger change, possibly associated with a transformation of the smooth muscle cell [223]. It would seem therefore that both atherogenesis and diffuse intimal thickening may involve primarily smooth muscle cell hyperplasia with increased production of collagen, but with little change in the phenotype expressed. Type V collagen containing both αA and αB chains is present throughout the vessel wall in diffusely thickened intima media and adventitia, as well as in the plaque, where a marked enrichment relative to interstitial collagen is noted [222]. This is presumed to reflect the relatively cellular nature of the atherosclerotic lesion. The αC chain of type V was detected in porcine but not in human aorta.

In addition to the major collagens, blood vessels contain type VI collagen, described by Furthmayr et al. as a short chain or intima collagen [224]. This collagen seems to be an integral part of a larger collagen-like glycoprotein isolated earlier from calf aorta and ligament [225,226]. Another collagen which was first isolated from the media of cultured endothelial cells, but has subsequently been found not to be restricted to the endothelium, is type VIII collagen [227]. This collagen is unusual with regard to the large size of its chains and because it is non-disulphide bonded and seems to lack non-helical domains at the C- and N-terminal ends.

Blood Vessels: Arteries and Veins

Arteries and veins are made up of collagen and elastin which contribute most significantly to their mechanical and structural properties. The nature of the composite varies from one location to another and is adapted to its physiological function by variations in diameter, collagen : elastin ratio, wall thickness, distribution of the fibrous proteins and smooth muscle cells.

Arteries exhibit three distinct morphological areas. The intima, which is in contact with the blood, consisting of a layer of endothelial cells which sit on a basement membrane, is a collagenous rich material (type IV collagen) associated with glycoproteins and proteoglycans. Below that is a layer of thin collagen, elastin and reticulin fibres. Then follows an elastic lamina which separates the intima from the media. This is a muscular layer populated by smooth muscle cells which generate concentric layers of elastin. The outer part of the vessel consists of woven connective tissue containing mostly collagen.

Veins are quite similar to arteries. They generally exhibit a smaller wall thickness and the media contains less elastin. They have a thicker adventitia. The correlation between the arrangement of collagen and elastin and its relationship to the function and elasticity of these structures is discussed by Fung [228].

Many studies have investigated the relative contributions of collagen and elastin to structural stability and elasticity. Roach and Burton studied vessel elasticity before and after removal of collagen and elastin by chemical or enzymatic means. They showed that the slopes of the distensibility curves of the trypsin-treated specimens (which removed collagen) were similar to the controls in the low stress region, reflecting the fact that elastin is the major contributor to function in this region. At high stresses, on the other hand, whether elastin was present or not did not make any difference. More recent studies have extended and confirmed these observations on vascular and non-vascular tissues. Hoffman et al. [71], studying bovine ligaments, also came to the conclusion that the initial portion of the stress – strain curves is mainly due to elastin following sequential enzymatic removal of the different structural components by collagenase, elastase and hyaluronidase plus β-glucuronidase (the latter enzymes remove the interfibrillar ground substance or proteoglycans) [71]. Hoffman's data suggest that the collagen and elastic fibre networks are kept somewhat apart and lubricated by the proteoglycan matrix, and that the elastic fibre network constrains the collagen network from slipping visco-elastically at both low and high strains.

On the other hand, studies performed in vitro on carotid, external iliac, internal iliac and common iliac arteries of man and dog treated with purified elastase and collagenase showed that elastase caused the vessels to dilate but otherwise remain intact. Treatment with collagenase led to ruptures leading to the conclusion that wall integrity ultimately depends on collagen. The common iliac arteries exhibited dramatically greater dilation after treatment with collagenase, corresponding to the greater tendency of aneurysms to develop in these arteries [229].

Heart Valves

Heart valves are thin, translucent structures containing mostly collagen and proteoglycans and small amounts of elastin which are subjected to continuous repetitive mechanical stresses for the lifespan of an individual. A variety of pathological processes can lead to heart valve malfunction. These include genetic diseases of the connective tissues where crosslinking of collagen is impaired, rheumatic fever, and a variety of infectious diseases. Dysfunction is usually associated with degenerative changes of the tissue substance which require surgical correction or replacement with a prosthesis.

A major cause of ultimate failure is calcification, a common sequela to problems involving the cardiovascular system. The pathogenesis of calcific aortic stenosis is still a matter of controversy. Calcification of the annulus fibrosus of the mitral valve is a frequent finding in older patients at necropsy. The possible mechanism of calcification of heart valves, vascular tissues and implanted prosthesis will be discussed below.

As mentioned above, collagen is a major component of heart valves. It comprises 50–70% of the dry weight of the tissue, depending on the species and age. It is almost completely insoluble in neutral salts, weak acids or protein denaturing solutions. Limited digestion with pepsin will dissolve between 30 and 50% of the collagen and allow its identification and characterization. The pepsin extract is usually purified by salt precipitation followed by column chromatography. Using this procedure Collins et al. found most of the collagen to be of type I, but with both of its component chains exhibiting an unusual chromatographic behaviour when compared to skin α1 and α2 chains, and also an increased content of hydroxylysine, supporting similar findings by previous investigators [230]. On the other hand, Bashey et al. using similar procedures for isolation but followed by polyacrylamide electrophoresis using bovine heart valves instead of porcine heart valves, found that type III collagen was also present [231]. This is not unexpected, since cardiovascular tissues usually contain relatively high quantities of type III collagen. Earlier, Mannschott et al. had also reported that heart valves contained type III collagen [232].

In addition, to be highly hydroxylated at the lysine position, heart valve collagen in the fibrillar form contains a preponderance of dehydro-dihydroxylysinonorleucine, a cross-link derived from two hydroxylysine residues present in adjacent molecules. This cross-link is usually found in hard tissues such as bone, in contrast to the dehydro-hydroxylysinonorleucine which is predominant in soft tissues such as dermis [230]. The more stable cross-link found in valvular tissue may be responsible for the insolubility of the collagen and essential for the function and durability of a tissue exposed to such constant stress. The ground substance of the cardiac valves is similar histochemically to that of aortic wall. It contains significant amounts of chondroitin sulphate and hyaluronic acid [233,234]. The physicochemical properties of heart valve hyaluronic acid are very similar to those obtained from other sources such as synovial fluid, suggesting that as in the latter it may serve as a lubricant. The continual displacement of the two zona fibrosa of a cusp during the normal pumping action of the heart would require such lubrication, and the hydrodynamic properties of hyaluronic acid are ideal for this purpose. On the other hand the chondroitin sulphate, by virtue of its strong negative charges, would tend to form a compact composite with the collagen network and thus provide a strong viscoelastic material with good flexing characteristics.

Biomechanical Modulation of Connective Tissue Metabolism

Many studies support the thesis that mechanical forces induce changes in the structure of connective tissues. Proteins, glycosaminoglycans, glycoproteins and other materials secreted into the environment by unstressed cells form a gelatinous coating which protects them from physical and chemical changes in the surrounding fluids. They function as mechanical cushions, hygroscopic agents, regulatory filters, adsorbents, ion-exchange medium, lubricants, cements and support structures. In sites where compression is very mild, the ground substance may integrate with the collagenous components to form boundaries, such as occurs in basement membranes which form under epithelial and endothelial cells [235].

The amount of collagen in a tissue and the pattern of weaving of the fibre are usually adequate to counteract the tensile forces in order to prevent rupture. The net amounts of collagen are generally sufficient to meet short periods of emergency loading which may be considerably greater than average. Sometimes the values are very marginal and it is only through the ability of the animal to repair minute fractures or tears that integrity is preserved.

The classical experiments of Weiss clarified the responsiveness of fibroblasts to tension [236]. Pins placed in a tissue culture of fibroblasts were slowly moved apart so that the materials of the culture were placed under tension. The cells were observed to become aligned along the lines of stress, and collagenous fibrils then appeared along these lines. These results suggest that tensile forces stimulate fibroblasts to produce and extrude collagenous fibrils and then arrange them so that the tension is borne by the rope-like strands rather than by the cells.

Evidence for the adaptation of collagen strength and direction to the operating forces have been documented in the skin and other organs, most clearly in the embryo where the subcutaneous collagenous fibres in the dermis become oriented along the lines of tension. Repeated biopsies of various sites of the skin reveal cleavage patterns which change characteristically with growth. Similarly, the lines of traction determine the orientation and direction of remodelling of fascia and tendons.

The quantity of collagen found in blood vessels appears to vary with tension, that is with the product of the blood pressure and the radius of the vessel. In vessels with low pressures, as in the elevated veins, collagen is present in very limited amounts. On the other hand veins in which the hydrostatic pressure is higher, have increased amounts of collagen. The quantity of collagen also increases with the radius of the vessel. These and other local adaptions in the amount of collagen to the tensile stresses provide support for the thesis that mechanical forces affect the extent of local development of collagen [237].

Collagen biosynthesis is increased in the aorta, mesenteric arteries and microvessels of the central nervous system of rats made hypertensive by treatment with deoxycorticosterone and in spontaneously hypertensive rats [238]. These changes can be reversed by antihypertensive agents.

It has also been shown that the proportions of collagen and elastin in the ascending aorta of the rabbit increase between birth and 2 months and correlate with the continuing rise in medial tension [239] – an observation that is in agreement with the fact that cyclic stretching of rabbit aortic medial cells grown in culture in elastic membranes also increases their synthesis of matrix components [240].

When homologous saphenous veins are implanted in the arterial circulation of dogs and explanted after several months the chemical composition of the explants are significantly changed, suggesting a molecular remodelling of the tissue [241]. The incorporation of lysine into elastin increased by a factor of ten, as compared to the non-grafted veins, and only small amounts of radioactivity were recovered in the polymeric collagen fraction. One can conclude from these experiments that the modified hemodynamic conditions provided by the arterial circulation behaved as a stimulus for a "redifferentiation" of the cellular elements of the venous wall. "Arteriolization", which has been documented histologically, is therefore accompanied by a shift in the ability of the smooth muscle cells to synthesize collagen and elastin, thus providing additional evidence for the modulating effects of the environment on matrix production.

Collagen, Platelet Aggregation and Thrombosis

Thrombosis is initiated when the non-thrombogenic vascular endothelium becomes detached and the underlying connective tissue is exposed to blood [242]. The thrombogenic and platelet aggregating activity of collagen is well known and the platelet–collagen system appears to be a good model in which to study the interactions of cell surfaces with collagen. The interactions of platelets with collagen which result in platelet aggregation can be easily monitored by the decreased turbidity of the suspension [243]. Usually type I collagen is used to test for the platelet aggregating activity, although type III is also a potent aggregator [243]. Both these collagens are major constituents of the media of the vascular wall. On the other hand, types IV and V collagens, which are associated with the endothelial cells that form the lining of blood vessels, are non-thrombogenic, and may contribute to providing the vascular system with a non-thrombogenic surface [244].

The process of blood coagulation is a complex one and many of the details are very well understood. When collagen types I and III become exposed, platelets become sticky and adherent, and begin to aggregate with one another and release vasoactive amines. Blood coagulation is initiated around the platelets and exposed collagen or damaged tissue, leading to thrombus formation. When the coagulation is initiated by surface contact (the intrinsic pathway) collagen fibres are not only able to activate platelets but also can activate the first of a long series of steps involving activation of factor XII (Hageman factor). Elastin appears not to react with platelets but may activate factor XII.

Activated platelets seem to be able to augment clot formation via this pathway by releasing factor V which in turn enhances the rate of activation of factor X, the last stage of the intrinsic pathway. The extrinsic pathway (initiated by tissue factors) is closely associated to the later stages of the intrinsic pathway and both lead to the final step in which prothrombin is converted to thrombin X in order to catalyze the conversion of fibrinogen to fibrin. As mentioned above, the collagen in the endothelium is non-thrombogenic as illustrated by experiments with human umbilical cord [245]. In these studies rings were prepared by sectioning these vessels, which were handled in such a way that the endothelium was exposed to heparinized, citrated or EDTA-anticoagulated blood. In all instances platelets were shown to adhere to the banded collagen fibres but not to the amorphous basement membrane. The basement membrane of the human umbilical cord morphologically resembles that of mammalian capillaries and heart valves, explaining why xenograft heart valves or vascular prostheses which retain such a structure are relatively non-thrombogenic. On the other hand, when these implants begin to degenerate, and presumably expose the subendothelial fibrillar collagens, they have been observed to react with platelets [246].

Platelets from patients implanted with porcine heart valves which were in stages of degeneration, showed signs of hyperactivity (cytoplasmic spreading) as well as changes in the differential platelet count. All such patients demonstrated in their explanted prosthetic valves platelet deposits on the surface of the degenerated bioprosthesis.

Although one of the main advantages of the bioprosthetic tissue derived valves relates to the fact that they do not require anticoagulation and that thromboembolic complications are rare, these studies, among others, suggest that degeneration of the matrix and exposure of interstitial collagens may provide a potential focus for thrombosis. The same caution applies to other types of cardiovascular prosthesis manufactured from fibrillar collagens.

Collagen as a Biomaterial

One of the earliest chemical modifications of collagen is associated with the process of leather tanning, a technology which has evolved over the ages. Heat-denatured collagen provides us with glues and gelatins. During the last 15 years, increased interest has developed in the use of collagen and collagen-containing tissues in the manufacturing of medical devices.

There are basically two fundamental approaches. One involves the use of collagen-rich tissues, usually structural in nature, which are treated chemically in order to transform them into implantable prostheses. Examples of these are heart valves, tendons, ligaments, blood vessels and pericardium. The handling and preservation of tissues is discussed below, with examples which have resulted in devices of significant value. The second approach involves the use of purified collagen, obtained from animal tissues (mostly from bovine skin), processed in a variety of ways to generate a large number of products which not only have applications in the medical field but also in the cosmetic industry.

Collagen is used in the form of native, soluble collagen, enzyme-degraded native collagen, soluble collagen reconstituted into fibres, microfibrillar collagen, collagen derived peptides, etc. Products manufactured from these sources began with chemically-tanned porcine heart valves. In 1969 it was found simultaneously by Carpentier in Paris and Hancock and Nimni in Southern California that porcine heart valves could be fixed with the dialdehyde glutaraldehyde, and that the cross-links introduced were chemically and biologically stable and could give rise to an essentially non-immunogenic graft. This resulted in the first stabilized glutaraldehyde-fixed porcine valve prosthesis, the Hancock valve, which was manufactured in the USA and which was implanted in humans that year. The author's decision to use glutaraldehyde followed the observation that formaldehyde-fixed porcine valves implanted into animals and humans exhibited a rapid rate of degeneration; they were rapidly degraded by the host and elicited an immune response. This was understandable since the methylene cross-links introduced by formaldehyde are not stable and the body fluids will remove the aldehyde from the tissues. In vitro studies proved that was the case. A simple preliminary experiment was done in which porcine heart valves were divided into three groups: fresh untreated, fixed with 1% formaldehyde, or with 0.2% glutaraldehyde at a pH of 7.4. These three sets of tissues were exposed to running tap water. Within a few days the fresh tissues disintegrated. The formaldehyde-fixed material took a little longer but began to disrupt within a couple of weeks, whereas the tissues fixed with glutaraldehyde maintained their structural integrity for years.

These simple but revealing experiments gave rise to the Hancock porcine valve bioprosthesis (Fig. 3.19) [247]. Glutaraldehyde was selected because it had been shown to restore cross-links which were chemically and thermally stable to collagen from animals treated with β-aminopropionitrile and D-penicillamine, agents that inhibit the formation of native cross-links in vivo and result in a very weak connective tissue framework [248]. Carpentier and his associates combined glutaraldehyde with sodium metaperiodate to destroy the interfibrillar ground substance (proteoglycans) and generate new sugar-derived

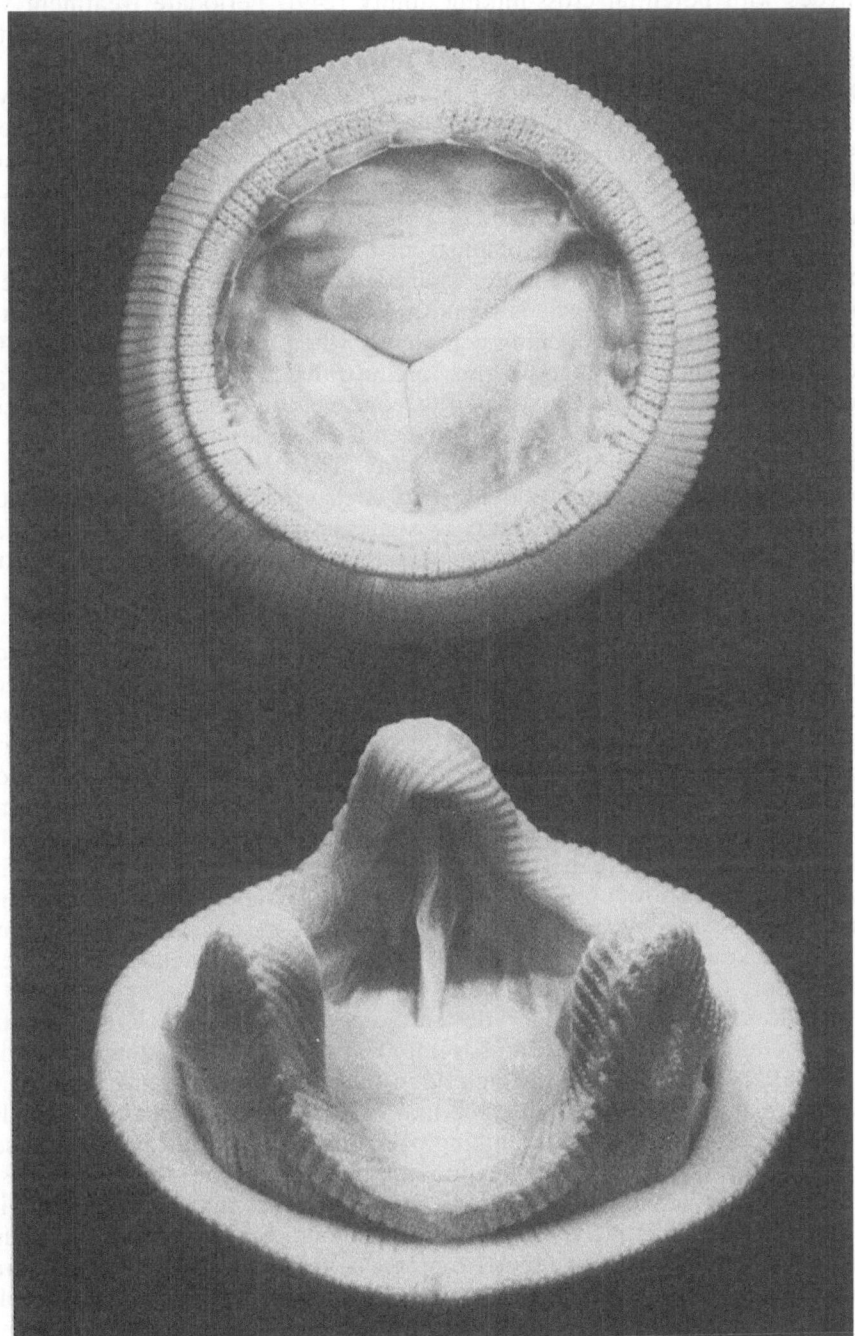

Fig. 3.19. Hancock aortic porcine heart valve prosthesis.

aldehydes with potential cross-linking ability [249]. Periodate treatment was subsequently abandoned since it seemed to contribute to the instability of the crosslinked matrix.

The author's studies used either glutaraldehyde alone or glutaraldehyde followed by sodium borohydride to stabilize the newly-formed synthetic cross-links. The latter step proved unnecessary and possibly damaging since small bubbles of nascent hydrogen could disrupt the structure of the connective tissues, and was therefore abandoned. Later, other tissues such as dura mater and pericardium were used to reconstruct heart valves. The advantage over porcine valves seemed to be a better hydrodynamic performance at the time of implant, since the porcine valves retain muscular tissues around their annulus which prevent them from opening completely when used as a heterograft. On the other hand, the advantages of the porcine valve at this time are the longer periods of observation and possibly the concave conformation of the native cusps, since they are supported by collagenous bundles which allow them to retain their natural shape much more readily. The pericardial tissue has to be "moulded" and fixed by glutaraldehyde. It is also thicker, and therefore more resistant to initial tears, but there is some uncertainty about its ultimate durability and performance. Nevertheless, both the porcine and pericardial reconstituted valves provide a useful prosthesis for hundreds of thousands of recipients.

About half of the valves implanted throughout the world are made from natural tissues crosslinked by glutaraldehyde, while the remainder are mechanical in nature and made out of synthetic materials (floating ball, tilting discs, etc.). Selection of a particular valve depends on many factors. In general, younger patients are more likely to receive machanical valves, while older individuals almost always are implanted with tissue valves. The major advantage of the mechanical valve is its proven durability. The advantages of the tissue valves are that the patients do not require anticoagulation, and that problems tend to show up gradually and allow for reoperation. Calcification around collagen is a recurrent problem in natural tissue valves and is more prevalent in younger people. The major problem of the mechanical valve is sudden failure due to thrombosis.

A significant effort is ongoing to devise the perfect valve, which may turn out to be a modified tissue valve. Improvement in flow characteristics, increasing the flexibility of the tissue through long-range cross-links, introduction of "lubricating macromolecules" into the matrix of the cusp, increased durability by alternate modalities of crosslinking, generation of antithrombogenic surfaces, and introduction of calcification inhibitors into the connective tissue matrix are being actively investigated. It is of interest that collagen in living adult tissues has a relatively very low turnover rate. Since crosslinking further reduces it hopefully to zero, adequate preservation of the collagen in the graft should yield a very durable implant. Other experimental approaches involve the use of synthetic polymer–collagen grafted composites, as well as valves manufactured entirely from reconstituted collagen, hydrogels, polyurethanes or other extruded polymers.

Crosslinking of Collagen by Glutaraldehyde

Glutaraldehyde is a valuable crosslinking agent which has been used to stabilize tissue heterografts and in the development of tissue bioprostheses such as heart valves, blood vessels and tendons [250,251]. It has long been used as a tanning agent in the leather and wool industries. Despite its wide use in electron microscopy, protein chemistry and immunochemistry, there have been few attempts made to understand the molecular nature of the products formed or the number and locations of the cross-links introduced. Since the raw biological materials used in most cases do not have uniform properties, it becomes difficult to use the physical strength of the final products to determine which fixation procedure is preferable. On the other hand, chemical analysis of the crosslinking entities formed by glutaraldehyde has not been completed due to the complexity and heterogeneity of the structures [252]. Therefore, the number of cross-links cannot yet be determined by chemical means.

Glutaraldehyde reacts primarily with amino groups of proteins in biological systems [253–255]. Tomimatsu et al. reported that only ε-amino groups of lysyl residues in proteins react with glutaraldehyde [256]. Bowes and Cater first reported the appearence of an UV absorption peak at 265 nm following the reaction of glutaraldehyde with amine compounds [257]. Richards and Knowles, as well as Monsan et al., proposed the Michael-addition reaction products of α,β-unsaturated Schiff's bases as the final stable products [258, 259]. However, Hardy et al. reported the isolation of a pyridinium-type compound following the reaction of glutaraldehyde with amines and suggested this structure as the stable cross-link [260]. They showed that this compound had an UV absorption maximum at 265 nm, consistent with the original observation of Bowes and Cater [257,260].

[3]H-Glycine and 6-aminohexanoic acid were used as model amine compounds and reacted with glutaraldehyde [261]. Based on the spectral characteristics and the molecular weights obtained from the reaction products, it was concluded that glutaraldehyde can modify amines to form an intermediate which absorbs at 300 nm and has a molecular weight of about 200 daltons. In the presence of excess glutaraldehyde, this intermediate is quickly converted to a much larger intermediate which absorbs strongly at 265 nm. The larger intermediates were finally altered to yield a strong absorption peak at 325 nm with no apparent change in the molecular weight. These results suggested that a process of polymerization is induced by the initial reaction of glutaraldehyde with amines. The glutaraldehyde–polymer amine complex is self-limiting in size and can undergo internal rearrangement to become chemically inert.

In another series of studies, collagen in three different states, i.e. native soluble molecules, denatured molecules and reconstituted fibres, was exposed to various concentrations of glutaraldehyde [262]. The degree of intramolecular and intermolecular cross-link formation was evaluated by measuring collagen solubility, chain formation, and resistance towards cleavage by CNBr or collagenase digestion. Modification of lysyl residues was measured by amino acid analysis. When dilute collagen solutions were reacted with low concentrations of glutaraldehyde, intramolecular cross-links were observed as the predominant cross-links. When the glutaraldehyde concentration was increased, the collagen became more insoluble, indicating the formation of intermolecular cross-links. When reconstituted collagen fibres were reacted with low concentrations of glutaraldehyde, intermolecular cross-links were formed, which prevented the material from being solubilized by CNBr. However, these materials could still be solubilized by collagenase. When the glutaraldehyde concentration was increased, the materials became resistant to collagenase, while there was only a small increase in the number of lysyl residues modified. This reflects an increase in the molecular length of the glutaraldehyde polymers extending from the initial glutaraldehyde and lysyl residue reaction sites rather than an increase in the actual number of cross-linking sites.

When dealing with fixation of tissues or of densely packed molecules such as collagen fibres, additional variables were introduced. Under these circumstances, penetration of the glutaraldehyde molecules and accessibility to the reactive group on the proteins became a significant issue [263]. When dealing with whole tissues this becomes even more so a matter of concern. Penetration at room temperature is definitely faster than in the cold. Glutaraldehyde (2%) penetrates into soft animal tissues (i.e. liver) 0.7 mm in 3 hours at room temperature, while its ability to produce adequate fixation lags behind since it reaches a depth of only 0.5 mm in the same period of time. After 24 hours, glutaraldehyde penetrates to a depth of 1.5 mm, while good fixation reaches to a depth of 1.0 mm. However, the maximum penetration of human liver by 4% glutaraldehyde in 24 hours at room temperature and in the cold was 4.5 mm and 2.5 mm, respectively [264]. Other investigators have also presented data on the penetration rate of glutaraldehyde into rat liver [265–267]. A mixture of glutaraldehyde (2%) and formaldehyde (2%) was shown to penetrate human liver to depths of 2.0, 2.5 and 5.0 mm in 4, 12 and 24 hours respectively [268].

This relatively slow rate of penetration and the uncertainty of its degree of reactivity as the distance from the surface increases can cause problems when fixing tissues for electron microscopy or for use as xenograft derived bioprostheses to be implanted in humans. Incomplete crosslinking of such tissues, in particular of the structural collagenous network, can lead to enhanced biodegradation, antigenicity and loss of mechanical function.

Studies using pericardium suggest that the initial fixation of collagen by glutaraldehyde occurs at the surfaces of the protein fibres, particularly when high concentrations of fixative are used [269]. This process is a very fast one associated with polymerization of the glutaraldehyde monomer. Based on previous work, this process seems to consume a large amount of free glutaraldehyde [270,271]. A slower time-dependent crosslinking process which can occur, at lower concentrations of glutaraldehyde, during fixation of tissues has also been identified [270,271]. These results emphasize the importance of the time of fixation and the concentration of glutaraldehyde in determining the nature of the crosslinking network generated. High concentrations may crosslink only the surface of the collagen fibres. This may be a result of too rapid polymerization at the site, and this event may impair the access of glutaraldehyde molecules to the interstitium of the larger collagen fibres by steric hindrance or by creating nucleation sites to which further glutaraldehyde molecules may attach.

Vascular Grafts

There is a significant need to replace damaged or degenerated blood vessels. Dacron grafts are satisfactory for the replacement of larger diameter blood vessels. Autologous veins, on the other hand, substitute very well for non-functional coronary vessels. In the latter case, the graft adapts to its new environment and responds to pulsation and the increased hydrostatic pressure by "arteriolizing". This can be evidenced histologically and biochemically, as shown by Moczar, Robert and associates in Paris, because the smooth muscle cells alter their biosynthetic pattern and begin to produce more elastin, a characteristic of arterial cells [272]. With the large, woven Dacron vessel substitutes initial leakage occurs which requires the graft to be pre-clotted before insertion. Binding of collagen and other macromolecules to the Dacron has been attempted to make this pretreatment unnecessary. It is reasonable to say that today we have adequate synthetic substitutes for the larger vessels. In the case of small diameter veins and arteries (less than 5 mm), we have to rely on autologous grafts, but if these fail or are unavailable, the patient has no other recourse available.

Attempts have also been made to extrude collagen, reconstitute it into tubular forms and use animal blood vessels as vascular grafts. Because of the antigenicity of xenografts, these are crosslinked with a variety of bifunctional reagents (dialdehyde starch, glutaraldehyde, etc.) to try and make them inert. Attempts are also made to select animal vessels of suitable diameter and sequentially solubilize the non-collagenous components, leaving behind the collagen framework. Examples are bovine aorta digested with the protease ficin, which removes the elastin and non-collagenous proteins, leaving behind essentially a collagen tube which is then crosslinked [273]. Some problems with these grafts are primarily related to the thrombogenicity of collagen. Even if this is overcome by adding a non-thrombogenic intima, a problem persists at the anastomosing site. It is always difficult to generate a suitable continuum where a synthetic material (or a non-viable collagenous matrix in this case), meets with living tissue. Surfaces which facilitate cellular ingrowth may be desirable. These could be made from biodegradable collagen, combined with permanent crosslinked collagen or a polyurethane scaffolding. In particular, the anastomosis region will have to be further developed so as to allow for ingrowth and attachments in order to generate a continuous interphase between host and graft. This is a major concern in the small diameter graft, since overgrowth in this instance causes narrowing of the lumen, intravascular thrombosis and finally leads to occlusion. Combinations of collagens of various degrees of crosslinking with cell attachment proteins such as fibronectin and laminin may prove to be of value and are worth investigating.

Relationship Between Surface Charge of the Vascular Interface and Thrombosis

It is generally accepted that the conventional woven, knitted, porous grafts will not function for extended periods of time when the diameter is less than 6 mm. Some prosthetic grafts, such as those made out of expanded polytetrafluoroethylene seem to do better, but they present with other problems such as difficulties in sewing, aneurysm formation, and questions about their long-term durability. Early work in this connection was reviewed by Sawyer et al. [274]. Collagen tubes of small diameter or modified animal blood vessels of small diameter present the same problems, particularly as they relate to thrombogenicity, which is not unexpected in view of the potent platelet aggregation activity and thrombogenicity of collagen. In spite of these problems, continued interest in the use of modified tissue grafts persists and many attempts are being made at introducing modifications which will generate a suitable prosthesis.

In 1951 Sawyer and his associates observed that the normal vascular interface appeared negative to a pair of searching electrodes placed across the blood vessel wall. Under normal conditions the interface always appears negative to an internal electrode; on the other hand reversal of the potential across the blood vessel by injury or by introducing a positively charged electrode produced local thrombosis. Following this observation, negatively charged bovine heterografts were developed [275,276]. The starting materials were bovine arteries which were treated with the protease ficin to remove most non-collagenous proteins, and then crosslinked with bifunctional reagents. Organic aliphatic acids were attached to the amino groups of collagen by acetylation, thus reducing the net positive charges of the exposed collagen surface. A multi-centre long-term evaluation of these grafts in animals and humans was published in 1980 [276].

Such studies, which encompassed a period of 12 years in experimental animals and 4.5 years of clinical experience with 134 grafts implanted in man, tended to confirm the earlier observation that the polarity of the blood intimal interface plays a major role in intravascular thrombosis. Negative charge density and distribution was determined by electrokinetic studies (electro-osmotic flow) and by colloidal iron staining visualized by scanning and transmission electron microscopy. In addition, fluorescamine ultraviolet fluorescence, which is increased around positively-charged areas and minimal on negatively-charged surfaces, was used to evaluate the efficacy of the charge modification. The biocompatibility studies were evaluated following removal from animals using microscopic and histological techniques. Patency in patients was monitored by Doppler pulse pressure measurements and by arteriograms in any case of doubt. Thrombogenesis appeared to be significantly decreased by the process of enhancement of the negative charges on collagen by chemical means. The mechanism of this inhibition of thrombogenesis is not yet understood, but these studies certainly point towards one approach that carries a certain degree of success and should stimulate other investigators to continue to modify the surface of collagen fibres to decrease their thrombogenicity, enhance their ability to allow endothelial cell attachment, and decrease its ability to act as a nucleus for calcification.

Calcification of Vascular Tissues

The morphological and biochemical changes of blood vessels associated with age are well documented. The theory that the loss of elasticity and weakening of the vessel wall are the primary factors that precipitate all subsequent intimal lesions is an old one. Some of the earlier ideas in this connection are summarized by Blumenthal et al. [277]. These investigators, looking at a large number of autopsy specimens, clearly demonstrated that calcification of the media of the aorta was primarily a function of age. They also showed that calcification of the media precedes the formation of intimal plaques and that these do not occur without medial calcification, as was the case of individuals of advanced age with syphilitic aortitis. Characteristic of this disease is the breakdown of the elastic and muscular components of the media (the targets of calcium deposition) and infiltration by scar tissue. As an example, the media of a 72-year-old subject with this disease (an age where extensive calcification normally occurs) showed calcium levels comparable to those of a child. This observation is of interest in considering how resorbtion of the connective tissue matrix of implanted xenografts is associated with low levels of ectopic calcification (see below).

By definition, extraskeletal calcification is pathological and can be subdivided into metastatic and distrophic. The former occurs in hypercalcaemic individuals, whereas the latter is found in normocalcaemic hosts, frequently in association with tissue necrosis. A comprehensive review of the tissue factors which may play a role in pathological calcification was provided by Kim [278].

As mentioned above, the vascular system is one of the most common sites of extraskeletal calcification, which begins in the second decade and increases with age. Aortic and valvular calcification follows tissue injury. In experimental anastomosis of piglet aorta, calcification occurred at the necrotic site of anastomosis and clamp injury [279]. Fascia lata autografts for replacement of aortic valves developed calcification accompanied by tissue necrosis [280]. Calcification of aortic valve allografts occurred with tissues sterilized in ethylene oxide, whereas fresh allografts had a much lower incidence of calcification [281,282]. Extensive aortic calcification was documented in primary aortitis [283] and following plastic sheathing of aorta in cholesterol-fed rats [284]. The importance of lipid deposition prior to aortic calcification has been pointed out. Rats fed high doses of vitamin D developed calcification, along with lipid deposition in the aorta [285]. In ageing human aortic valve, calcification characteristically occurred along a zone of lipid deposition [286]. In studies of human aortic valve and aorta obtained from autopsies performed immediately after death, calcification was found to take place in association with cellular degradation products that apparently had originated from senescent and degenerate fibrocytes and smooth muscle cells [287,288].

Calcification of the aorta has several features in common with cartilage calcification. In both, membranous vesicles are the initial loci of calcification and calcification occurs in extracellular space that is rich in proteoglycans. Both tissues are avascular. Although calcification of the epiphyseal cartilage occurs in close apposition to the bone, which is rich in vascularity, calcification of the matrix vesicles occurs in the avascular zone of the cartilage. It has been postulated that this avascularity and the lack of scavenging are responsible for the accumulation of the calcifying vesicles in the tissue [289].

Kim and associates have performed some interesting studies which may shed significant light on the mechanisms of calcification of vascular tissues and vascular prosthesis. Using Millipore chambers to isolate the vascular tissue or purified elastic fibres from the host, which prevented diffusion and scavenging of tissue degradation products, they observed that it was these degradation products that became calcified. It seems as if aortic calcification does not require live cells and may not be energy dependent, and that elastin per se is not a nucleus for calcification but may become involved only after calcification is initiated in the vicinity, probably as a result of the presence of vesicles. It appears as if cellular degradation products, which may give rise to such vesicles, are the nidi of calcification, and that the lipids seen at the light microscopic level by Irving at the calcification front and the cellular degradation products seen at the electron microscopic level by Kim correspond to the same materials.

Mechanisms of Calcification

Some thoughts have already been expressed in the discussion of the normal and pathological calcification of the vascular media. The vesicles described, rich in phospholipids, seem to be able to concentrate calcium (and phosphate as a counterion) and by exceeding the solubility product within the vesicle cause the formation of hydroxyapatite crystals. Type I collagen has been shown to have a particular affinity for lipids and under certain pathological circumstances this may be enhanced [290]. Normally collagen fibres seem to lie in close association with proteoglycans and these negatively-charged macromolecules may prevent lipids from associating with collagen. During the process of tissue degeneration or following injury, as well as during the early stages of normal mineralization of bone (endochondral ossification), proteoglycans are removed or turned over very rapidly and the lipid-coated vesicles may find it easier to approach the denuded collagen fibres.

Theories developed by Neuman, Glimcher and their associates suggest that components of the organic matrix (collagen, proteoglycans) are responsible for the initial nucleation and growth of the hydroxyapatite crystals. For a detailed discussion of these concepts the reader is referred to reviews by Wadkins et al. [291] and Boskey [292]. Collagen and proteoglycans are not ubiquitous to bone, but are present in many connective tissues that normally do not calcify, so even though collagen is able to nucleate and cause hydroxyapatite crystals to grow when added to a saturated solution of calcium and phosphate ions, this does not explain why calcification occurs at some sites and not at others. On the other hand the negatively-charged polyelectrolytes such as the glycosaminoglycans are potent in vitro inhibitors of crystal nucleation. It is of interest in this connection that cortical bone has only small amounts of these substances but has other proteins and glycoproteins such as the β-carboxyglutamic acid-containing polypeptide osteocalcin and a sialoglyco-protein, both of which have a strong affinities for calcium and are able to inhibit nucleation in vitro. So it seems as if a delicate balance between pro-motors and inhibitors is present in connective tissues, some conditions enhanc-ing and others inhibiting calcification.

Calcification of Collagen-Based Cardiovascular Prostheses

Although the use of collagen-derived prostheses such as porcine aortic valve heterografts crosslinked with glutaraldehyde are of significant value in restor-ing cardiac function there are circumstances that limit their durability and can lead to failure. Explanted valves sometimes show signs of degeneration of the connective tissue matrix, suggesting that fixation with glutaraldehyde has not rendered the prosthesis completely inert or that mechanical wear and tear will eventually destroy the collagenous network.

A detailed ultrastructural study performed by Ferrans and his associates clearly documented a progressive disruption of collagen fibrils, erosion of the valve surfaces, formation of aggregates of platelets and accumulation of lipid [293]. Calcific deposits were also found. Earlier studies had already reported calcification of the cusps, a problem which was more acute when the porcine heterografts were implanted in children. The reason for this is not known but it is suspected to be associated with higher levels of calcium and the increased metabolic turnover of this element in the tissues and body fluids of growing individuals. Higher rates of calcification of implants in calves may be related to the same phenomena. Levy and associates have shown that the process of calcification of bioprosthetic heart valves is accompanied by the accumulation of osteocalcin, a protein which depends on the presence of vitamin K for its post-translational modification [294]. It is of interest that attempts to inhibit osteocalcin synthesis by warfarin, used at levels which provided anticoagulant activity, did not prevent calcification or accumulation of osteocalcin at the sites of calcification.

Experiments completed in the author's laboratory are in good agreement with the findings of Levy. Rats implanted subcutaneously with glutaraldehyde fixed pericardium showed a progressive accumulation of calcium at the implant. As observed by Levy this effect is more pronounced when young rats are used, in good agreement with the clinical observation that children receiving porcine valve bioprostheses are more likely to show calcification than adults.

Also, it is of interest that fresh bovine pericardium when implanted in rats does not calcify but of course it is gradually resorbed and will disappear after several months. Is there some analogy between this observation and that reported earlier showing that arteries of elderly people suffering from syphilitic aortitis failed to show age-related calcific deposits? It seems that for calcification to occur well crosslinked collagen together with some stimulus associated with injury or degeneration are required. There is no doubt that a full understanding of the mechanism and sequence of events associated with normal and dystrophic calcification and the role of the macromolecules involved is slowly being achieved. It is also very likely that this information will allow us to design chemically-modified bioprostheses that will be more durable, where the collagen will not degenerate, and where calcification will not be an unavoidable sequela.

References

1. Nimni ME. Collagen: structure, function and metabolism in normal and fibrotic tissues. Semin Arthritis Rheum 1983;XIII(1):1–86
2. Bertelsen S. In: Sandler M, Bourne GF (eds) Atherosclerosis and its origin. Academic Press, New York, 1963, pp 119–165
3. Bashey RI, Torii S, Angrist A. Age-related collagen and elastin content of human heart valves. Geront J 1967;22(2):203–208
4. Baig MM, Daicoff GR, Ayoub EM. Comparative studies of the acid mucopolysaccharide composition of rheumatic and normal heart valves in man. Circ Res 1978;42(2):271–275
5. Ramachandran GN. Treatise on collagen. Chemistry of collagen. Academic Press, New York, 1967, p 103
6. Rich A, Crick FHC. The molecular structure of collagen. J Mol Biol 1961;3:483
7. Petruska JA, Hodge AJ. A subunit model for the tropocollagen macromolecule. Proc Natl Acad Sci USA 1964;51:871
8. Kuhn K. Relationship between amino acid sequence and higher structures of collagen. Connect Tissue Res 1982;10:5–10
9. Veis A. Collagen fibrillogenesis. Connect. Tissue Res 1982;10:11–24
10. Piez KA. Structure and assembly of the native collagen fibril. Connect Tissue Res 1982;10:25–36
11. Timpl R, Glanville RW. The amino-peptide of collagen. Clin Orthop Relat Res 1981;158:224–242
12. Becker U, Helle O, Timpl R. Characterization of the aminoterminal segment in procollagen p 2 chain from dermatosporactic sheep. FEBS Lett 1977;73:197–200
13. Curran S, Prockop DJ. Isolation and partial characterization of the amino-terminal propeptide of type II procollagen from chick embryos. Biochemistry 1982;21:1482
14. Pesciotta DM, Silkowitz MH, Fietzek PP, Graves PN, Berg RA, Olsen BR. Purification and characterization of the amino-terminal propeptide of pro α1 (I) chains from embryonic chick tendon procollagen. Biochemistry 1980;19:2447–2454
15. Novak H, Olsen BR, Timpl R. Characterization of the amino-terminal segment in type III procollagen. Eur J Biochem 1976;70:205–216
16. Fessler LI, Fessler JH. Characterization of type III procollagen from chick embryo blood vessels. J Biol Chem 1979;254:239–244
17. Olsen BR, Guzman NA, Engel J, Condit C, Aase S. Purification and characterization of a peptide from the carboxyterminal region of chick tendon procollagen type I. Biochemistry 1978;17:2948–2954
18. Clark CC, Kefalides NA. Carbohydrate moieties of procollagen: incorporation of isotopically labeled mannose and glucosamine into propeptides of procollagen secreted by matrix-free chick embryo tendon cells. Proc Natl Acad Sci 1976;73:34–38
19. Prockop DJ, Kivirikko KI, Tuderman L, Guzman NA. The biosynthesis of collagen and its disorders. N Engl J Med 1979;301:13–23

20. Pesciotta DM, Dickson LA, Showalter AM, Eikenberry EF, de Crombrugghe B, Fietzek PP, Olsen BR. Primary structure of the carbohydrate-containing regions of the carboxyl propeptides of type I procollagen. FEBS Lett 1981;125:2:170–174

21. Hart GW, Brew K, Grant GA, Bradshaw RA, Lennarz WJ. Primary structural requirements for the enzymatic formation of the N-glycosidic bond in glycoproteins. J Biol Chem 1979;254:9747–9753

22. Sundar Raj CV, Church RL, Klobutcher LA, Ruddle FH. Genetics of the connective tissue proteins. Assignment of the gene for human type i procollagen to chromosome 17 by analysis of cell hybrids and microcell hybrids. Proc Natl Acad Sci USA 1977;74:4444–4448

23. Church RL, Chromosome mapping of connective tissue protein genes. Int Rev Connect Tissue Res 1981;9:99–150

24. Frischauf AM, Lerach H, Rosner C, Boedtker H. Procollagen complementary DNA, a probe for messenger RNA purification and the number of type I collagen genes. Biochemistry 1978;17:3243–3249

25. De Crombrugghe B, Pastan I. Structure and regulation of a collagen gene. TIBS 1982;7:11–13

26. Wozney J, Hanahan D, Tate V, Boedtker H, Doty P. Structure of the pro α2(I) collagen gene. Nature 1981;294:129–135

27. Nimni ME, Collagen: its structure and function in normal and pathological connective tissues. Semin Arthritis Rheum 1974;4:95–150

28. Vuust J, Piez KA. A kinetic study of collagen biosynthesis. J Biol Chem 1972;247:856–862

29. Cardinale GJ, Udenfriend S. Prolyl hydroxylase. Adv Enzymol 1974;41:245–300

30. Berg RA, Kedersha NL, Guzman NA. Purification and partial characterization of the two non-identical subunits of prolyl hydroxylase. J Biol Chem 1979;254:3111–3118

31. Turpeenniemi TM, Puistola U, Anttinen H, Kivirikko KI. Affinity chromatography of lysyl hydroxylase on concanavalin a-agarose. Biochim Biophys Acta 1977;483:215-219

32. Majamaa K. Effect of prevention of procollagen triple-helix formation on proline 3-hydroxylation in freshly isolated chick-embryo tendon cells. Biochem J 1981;196:203–206

33. Schofield JD, Uitto J, Prockop DJ. Formation of interchain disulfide bonds and helical structure during biosynthesis of procollagen by embryonic tendon cells. Biochemistry 1974;13:1801–1806

34. Uitto J, Prockop DJ. Biosynthesis of cartilage procollagen: influence of chain association and hydroxylation of prolyl residues on the folding of the polypeptides into the triple-helical conformation. Biochemistry 1974;13:4586–4591

35. Williams IF, Harwood R, Grant ME. Triple helix formation and disulphide bonding during the biosynthesis of glomerular basement membrane collagen. Biochem Biophys Res Commun 1976;70:200–206

36. Dehm P, Prockop DJ. Time lag in the secretion of collagen by matrix-free tendon cells and inhibition of the secretory process by colchicine and vinblastine. Biochim Biophys Acta 1972;264:375–382

37. Dehm P, Prockop DJ. Biosynthesis of cartilage procollagen. Eur J Biochem 1973;35:159–166

38. Clark CC, Tomichek EA, Koszalka TR, Minor RR, Kefalides NA. The embryonic rat parietal yolk sac. The role of the parietal endoderm in the biosynthesis of basement membrane collagen and glycoprotein in vitro. J Biol Chem 1974;250:5259–5267

39. Uitto VJ, Uitto J, Kao WWY, Prockop DJ. Procollagen polypeptides containing cis-4-hydroxy-1-proline are overglycos⁰lated and secreted as nonhelical pro-α-chains. Arch Biochem Biophys 1978;185:214–221

40. Kivirikko KI, Myllyla R. Collagen glycosyltransferases. Int Rev Connect Tissue Res 1981;9:23–72

41. Risteli L, Myllyla R, Kivirikko KI. Affinity chromatography of collagen glycosyltransferases on collagen linked to agarose. Eur J Biochem 1976;67:197–202

42. Clark CC, Kefalides NA. Localization and partial composition of the oligosaccharide units on the propeptide extensions of type I procollagen. J Biol Chem 1978;253:47–51

43. Olsen BR, Guzman NA, Engel J, Condit C, Aase S. Purification and characterization of a peptide fom the carboxyterminal region of chick tendon procollagen type I. Biochemistry 1977;16:3030–3036

44. Sharon N, Lis H, Glycoproteins. In: Neurath H, Hill RE (eds) The proteins. Academic Press, New York, 1982, pp 1–144

45. Harwood R, Grant ME, Jackson DS. The subcellular location of inter-chain disulfide bond formation during procollagen biosynthesis by embryonic chick tendon cells. Biochem Biophys Res Commun 1973;55:1188–1196

46. Brownell AG, Veis A. Triple-helix formation on ribosome-bound nascent chains of procollagen: deuterium-hydrogen exchange studies. Proc Natl Acad Sci USA 1977;74:902–905

47. Rosenbloom J, Endo R, Harsch M. Termination of procollagen chain synthesis by puromycin. Evidence that assembly and secretion require a cooh-terminal extension. J Biol Chem 1976;251:2070–2076

48. Bachinger HP, Fessler LI, Timpl R, Fessler JH. Chain assembly intermediate in the biosynthesis of type III procollagen in chick embryo blood vessels. J Biol Chem 1981;256:13193–13199

49. Gelman RA, Poppke DC, Piez KA. Collagen fibril formation in vitro. J Biol Chem 1979;254:11741–11745

50. Kornberg A. Structure and functions of DNA and binding and unwinding proteins and topoisomerases in DNA replication. WH Freeman and Co, San Francisco, 1980

51. Bruckner P, Eikenberry EF, Prockop DJ. Formation of the triple helix of type I procollagen in cellulo. A kinetic model based on cis–trans isomerization of peptide bonds. Eur J Biochem 1981;118:607–613

52. Fessler LI, Timpl R, Fessler JH. Assembly and processing of procollagen type III in chick embryo blood vessels. J Biol Chem 1981;256:2531–2537

53. Blobel G. In: Brinkley BB, Porter KR (eds) International cell biology. Rockefeller University Press, New York, 1976, p 318

54. Kleine TO. Biosynthesis of proteoglycans. An approach to locate it in different membrane systems. Int Rev Connect Tissue Res 1981;9:27–98

55. Cheah KSE, Grant ME, Jackson DS. Translation of embryonic-chick tendon procollagen messenger ribonucleic acid in two cell-free protein-synthesizing systems. Biochem J 1979;182:81–93

56. Bonatti S, Blobel G. Absence of a cleavable signal sequence in sindbis virus glycoprotein PE_2. J Biol Chem 1979;254:12261–12264

57. Meyer DI. The signal hypothesis – a working model. TIBS 1982;7:320–321

58. Tanzer ML. Collagen biosynthesis and degradation. Disorders Min Metab 1982;2:237–270

59. Hedman K, Alitalo K, Lehtinen S, Timpl R, Vaheri A. Deposition of an intermediate form of procollagen type III (pN-collagen) into fibrils in the matrix of amniotic epithelial cells. Embo J 1982;1:47–52

60. Fleishmajer R, Timpl R, Tuderman L, Raisher L, Wiestner M, Perlish JS, Graves PN. Ultrastructural identification of extension aminopropeptides of type I and III collagens in human skin. Proc Natl Acad Sci USA 1981;78:7360–7364

61. Veis A, Anesey J, Yuan L, Levy SJ. Evidence for an amino-terminal extension in high-molecular-weight collagens from mature bovine skin. Proc Natl Acad Sci USA 1973;70:1464–1467

62. Siegel RC. Lysyloxidase. Int Rev Connect Tissue Res 1978;6:73–118

63. Pinnell SR, Martin GR. The crosslinking of collagen and elastin: enzymatic conversion of lysine in peptide linkage to α-aminoadipic-α-semialdehyde (allysine) by an extract from bone. Proc Natl Acad Sci USA 1968;61:708–714

64. Frazer RDB, Macrae TP, Suzuki E. The molecular and fibrillar structure of collagen in fibrous proteins. In: Parry DAD, Creamer LK (eds) Industrial and medical aspects. Academic Press, London, 1979, vol 1, pp 179–206

65. Brodsky B, Eikenberry EF. Characterization of fibrous forms of collagen. In: Cunningham LW, Fredericksen W (eds) Methods in enzymology. Academic Press, London, 1982, vol 28, part 1, pp 127–174

66. Bornstein P, Traub W. The chemistry and biology of collagen. In: Neurath H, Hill RL (eds) The proteins. Academic Press, London, 1979, vol 4, pp 411–632

67. Smith JW, Molecular pattern in nature collagen. Nature 1968;219:157–158

68. Piez KA, Trus Bl. A new model for packing of type I collagen molecules in the native fibril. Bioscience Reports 1981;1:801–810

69. Hulmes DJS, Miller A. Quasi-hexagonal molecular packing in collagen fibrils. Nature 1979;2:878–880

70. Silver FH. A molecular model for linear and lateral growth of type I collagen fibrils. Coll Res 1982;2:219–229
71. Hoffman H, Kuhn K. Packing models for collagen types I and III molecules based on the calculation of an interaction score and distinct sequence regularities. In: Structural aspects of recognition and assembly in biological macromolecules. Rehoboth, Philadelphia, 1981, 427–440
72. Kuhn K. Segment-long-spacing crystallites, a powerful tool in collagen research. Coll Res 1982;2:61–80
73. Helseth DLJr, Veis A. Collagen self-assembly in vitro. J Biol Chem 1981;256:7118–7128
74. Trelstad RL, Coulombre AJ. Morphogenesis of the collagenous stroma in the chick cornea. J Cell Biol 1971;50:840–858
75. Weinstock M. Collagen formation: observations on its intracellular packaging and transport. Z Zellforsch Mikrosk Anat 1972;129:455–470
76. Trelstad RL, Hayashi K. Tendon fibrillogenesis: intracellular collagen subassemblies and cell surface changes associated with fibril growth. Dev Biol 1979;71:228–242
77. Bruns RR, Hulmes DJS, Therrien SF, Gross J. Procollagen segment-long-spacing crystallites: their role in collagen fibrillogenesis. Proc Natl Acad Sci USA 1979;76:313–317
78. Renteria VG, Ferrans VJ. Intracellular collagen fibrils in cardiac valves of patients with the hurler syndrome. Lab Invest 1976;34:263–272
79. Wood GC, Keech MK. The formation of fibrils from collagen solutions. I. The effect of experimental conditions: kinetic and electron-microscope studies. Biochem J 1960;75:588–598
80. Gelman RA, Piez KA. Collagen fibril formation in vitro. J Biol Chem 1980;255:8098–8102
81. Silver FH. Type I collagen fibrillogenesis in vitro: additional evidence for the assembly mechanism. J Biol Chem 1981;256:4972–4977
82. Helseth DL, Veis A. Collagen self-assembly in vitro. J Biol Chem 1981;256:7118–7128
83. Trelstad RL, Silver FH. Matrix assembly. In: Hay ED (ed) Cell biology of the extracellular matrix. Plenum Publishing Corporation, New York, 1981, pp 179–215
84. Trelstad RL. Multistep assembly of type I collagen fibrils. Cell 1982;28:197–198
85. Revel JP, Hay ED. An autoradiographic and electron microscopic study of collagen synthesis in differentiating cartilage. Z Zellforsch Mikrosk Anat 1963;61:110–144
86. Weinstock M, Leblond CP. Synthesis migration and release of precursor collagen by odontoblasts as visualized by radioautography after [^{3}H] proline administration. J Cell Biol 1974;60:92–127
87. Hay ED, Revel JP. Fine structure of the developing avian cornea. In: Wolsky A, Chen PS (eds) Monographs in developmental biology. Karger, Basel, vol 1, 1969
88. Kuhn K, Wiestner T, Krieg T, Muller PK. Structure and function of the aminoterminal propeptide of type I and III collagen. Conn Tiss Res 1982;10:43–50
89. Veis A. Characterization of soluble collagens by physical techniques. In: Cunningham LW, Frederiksen DF (eds) Methods in enzymology. Academic Press, London, 1983, pp 186–217
90. Miller EJ. Collagen: an overview. In: Cunningham LW, Frederiksen DF (eds) Methods in enzymology. Academic Press, London, 1982, pp 3–64
91. Benya P, Padilla S, Nimni ME. The progeny of rabbit articular chondrocytes synthesize collagen types I and III and type I trimer, but not type II. Verification by cyanogen bromide peptide analysis. Biochemistry 1977;16:865–872
92. Miller EJ, Epstein EHJr, Piez KA. Identification of three genetically distinct collagens by cyanogen bromide cleavage of insoluble human skin and cartilage collagen. Biochem Biophys Res Commun 1971;42:1024–1029
93. Cheung E, Miller EJ. Collagen polymorphism, characterization of molecules with the chain composition [alfa 1(III)]$_3$ in human tissues. Science 1974;183:1200–1201
94. Epstein EHJr. [a1(III)]$_3$ human skin collagen. J Biol Chem 1974;249:3225–3231
95. Gabbiani G, Le Lous M, Bailey AJ, Bazin S, Delaunay A. Collagen and myofibroblasts of granulation tissue. Virchows Arch [Cell Pathol] 1976;21:133–145
96. Shuttleworth CA, Forrest L. Changes in guinea-pig dermal collagen during development. Eur J Biochem 1975;55:391–395
97. Cheung DT, DiCesare P, Benya PD, Libaw E, Nimni ME. The presence of intermolecular disulfide crosslinks in type III collagen, J Biol Chem 258(12):7774–7778

 98. Epstein EHJr, Munderloh NH. Human skin collagen: presence of type I and type III at all levels of the dermis. J Biol Chem 1978;253:1336–1337
 99. Gay S, Muller PK, Meigel WN, Kuhn K. Hautarzt 1976;27:196–205
100. Becker U, Nowack H, Gay S, Timpl R. Production and specificity of antibodies against the aminoterminal region in type III collagen. Immunology 1976;31:57–65
101. Tajima S, Nagai Y. Distribution of macromolecular components in calf dermal connective tissue. Connect Tiss Res 1980;7:65–71
102. Lapiere CM, Nusgens B, Pierard GE. Interactions between collagen type I and type III in conditioning bundles organization. Connect Tiss Res 1977;5:21–29
103. Byers PH, McKenney KH, Lichtenstein JR, Martin GR. Preparation of type III procollagen and collagen from rat skin. Biochemistry 1974;13:5243–5248
104. Chandrarajan J. Separation of type III collagen from type I collagen and pepsin by differential denaturation and renaturation. Biochem Biophys Res Commun 1978;83:180–186
105. Macek K, Deyl Z, Coupek J, Sanitrak J. Separation of collagen types I and II by high-performance column liquid chromatography. J Chromatogr 1981;222:284–290
106. Goldberg B. Kinetics of processing of type I and type III procollagens in fibroblast cultures. Proc Natl Acad Sci USA 1977;74:3322–3325
107. Wu CH, Rojkind M, Rifas L, Seifter S. Biosynthesis of type I and type III collagens by cultured uterine smooth muscle cells. Arch Biochem Biophys 1978;188:294–300
108. Robins SP. Metabolism of rabbit skin collagen. Biochem J 1979;181:75–82
109. Fietzek PP, Allmann H, Rauterberg J, Henkel W, Wachter E, Kuhn K. The covalent structure of calf skin type III collagen. Hoppe-Seyler's Z Physiol Chem 1979;360:809–868
110. Bornstein P, Sage H. Structurally distinct collagen types. Ann Rev Biochem 1980;49:957
111. Morton LF, Barnes MJ. Collagen polymorphism in the normal and diseased blood vessel wall. Atherosclerosis 1982;42:41–51
112. Rauterberg J, Allam S, Brehmer V, Wirtz W, Hauss WH. Characterization of the collagen synthesized by cultured human smooth muscle cells from fetal and adult aorta. Hoppe-seyler's Z physiol Chem 1977;358:401
113. McCullagh KG, Balian G. Collagen characterization and cell transformation in human atherosclerosis. Nature 1975;258:73–79
114. Morton LF, Barnes MJ. Collagen polymorphism in the normal and deseased blood vessel wall. Investigation of collagen types I, III and V. Atherosclerosis 1982;42:41–51
115. Aumailley M, Bricaud H. Collagen synthesis in organ culture of normal and atherosclerotic aortas. Atherosclerosis 1981;39:1
116. Meikle MC, Heath JK, Hembry RM, Reynolds JJ. Rabbit cranial suture fibroblasts under tension express a different collagen phenotype. Arch Oral Biol. 1982;27:609–613
117. Timpl R, Martin GR. Immunochemistry of the extracellular matrix, Volume II. CRC Press Inc., Boca Raton, Florida, 1982.
118. Mayne R, Wiedemann H, Dessau W, Von Der Mark K, Bruckner P. Structural and immunological characterization of type IV collagen isolated from chicken tissues. Eur J Biochem 1982;126:417–423
119. Kuehn K, Schoene H, Timple R. (eds) New trends in basement membrane research (10th workshop conference) Hoechst, 1982.
120. Butkowski RJ, Brungardt GS, Grantham JJ, Hudson BG. Characterization of the collagenuous domain of tubular basement membrane. J Biol Chem 1981;256:7603–7609
121. Kefalides NA, Alper R, Clark CC. Biochemistry and metabolism of basement membranes. Int Rev Cytol 1979;61:167
122. Krakower CA, Greenspon SA. The isolation of basement membranes. In: Kefalides NA (ed) Biology and chemistry of basement membranes. Academic Press, New York, 1978, p 1
123. Kefalides NA. Isolation of collagen from basement membrane containing three identical α-chains. Biochem Biophys Res Commun 1971;45:226
124. Kefalides NA. Structure and biosynthesis of basement membranes. Int Rev Connect Tiss Res 1973;6:63
125. Hudson BG, Spiro RG. Fractionation of glycoprotein components of the reduced alkylated renal glomerular basement membrane. J Biol Chem 1972;247:4239
126. Sato T, Spiro RG. Studies on the subunit composition of the renal glomerular basement membrane. J Biol Chem 1976;251:4062
127. Spiro RG. Nature of the glycoprotein components of basement membranes. Ann NY Acad Sci 1978;312:106

128. Spiro RG. Studies on the renal glomerular basement membrane. Nature of the carbohydrate units and their attachment to the peptide portion. J Biol Chem 1967;242:1923

129. Levine MJ, Spiro RG. Isolation from glomerular basement membrane of a glycopeptide containing both asparagine-linked and hydroxylysine-linked carbohydrate units. J Biol Chem 1979;254:8121

130. Schuppan D, Timpl R, Glanville RW. Discontinuities in the triple helical sequence gly-X-Y of basement membrane (type IV) collagen. FEBS Lett. 1980;115:297

131. Timpl R, Martin GR, Bruckner P, Wick G, Wiedemann H. Nature of the collagenous protein in a tumor basement membrane. Eur J Biochem 1978;84:43

132. Olsen BR, Alper R, Kefalides NA. Structural characterization of a soluble fraction fromlens capsule basement membrane. Eur J Biochem 1973;38:220

133. Gay S, Miller EJ. Characterization of lens capsule collagen: evidence for the presence of two unique chains in molecules derived from major basement membrane structures. Arch Biochem Biophys 1979;198:370

134. Gehron RP, Martin GR. Type IV collagen contains two distinct chains in separate molecules. Coll Res 1981;1:27

135. Schwartz D, Chin-quee T, Veis A. Characterization of bovine anterior lens capsule basement membrane collagen. 1. Pepsin susceptibility, salt precipitation and thermal gelatin: a property of non-collagen component integrity. Eur J Biochem 1980; 103:21

136. Schwartz D, Veis A. Characterization of bovine anterior-lens-capsule basement-membrane collagen. 2. Segment-long-spacing precipitates: further evidence for large N-terminal and C-terminal extensions. Eur J Biochem 1980;103:29

137. Reid KBM. Complete amino acid sequences of the three collagen-like regions present in subcomponent clq of the first component of human complement. Biochem J 1979;179:367

138. Kleinman HK, McGarvey ML, Liotta LA, Robey PG, Tryggvason K, Martin GR. Isolation and characterization of type IV procollagen, laminin, and heparan sulfate proteoglycan from the ehs sarcoma. Biochemistry 1982;21:6188–6193

139. Burgeson RE, El Adli FA, Kaitila II, Hollister DW. Fetal membrane collagens: identification of two new collagen alpha chains. Proc Natl Acad Sci USA 1976;73:2579

140. Chung E, Rhodes RK, Miller EJ. Isolation of three collagenous components of probable basement membrane origin from several tissues. Biochem Biophys Res Commun 1976;71:1167

141. Von Der Mark H, Von Der Mark K. Isolation and characterization of collagen a and b chains from chick embryos. FEBS Lett 1979;99:101

142. Rhodes RK, Miller EJ. Physiochemical characterization and molecular organization of the collagen a and b chains. Biochemistry 1978;17:3442

143. Hong BS, Davison PF, Cannon DJ. Isolation and characterization of a distinct type of collagen from bovine fetal membranes and other tissues. Biochemistry 1979;18:4278

144. Sage H, Bornstein P. Characterization of a novel collagen chain in human placenta and its relation to ab collagen. Biochemistry 1979;18:3815

145. Brown RA, Shuttleworth A, Weiss JB. Three new α-chains of collagen from a non-basement membrane source. Biochem Biophys Res Commun 1978;80:866

146. Bentz H, Bachinger HP, Glanville R, Kuhn K. Physical evidence for the assembly of A and B chains of human placental collagen in a single triple helix. Eur J Biochem 1978;92:563

147. Welsh C, Gay S, Rhodes RK, Pfister R, Miller EJ. Collagen heterogeneity in normal rabbit cornea. I. Isolation and biochemical characterization of the genetically-distinct collagens. Biochim Biophys Acta. 1980;625:78–88

148. Bailey AJ, Shellswell GB, Duance VC. identification and change of collagen types in differentiating myoblasts and developing chick muscle. Nature 1979;278:67–69

149. Gay S, Rhodes RK, Gay RE, Miller EJ. Collagen molecules comprised of α_1(V)-chains (b-chains): an apparent localization in the exocytoskeleton. Coll Res 1981;1:53–58

150. Martinez-hernandez A, Gay S, Miller EJ. Ultrastructural localization of type V collagen in rat kidney. J Cell Biol 1982;92:343–349

151. Leblond CP, Glegg RE, Eidinger D. Presence of carbohydrates with free 1, 2-glycol groups in sites stained by the periodic acid-schiff technique. J Histochem Cytochem 1957;5:445

152. Timpl R, Rohde H, Gehron Robey P, Rennard SI, Foidart JM, Martin GR. Laminin – a glycoprotein from basement membranes. J Biol Chem 1979;254:9933

153. Foidart JM, Bere EW, Yaar M, Rennard SI, Gullino M, Martin GR, Katz SI. Distribution and immunoelectron microscopic localization of laminin, a non-collagenous basement membrane glycoprotein. Lab Invest 1980;42:336

154. Timpl R, Rohde H, Ott-Ulbricht U, Risteli L, Bachinger HP. Chemical characterization of laminin, a major glycoprotein of basement membranes. In: Schauer R, Boer P, Buddecke E, Kramer MF, Vliegenthart JFG, Wiegandt H (eds) Glycoconjugates, George Thieme, Stuttgart, 1979, p 145

155. Sakashita S, Engvall E, Ruoslahti E. Basement membrane glycoprotein laminin binds to heparin. FEBS Lett 1980;116:243

156. Terranova VP, Rohrbach DH, Martin GR. Role of laminin in the attachment of PAM 212 (epithelial) cells to basement membrane collagen. Cell 1980;22:719

157. Ruoslahti E, Vaheri A. Novel human serum protein from fibroblast plasma membranes. Nature 1974;248:789

158. Ruoslahti E, Vaheri A. Interaction of soluble fibroblast surface antigen with fibrinogen and fibrin. Identity with cold-insoluble globulin of human plasma. J Exp Med 1975;141:497

159. Mosesson MW, Umfleet RA. The cold-insoluble globulin of human plasma. J Biol Chem 1970;245:5728

160. Vaheri A, Mosher DF. High molecular weight, cell surface associated glycoprotein (fibronectin) lost in malignant transformation. Biochim Biophys Acta 1978;516:1

161. Wartiovaara J, Leivo I, Vaheri A. Expression of the cell surface-associated glycoprotein, fibronectin, in the early mouse embryo. Dev Biol 1979;69:247

162. Stenman S, Vaheri A. Distribution of a major connective tissue protein, fibronectin, in normal human tissue. J Exp Med 1978;147:1054

163. Engvall E, Ruoslahti E, Miller EJ. Affinity of fibronectin to collagens of different genetic types and to fibrinogen. J Exp Med 1978;147:1584

164. Dessau W, Adelmann BC, Timpl R, Martin GR. Identification of the sites in collagen α-chains that bind serum anti-gelatin factor (cold-insoluble globulin). Biochem J 1978;169: 55

165. Jilek F, Hormann H. Cold-insoluble globulin (fibronectin): affinity to soluble collagen. Thromb Res 1981;21:265–272

166. Kleinman HK, McGoodwin EB, Martin GR, Klebe RJ, Fietzek PP, Woolley DE. Localization of the binding site for cell attachment in the α1(I) chain of collagen. J Biol Chem 1978;253:5642

167. Kleiman HK, Wilkes CM, Martin GR. Interaction of fibronectin with collagen fibrils. Biochemistry 1981;20:2325–2330

168. Balian G, Click EM, Bornstein P. Location of a collagen-binding domain in fibronectin. J Biol Chem 1980;255:3234–3236

169. Menzel EJ, Smolen JS, Liotta L, Reid KBM. Interaction of fibronectin with clq and its collagen-like fragment (CLF). FEBS Lett 1981;129:188–192

170. Hay ED, Meier S. Glycosaminoglycan synthesis by embryonic inductors: neural tube, notochord and lens. J Cell Biol 1974;62:889

171. Conn RH, Bannerjee SD, Bernfield MR. Basal lamina of embryonic salivary epithelia. J Cell Biol 1977;73:464

172. Kanwar YS, Farquhar MG. Anionic sites in the glomerular basement membrane. in vivo and in vitro localization to the laminae rarae by cationic probes, J Cell Biol 1979;81:137

173. Kanwar YS, Farquhar MG. Presence of heparan sulfate in the glomerular basement membrane. Proc Natl Acad Sci USA 1979;76:1303

174. Cohen MP, Glycosaminoglycans are integral constituents of renal glomerular basement membrane. Biochem Biophys Res Commun 1980;92:343

175. Hassell JR, Gehron Robey P, Barrach HJ, Wilczek J, Rennard SI, Martin GR. A basement membrane proteoglycan isolated from the ehs sarcoma. Proc Natl Acad Sci USA 1980;77:4494

176. Hay ED, Extracellular matrix. J Cell Biol 1981;91:205s–223s

177. Tomasek JJ, Hay ED, Fujiwara K. Collagen modulates cell shape and cytoskeleton of embryonic corneal and fibroma fibroblasts: distribution of actin, α-actinin, and myosin. Dev Biol 1982;92:107–122

178. Hay ED, Revel JP. Fine structure of the developing avian cornea. Karger, Basel, 1969

179. Gauss-muller V, Kleinman HK, Martin GR, Schiffmann E. Role of attachment factors and attractants in fibroblast chemotaxis. J Lab Clin Med 1980;1071–1078

180. Goldberg B, Binding of soluble type I collagen molecules to the fibroblast plasma membrane. Cell 1979;16:265–275

181. Sugrue SP, Hay ED. Interaction of embryonic corneal epithelium with exogenous collagen, laminin, and fibronectin: role of endogenous protein synthesis. Dev Biol 1982;92:97–106
182. Trotter JA, Corbett K, Avner BP. Structure and function of the murine muscle–tendon junction. Anat Rec 1981;201:293–302
183. Ross R, Odland G. Fine structure observations of human skin wound and fibrogenesis in repair and regeneration. In: Dunphy JE, Van Winkle W (eds) McGraw Hill, New York; 1968, pp 101–116
184. Cohen IK, Moore CD, Diegelmann RF. Proc Soc Exp Biol Med 1979;160:458
185. Bailey AJ, Sims TJ, Lelous M, Bazin S. Collagen polymorphism in experimental granulation tissue. Biochem Biophys Res Commun 1975;66:1160
186. Gay S, Viljanto J, Raekallio J, Penttinen R. Collagen types in early phases of wound healing in children. Acta Chir Scand 1978;144:205
187. Clore JN, Cohen IK, Diegelmann RF. Quantitative of collagen types I and III during wound healing in rat skin. Proc Soc Exp Biol Med 1979;161:337
188. Barnes MJ, Morton LF, Bennett RC, Bailey AJ, Sims TJ, presence of type III collagen in guinea-pig dermal scar. Biochem J 1976;157:263–266
189. Forrest L, Shuttleworth A, Jackson DS, Mechanic G. A comparison between the reducible intermolecular crosslinks of the collagens from mature dermis and young dermal scar tissue of the guinea pig. Biochem Biophys Res Commun 1972;46:1776–1781
190. Bailey AJ, Robins SP. Embryonic skin collagen. Replacement of the type of aldimine crosslinks during the early growth period. FEBS Lett. 1972;21, 330–334
191. Cohen IK, Diegelmann RF, Wise WS. Biomaterials and collagen synthesis. J Biomed Mater Res. 1976;10:965–970
192. Gayou R, Rudolph R. Capsular contraction around silicone mammary prostheses. Ann Plast Surg. 1979;2:2–10
193. Vistnes LM, Ksander GA. Tissue response to soft silicone prostheses: capsule contracture and other sequelae. In: Rublin LR (ed) Biomaterials in reconstructive surgery. Mosby, St. Louis, 1981
194. Ksander GA, Vistnes LM, Kosek JC. The effect of implant location on compressibility and capsule formation around mini-prostheses in rats and the occurence of experimental capsule contracture. Ann Plast Surg, 1981;6:182
195. Ginsbach G, Busch Luder C, Wolfgang K. The nature of the collagenous capsules around breast implants. Plast Reconstr Surg, 1979;64:4
196. Ksander GA, Vistness LM. Collagen and glycosaminoglycans in capsules around silicone implants. J Surg Res 1981; 31, 433–439
197. Guber S, Rudolph R. The myofibroblast. Surg Gynecol Obstet 1978;146:641
198. Gross J, Lapiere CM. Collagenolytic activity in amphibian tissues. A tissue culture assay. Proc Natl Acad Sci USA 1962;408:1014
199. Kang AH, Nagai Y, Piez K, Gross J. Studies on the structures of collagen utilizing a collagenolytic enzyme from tadpole. Biochemistry 1966;5:509
200. Woolley DE, Evanson JM (eds) Collagenase in normal and pathological connective tissue. J Wiley and Sons, Chichester, 1980
201. Harris ED Jr. Role of collagenases in joint destruction. Joints and Synovial Fluid 1978;10:243–272
202. Harper E. Collagenases. Ann Rev Biochem 1980;49:1063–1078
203. Tschesche H, Macartney HW. A new principle of regulation of enzymic activity. Eur J Biochem 1981;120:183–190
204. Woessner JF Jr. Mammalian collagenases. Clin Orthop 1973;96:310–326
205. Harris ED Jr, Cartwright EC. Proteinases in mammalian cells and tissues. Elsevier, New York, 1977, p 249
206. Harris ED Jr, Farrell ME. Resistance to collagenase: a characteristic of collagen fibrils cross-linked by formaldehyde. Biochim Biophys Acta 1972;278:133–141
207. Vater CA, Harris ED Jr, Siegel RC. Native cross-links in collagen fibrils induce resistance to human synovial collagenase. Biochem J 1979;181:639–645
208. Cheung D, Nimni ME. Mechanism of crosslinking of proteins by glutaraldehyde. II: reaction with monomeric and polymeric collagen. Connect Tissue Res 1982;10:210–216
209. Zwolinski RJ, Hamilin CR, Kohn R. Age related lateration in human heart collagen. Proc Soc Exp Biol Med 1976;152:362–365

210. Siegel RC, Pinnell SR, Martin GR. Crosslinking of collagen and elastin. Properties of lysyl oxidase. Biochemistry 1970;9:4486
211. Rojkind M, Blumenfeld OO, Gallop PM. Isolation of an aldehyde-containing peptide from tropocollagen. Biochem Biophys Res Commun 1964;17:320
212. Bornstein P, Piez KA. The nature of the intermolecular cross-links in collagen. Biochemistry 1966;5:3460
213. Deshmukh A, Deshmukh K, Nimni ME. Synthesis of aldehydes and their interactions during the in vitro aging of collagen. Biochemistry 1971;10:2337
214. Siegel RC. Lysyloxidase. Int Rev Connect Tissue Res 1981;9:73–118
215. Deshmukh K, Nimni ME. Characterization of the aldehydes present on the cyanogen bromide peptides from mature rat skin collagen. Biochemistry 1971;10:1640
216. Fukae M, Mechanic GH. Maturation of collagenous tissue, temporal sequence of formation of peptide lysine derived cross-linking aldehydes and cross-links in collagen. J Biol Chem 1980;255, 6511–6518
217. Harkness RD, Harkness M. An effect of cyanide and nitriles on connective tissue. Nature 1965;205:912–913
218. Harkness RD, Nimni ME. Chemical and mechanical changes in the collagenous framework of skin induced by thiol compounds. Acta Physiol Acad Sci Hung 1968;33:325–343
219. Tanzer ML, Stimler NP. Isolation and characterization of a double chain intermolecular crosslinked peptide from insoluble calf bone collagen. J Biol Chem 1968;243:4045
220. Bailey AJ, Peach CM. Isolation and structural identification of a labile intermolecular crosslink in collagen. Biochem Biophys Res Commun 1968;33:812
221. Tanzer ML. Crosslinking of collagen. Science 1973;180:561
222. Barnes MJ, Morton LF. Collagen polymorphism in the normal and diseased blood vessel wall. Atherosclerosis 1982;42:41
223. McCullagh KG, Balian G. Collagen characterisation cell transformation in human atherosclerosis. Nature 1975;258:73
224. Furthmayr H, Wiedemann H, Timpl R, Odermatt E, Engel J. Electron-microscopical approach to a structural model of intima collagen. J Biochem 1983;1:303
225. Gibson MA, Cleary EG. A collagen-like glycoprotein from elastin-rich tissues. Biochem Biophys Res Commun 1982;29:1288
226. Jander R, Troyer D, Rauterberg J. A collagen-like glycoprotein of the extracellular matrix is the undegraded form of type VI collagen. Biochemistry 1984;31:3675
227. Sage H, Trueb B, Bornstein P. Biosynthetic and structural properties of endothelial cell type VIII collagen. J Biol Chem 1983;258:13391
228. Fung YC. Biomechanics. Springer, Berlin, Heidelberg, New York, 1984, p 183
229. Dobrin PB, Baker WH, Gley WC. Elastolytic and collagenolytic studies of arteries. Arch Surg 1984;119:405
230. Collins D, Lindberg K, McLees B, Pinnell S. The collagen of heart valve. Biochim Biophys Acta 1977;495:129
231. Bashey RI, Bashey HM, Jimenez SA. Characterization of pepsin-solubilized bovine heart-valve collagen. Biochem J 1978;173:885
232. Mannschott P, Herbage D, Weiss M, Buffevant C. Collagen heterogeneity in pig heart valves. Biochim Biophys Acta 1976;434:177
233. Lowther DA, Toole B, Meyer FA. Extraction of acid mucopolysaccharides from the bovine heart valves. Arch Biochem Biophys 1967;118:1
234. Meyer FA, Preston BN, Lowther DA. Isolation and properties of hyaluronic acid from bovine heart valves. Biochem J 1969;113:559
235. Rodbard S, Negative feedback mechanisms in the architecture and function of the connective and cardiovascular tissues. Perspect Biol Med 1969–70;13:597
236. Weiss P. Cellular dynamics. Rev Mod Phys 1959;31:11–20
237. Kemp NE, Quinn BL. Morthogenesis and metabolism of amphibian larvae after excision of heart. Anat Rec 1954;118:773–788
238. Ooshima A, Fuller GC, Cardinale GJ, Spector S, Udenfriend S. Increased collagen synthesis in blood vessels of hypertensive rats and its reversal by antihypertensive agents. Proc Natl Acad Sci USA 71:3019, 1074
239. Leung DYM, Glagov S, Mathews MB. Elastin and collagen accumulation in rabbit ascending aorta and pulmonary trunk during postnatal growth. Circ Res 1977;41:316

240. Leung DYM, Glagov S, Mathews MB. Cyclic stretching stimulates synthesis of matrix components by arterial smooth muscle cells in vitro. Science 1976;191:475
241. Moczar M, Allard R, Robert L, Loisance D, Derouette S, Cachera JP. Biosynthesis of elastin and other matrix-macromolecules in veinous arterial prosthesis. Path Biol 1976;24:37
242. Stemerman MB, Spaet TH. The subendothelium and thrombogenesis. Bull Acad Med NY 1972;48:289–301
243. Santoro SA, Cunningham, LW. Platelet–collagen adhesion. Methods Enzymol 1982;82:509
244. Madri JA, Dreyer B, Pitlick FA, Furthmayr H. The collagenous components of the subendothelium: Correlation of structure and function. Lab Invest 1980;43:303
245. Gloster ES, Stemerman MB, Spaet TH. Platelet interaction with human umbilical cord vascular basement membrane. Blood Vessels 1976;13:267
246. Riddle JM, Magilligan DJ, Stein PD. Platelet reactivity in patients with degenerated porcine bioprosthetic valves. Thromb Res 1981;22:185
247. Strawich E, Hancock WD, Nimni ME. Chemical composition and biophysical properties of porcine cardiovascular tissues. Biomater Med Dev Artif Organs 1975;3:309
248. Nimni ME. A deffect in the intramolecular and intermolecular cross-linking of collagen caused by penicillamine. I. Metabolic and functional abnormalities in soft tissues. J Biol Chem 1968;243:1456
249. Carpentier A, Lemaigre G, Robert L, Carpentier S, Dubost C. Biological factors affecting long term results of valvular heterografts. J Thorac Cardiovasc Surg 1969;58:467
250. Nimni ME. The molecular organization of collagen and its role in determining the biophysical properties of the connective tissues. Biorheology 1980;17:51
251. Nimni M, Strawich E, Hancock WD. Chemical composition and physical properties of porcine cardiovaxcular tissues. Symposium on Polymedical Materials in Artificial Organs. California Institute of Technology, Pasadena 1971, p 17
252. Cheung DT, Nimni ME. Mechanism of crosslinking of proteins by glutaraldehyde I. Reaction with monomeric and polymeric collagen. Connect Tissue Res 1982;10:201–216
253. Hopwood D. The reactions of glutaraldehyde with nucleic acids. J Histochem 1975;7:267
254. Levy WA, Herzog I, Suzuki, Katzman H, Scheinberg L. Methods for combined ultrastructural and biochemical analyses of neural tissue. J Cell Biol 1965;27:119
255. Cater CW. The evaluation of aldehydes and other difunctional compounds as cross-linking agents for collagen. J Soc Leather Trade Chemists. 1963;43:203
256. Tomimatsu U, Jansen EF, Garffield W, Olsen AC. Physical and chemical observations on the alpha-chymotrypsin glutaraldehyde system during formation of an insoluble derivate. J. Colloid Interface Sci 1971;36:51
257. Bowes JH, Cater CW. The interaction of aldehydes with collagen. Biochim Biophys Acta 1968;168:341
258. Richards FM, Knowles JR. Glutaraldehyde as a protein cross-linkage reagent. J Mol Biol 1968;37:231
259. Monsan P, Puzo G, Mazarquil. Mechanism of glutaraldehyde-protein bond formation, Biochemie 1975;57:1281
260. Hardy P, Hughes GJ, Rydon HN. The nature of the cross-linking of proteins by glutaraldehyde. J Chem Soc. 1976;[Perkin I]:958
261. Cheung DT, Nimni ME. Mechanism of crosslinking of proteins by glutaraldehyde I. Reaction with model compounds. Connect Tissue Res 1982;10:187
262. Cheung DT, Nimni ME. Mechanism of crosslinking of proteins by glutaraldehyde II. Reaction with monomeric and polymeric collagen. Connect Tissue Res 1982;10:201
263. Hayat MA. Fixation for electron microscopy. Academic Press, New York 1981, p 66
264. Chambers RW, Bowling MC, Grimley PM. Glutarladehyde fixation in routine histopathology. Arch Pathol 1968;85:18
265. Hopwood DJ. Some aspects of fixation with glutaraldehyde. A biochemical and histochemical comparison of the effects of formaldehyde and glutaraldehyde fixation on various enzymes and glycogen, with a note on penetration of glutaraldehyde into liver. J Anat 1967; 101:83
266. Hopwood DJ. Theoretical and practical aspects of glutaraldehyde fixation. Histochem J 1972;4:267
267. Ericsson JLE, Biberfield P. Studies on aldehyde fixation. Fixation rates and their relation to fine structure and some histochemical reactions in liver. Lab Invest 1967;17:281

268. McDowell EM, Trump BF. Histologic fixatives suitable for diagnostic light and electron microscopy. Arch Pathol Lab Med 1976;100:405

269. Cheung DT, Perelman N, Ko EC, Nimni ME. Mechanism of crosslinking of proteins by glutaraldehyde III. reaction with collagen in tissues. Connect Tissue Res 1985;13:109

270. Cheung DT, Nimni ME. Mechanism of crosslinking of proteins by glutaraldehyde II. Reaction with monomeric and polymeric collagen. Connect Tissue Res 1982;10:201

271. Cheung DT, Nimni ME. Mechanism of crosslinking of proteins by glutaraldehyde I: Reaction with mode compounds. Connect Tissue Res 1982;10:187

272. Moczar M, Allard R, Robert L, Loisance D, Derouette S, Cachera J-P. Biosynthesis of elastin and other matrix-macromolecules in veinous arterial prosthesis. Pathol Biol 1976;24 (Suppl. 37):37–41

273. Rosenberg N, Hendersen J, Douglas JF, Lord GH, Gaughran ERL. The use of arterial implants prepared by enzymatic modification of arterial grafts. II. The physical properties of the elastic and collagen components of the arterial wall. Arch Surg 1957;74:89

274. Sawyer PN, Stanczewski B, Lucas TR, Kirschenbaum D, Newman M, Taylor R, Kaplitt MJ, Vagnini FJ, Frantz S. Experimental and clinical evaluation of a new negatively charged bovine heterograft for use in peripheral and coronary revascularization. Vascular Grafts 1977;27:282

275. Sawyer PN. The relationship between surface charge (Potential Characteristics) of the vascular interface and thrombosis. Ann NY Acad Sci 1983; 415:561–583

276. Sawyer PN, Adamson R, Butt K, Fitzgerald J, Haque S, Landi J, Malik L, Mistry F, Ramasamy N, Reddy K, Stanczewski B, Kirschenbaum D. Long-term function of NCGT vascular conduits in a multicenter trial: Evaluation of physical chemical parameters. Biomater Med Devices Artif Organs 1980;8:345

277. Blumenthal HT, Lansing AI, Wheeler PA. Calcification of the media of the human aorta and its relation to intimal arteriosclerosis, aging and disease, Am J Pathol 1944;20:665

278. Kim KM. Pathological calcification. In: Kim KM (ed.) Pathobiology of cell membranes. Academic Press, London 1983 vol 3, pp 117–155

279. Berry CL, Starl J, Anderson C, Histopathological changes after aortic anastomosis: Their effects on the assessment of suture materials. J Pathol 1970;102:213

280. Gersbach Ph, Wegman W. Aorta valve replacement using autologous fascia lata transplants. Late morphological changes, an electron microscopic study. Virchows Arch A: Pathol Anat Histol 1974;364:235

281. Brock L. Long-term degenerative changes in aortic segment homografts, with particular reference to calcification. Thorax 1968;23:249

282. Missen GAK, Roberts CI. Calcification and cusp-rupture in human aortic-valve homografts sterilised by ethylene oxide and freeze-dried. Lancet 1970;ii:962

283. Choube BS. Extensive aortic calcification in a case of primary arteritis. Angiology 1972; 23:628

284. Meesen H, Kojimahara M, Franken T, Rhedin P, Huth F. Beitr Pathol 1975;154:218

285. Irving JT, Shibler D, Fleisch H. Effect of condensed phosphates on vitamin-D induced aortic calcification in rats. Proc Soc Exp Biol Med 1966;122:852

286. Kim KM, Huang SN. Ultrastructural study of calcification of human aortic valve. Lab Invest 1971;25:357

287. Kim KM. Calcification of matrix vesicles in human aortic valve and aortic media. Fed Proc Fed Am Soc Exp Biol 1976a;35:156

288. Kim KM, Trump BF. Amorphous calcium precipitations in human aortic valve. Calcif Tissue Res 1975;18:155

289. Kim KM, Valigorsky JM, Mergner WJ, Jones RT, Penergrass RE, Trump BF. Aging changes in the human aortic valve in relation to dystrophic calcification. Hum Pathol 1976; 7:47

290. Lous MLe, Boudin D, Salmon S, Polonovski J. The affinity of type I collagen for lipid in vitro. Biochim Biophys Acta 1982;708:26

291. Wadkins Cl, Luben R, Thomas M, Humphreys R. Physical biochemistry of calcification. Clin Orthop 1974;99:246

292. Boskey AL. Current concepts of the physiology and biochemistry of calcification. Clin Orthop 1981;157:225

293. Ferrans VJ, Spray TL, Billingham ME, Roberts WC. Structural changes in glutaraldehyde-treated porcine heterografts used as substitute cardiac valves. Am J Cardiol 1978;41:1159
294. Levy RJ, Zenker JA, Bernhard WF. Porcine bioprosthetic valve calcification in bovine left ventricle-aorta shunts: Studies of the deposition of vitamin K-dependent proteins. Ann Thorac Surg 1983;36: 187

Chapter 4

Biostability of Vascular Prostheses

R.G. Guidoin, R.W. Snyder, J.A. Awad and M.W. King

Introduction

Arteries which become occluded threaten the survival of the affected limb or organ, or result in an incapacity which might affect the quality of life of the patient. Replacement of these arteries by other vessels, whether biological or synthetic has, for many years, resulted either in the saving of the organ affected or has produced enough improvement of the circulation to make the patient relatively autonomous [1–3]. The fate of these bypasses can be affected by the progression of the arteriosclerosis, the presence of associated diseases and other risk factors [4,5]. These other factors include those which affect the thrombotic and haematological constituents of the blood, the haemodynamic aspect of the bypass itself and the type and quality of the arterial substitute chosen. In terms of the latter risk factor:

1. The durability of the implant should be superior to the life expectancy of the host.
2. The insertion of the graft should not cause undesirable reactions beyond the capacity of the host to handle and correct them.

Thrombosis has been observed in every type of graft. In the early postoperative period it may be due to technical error, while late thrombosis is usually due to extension of the disease or increased vascular resistance distally. In addition to thrombosis, some vascular prostheses have exhibited other complications which are more related to the prosthesis than to the host. Hence, a close examination of current prostheses and their weaknesses might be in order and could result in important improvements [6].

The most common complications we have observed with various arterial prostheses are:

1. The relatively rapid ageing of the genuine biological prosthesis, i.e. venous autologous and homologous grafts. The healing capacity of the autologous saphenous vein is limited [7] and the homologous saphenous vein deteriorates very rapidly [8].
2. The degeneration of processed biological prostheses such as bovine heterografts [9] or processed human umbilical vein, which may be invaded by lipids shortly after implantation [10].

3. Infections of the prostheses, especially in the synthetic group. The luminal surface is coated by a biofilm quite often incorporating a bacteraemic colonization [11].
4. Dilatation and rupture of the light polyester grafts [12].

Current Vascular Prostheses

Unprocessed Biological Prostheses

To date, genuine biological grafts are for all practical purposes limited to saphenous veins, the autologous mammary artery being used only for aorto-coronary bypasses and other veins only when the saphenous vein is unsuitable or unavailable.

Autologous Saphenous Vein

This is, to date, the prosthesis which comes the nearest to the ideal whenever a vessel of between 4 and 6 mm diameter is needed [13]. In the case of the reversed saphenous vein, careful dissection and anastomosis is important [14]. On the other hand, in veins left in situ, valve destruction is critical [15,16]. It might be very useful to control the quality of the inner surface by means of a specially designed endoscope after dilatation of the site of destruction of the valves. It is important that veins to be grafted are handled with caution.

Venous Homograft

On some occasions, veins which have been obtained by stripping from patients have been used as a secondary access in haemodialysis, for femoropopliteal and for aorto-coronary bypass [17]. The results have, however, been inconsistent. They have been reported as giving excellent results but, at other times, their implantation has been disastrous, resulting in aneurysmal formation and stenosis [18,19]. Thus, the mechanical properties of each stripped vein would have to be tested individually [20,21]. It might also be interesting to measure the electrical impedance in these veins. On the other hand, more than 35% of stripped veins have been shown to be contaminated with various bacteria [22]. The venous homograft also provokes a type of immunological reaction in the host [23]; freezing alone has not been able to completely eliminate this reaction [24]. Veins removed from cadavers offer another more interesting possibility since only normal veins would be removed [25]. Each should still be evaluated individually for possible defects. The authors believe that venous transplantation should, at this time, be limited to aorto-coronary bypass and only when removed from a near parent, after typing. Their use should be in conjunction with cyclosporin administration [26].

Processed Biological Prostheses

Prostheses of biological tissues which have been processed chemically and tanned, thus becoming a form of leather, have been used. These grafts have come from two sources, bovine carotid and human umbilical vein. Other sources such as the canine carotid have been explored.

Bovine Heterografts

Bovine heterografts are prepared from bovine carotid arteries (Fig. 4.1). The cellular content is digested enzymatically and the remaining material (mostly collagen) is crosslinked [27–29]. They have been shown to have numerous structural weaknesses [30]. All models have in time shown marked degeneration and a tendency for lipid absorption. The possibility of improving these grafts is unfortunately limited [31].

Processed Human Umbilical Vein

The umbilical veins of human newborns are removed and processed no more than 24 h after birth. The vein has no side branches. A mandrel is inserted in the lumen to straighten the vein and it is then fixed in either glutaraldehyde or a starch dialdehyde [32,33]. Whether a synthetic net is used to reinforced them or not, they all eventually undergo a marked degeneration about 5 years after implantation [34]. Treatment with heparin might improve the thrombogenicity of these grafts on a short-term basis [35] but it is unfortunately unlikely to prevent the resorption of the vessel wall [10,36].

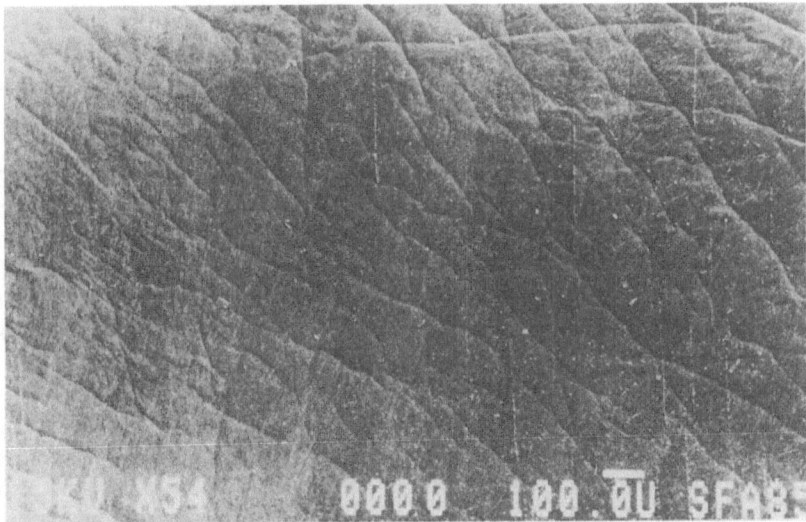

Fig. 4.1. Example of a processed biological prosthesis, the Solcograft® (×54).

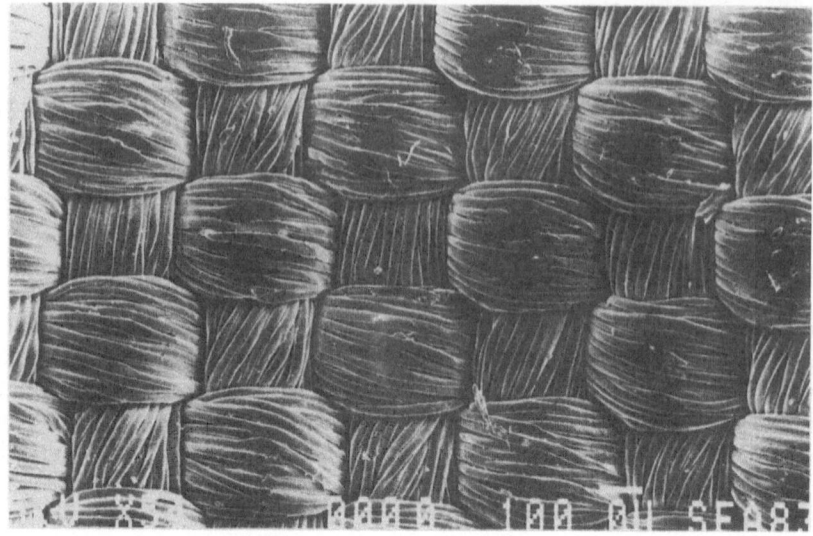

Fig. 4.2. A Bard Woven PTFE graft 19 years after implantation as an aortofemoral bifurcation (×54).

The Synthetic or Alloplastic Prostheses

Of the various synthetic materials, only polytetrafluoroethylene (PTFE, i.e. Teflon) and poly(ethylene terephthalate) (PET, i.e. Dacron) have proved to be sufficiently resistant to degradation in the body [37]. Nylon, Orlon and Ivalon (among others) now belong to history [38,39].

PTFE Grafts

Two forms have been used as prostheses. The textile type and the microporous graft.

PTFE textiles. PTFE textiles can either be woven (as shown in Fig. 4.2) or knitted, as suggested by Edwards [40] nearly 30 years ago. The main objection to these grafts have been their tendency to fray at the cut edges, i.e. at the anastomotic line [41]. However, some of the cases of disruption at the anastomotic line may have been due to the silk suture material used, which is partially biodegradable. PTFE as such does not deteriorate and thus the use of this material especially as warp knit should be reconsidered [42].

Microporous PTFE. Microporous PTFE was introduced commercially in the seventies and has become increasingly popular for femoropopliteal and axillo-femoral bypasses (43–45). Microporous or expanded PTFE consists of nodules of PTFE interconnected by fibrils as shown in Fig. 4.3. At present, the most popular is the reinforced Gore-Tex, which has an outer wrap of microporous

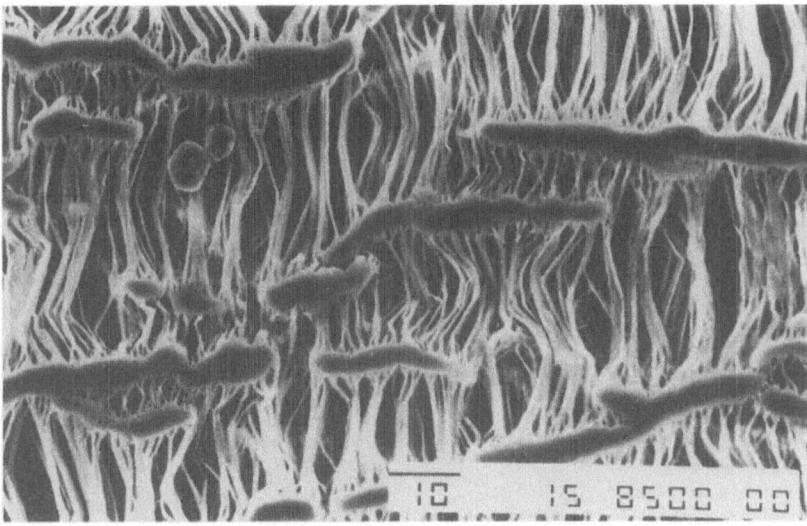

Fig. 4.3. Typical expanded PTFE structure (Bard PTFE; ×2700).

PTFE tape for strength. The tape has a much lower porosity than the body, which may modify tissue ingrowth. Although the results of bypasses with these grafts have been very satisfactory (46–48), this material appears to function against all logic. It lacks compliance, it heals very little or not at all [49] and very often it presents on its inner surface a biofilm of glycocalyx frequently incorporating some bacterial colonies capable of being reactivated under special conditions [50]. The numerous attempts to correct these deficiencies have proved disappointing. When made hydrophilic, the grafts show a fibrous proliferation and when treated with carbon or reinforced with external rings, they tend to become calcified (R. Guidoin, unpublished data). On the other hand, the in situ stability of reinforced Gore-Tex is impressive if manipulated with care. The ruptures and tears occasionally observed in some of these grafts are most likely due to indiscriminate use of surgical clamps [51].

Polyester or PET Grafts

These are the most popular prostheses, at least for replacement of large and medium-sized vessels. They have endured the test of time, although a large number of types and various forms have been devised or proposed to improve the clinical results. For a more complete description of these grafts, see King et al. [52].

Type I PET Grafts. Type I PET grafts are low porosity grafts designed primarily for use in cases where porosity is a concern, e.g. heavily anticoagulated patients, patients with bleeding disorders, and patients who cannot accept transfusions. These grafts are primarily of woven construction (Fig. 4.4) and are more difficult to handle and suture than knitted grafts. In general, how-

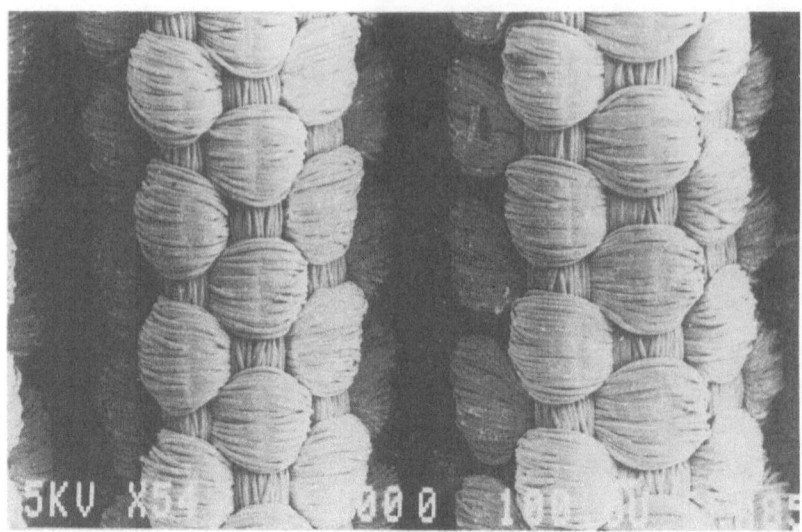

Fig. 4.4. Bard DeBakey extra low porosity PET prostheses, typical of the woven structures (×54).

ever, woven grafts are stronger than other types. The low porosity is believed to restrict tissue ingrowth. However, woven grafts have functioned successfully for up to 20 years after implantation [53].

Type II PET Grafts. Type II PET grafts centre on the importance of the porosity factor (i.e. permeability to water), also known as the Wesolowski concept [54]. The first grafts, whether woven or knitted (tight knit or warp knit), occasionally resulted in calcification when inserted in the growing pig [55]. Wesolowski then suggested increasing the porosity or permeability to water in order to produce better encapsulation and provoke a superior healing reaction [56]. Lighter PET grafts were then produced. Although the resistance to rupture of these light grafts proved superior to the human aorta, they eventually showed frequent areas of deformities (either slipped stitch patterns or yarn rupture) due probably to the repeated hammering of the pulsatile blood flow. At present, this concept has been definitely discarded [57].

Type III PET Grafts. Type III PET grafts concentrate mainly on the knit pattern with the idea of producing a complete healing with endothelialization of the inner surface. The new designs were based on the weft and warp knit designs shown in Fig. 4.5. The straight fibres were changed to a texturized type and additional yarns were added as velour loops to form anchoring sites as proposed by DeBakey [58] (Fig. 4.6). Sauvage then became the main proponent of this concept [59], although it has not been confirmed clinically. However, the external velour types resulted in better anchoring of the graft. Double velour grafts (inner and outer surface) also were made available (Fig. 4.7) [60]. They consisted of two fibres. The first had cylindrical filaments, while the second was made of trilobal filaments. The type III PET grafts improved the haemostatic properties of the grafts during placement but showed some

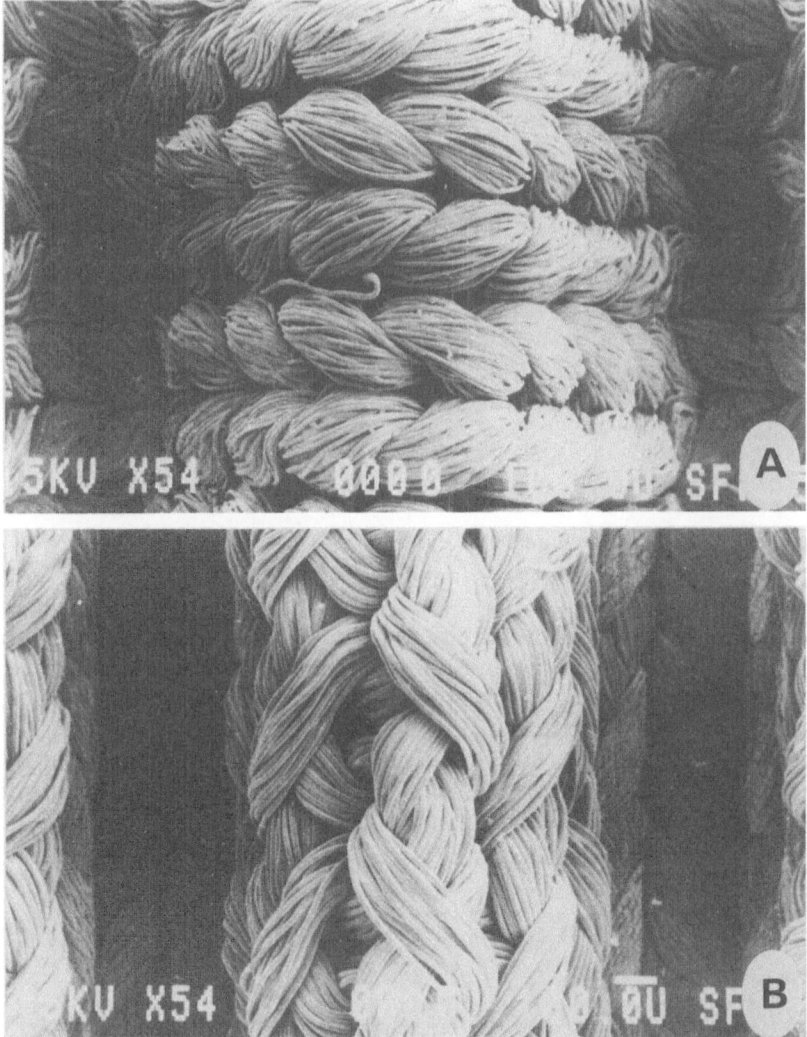

Fig. 4.5. a Bard DeBakey Standard knit PET graft, a weft-knit construction (×54). **b** Meadox Cooley Weavenit PET graft, a warp-knit structure (×54).

mechanical instability and tended to fray. The concept of endothelializing the inner surface of prostheses appears now somewhat less important. In general, humans do not develop extensive endothelial linings on grafts.

Type IV PET Grafts. Type IV PET grafts revolved around the strength of the prostheses. Following a number of reports of dilatation and even rupture of some PET grafts, which appeared in the literature of the late 1970s [61–63], the manufacturers proposed to increase the strength of these prostheses by introducing or reintroducing different forms of woven grafts or by strengthening the warp-knitted grafts. The modifications made on the woven grafts were

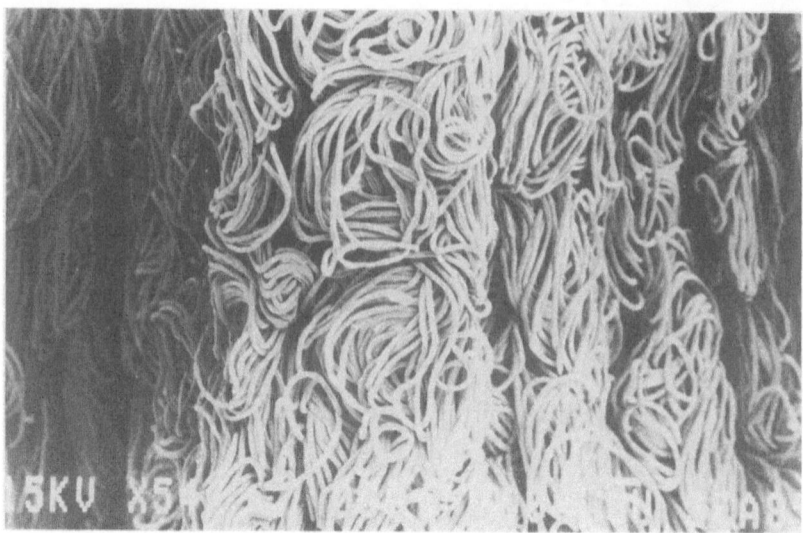

Fig. 4.6. Luminal surface of the Bard DeBakey Vasculour D (×54).

not always desirable. The woven velours (Fig. 4.8) and the excessively porous woven grafts tend to fray at the anastomotic line and have to be cauterized. On the other hand, the regular woven grafts and those with low porosity present a high degree of compaction and can thus be anastomosed without danger. The warp-knitted prostheses have become more and more popular since they frequently incorporate texturized fibres, resulting in better anchorage of the graft without affecting mechanical stability [64].

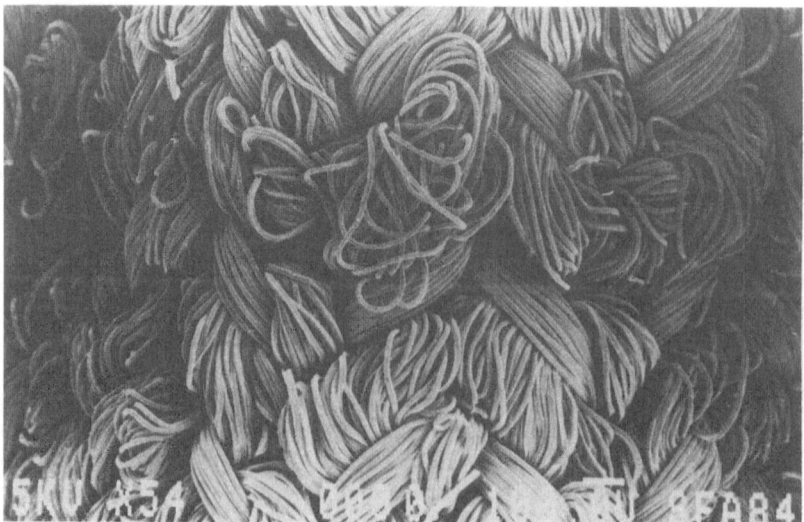

Fig. 4.7. Luminal surface of the Meadox Cooley Double Velour (×54).

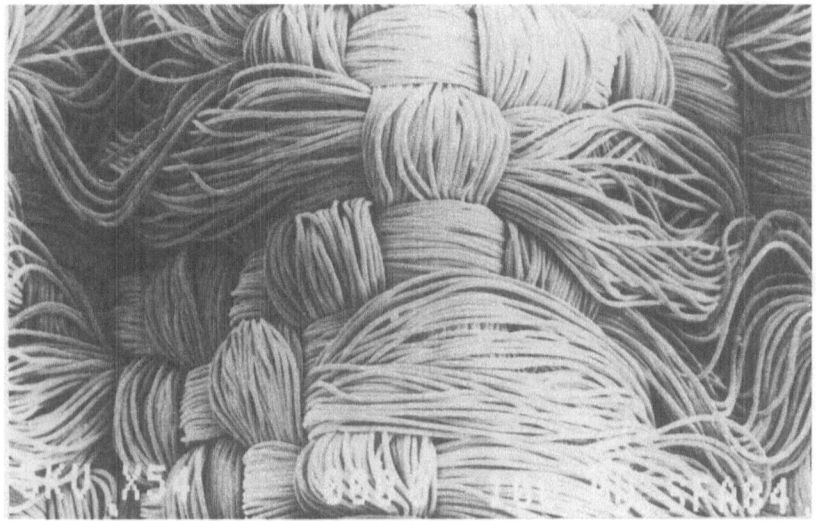

Fig. 4.8. Luminal surface of the Meadox Woven Velour (×54).

Type V Grafts. Type V grafts are the composite of hybrid prostheses. The main purpose here is to ensure the best chances of healing in order to prevent eventual and long-term complications.

1. *Cellular Seeding of Prostheses.* Endothelial cells obtained from veins either mechanically [65] or enzymatically [66] or mesothelial cells from the peritoneum [67] are spread on the inner thrombotic layer during pre-clotting. Healing of the prostheses in dogs has been very impressive. However, the technique is difficult and is restricted to a few selected centres [68].
2. *Composite Prostheses.* In composite prostheses the wall of the polyester graft is impregnated with a biodegradable material, either collagen [69] or albumin [70], these prostheses do not require pre-clotting. Eventually, they could be used to incorporate antibiotics [71] or growth-stimulating factors [72].

Sparks Mandrel

With the Sparks mandrel, the tissue from the host is induced to produce a graft. This device is produced by inserting a mandrel under the skin of the host in the area of the vessel to be bypassed. Tissue from the host grows on two polyester nets inserted over the mandrel which, in most cases, is made of siloxane elastomer. After maturation, the mandrel is removed and the conduit formed is anastomosed at both ends to the vessel to be bypassed [73]. This concept has now been completely abandoned because of the disastrous results, mainly thrombosis of the graft, aneurysmal dilatation and haemorrhage. Most of these complications are due to the fact that the graft wall does not incorporate either smooth muscle or elastic fibres. Thus, as long as our knowledge of the growth factors and of the angiogenesis involved remains at its present level, this concept must not be reintroduced, however fascinating it appears [74].

Biological Response

Biological Grafts

In general, unprocessed biological grafts are partially or totally devoid of endothelial cells, and lead to different levels of healing [75]. The umbilical vein graft, like the bovine heterograft, shows more debris than the homologous vein graft. Little ingrowth or native lining appears to form on these grafts [76] (Fig. 4.9).

PET Vascular Prostheses

In the dog, PET textile grafts are eventually completely encapsulated [77]. They are usually lined with endothelial cells, as seen in Fig. 4.10. In humans, these grafts are lined with a pseudointima composed of compacted fibrin (Fig. 4.11). However, in diabetic patients, the inner surface of the graft may be bare, exposing PET to the blood stream (Fig. 4.12) [6].

PTFE Vascular Prostheses

PTFE grafts, explanted from humans, show thinner linings than PET grafts. Again, this is not a genuine pseudointima. Occasionally, bacterial colonies are found within this material [42].

Long-Term Failure Modes

Vascular prostheses suffer from two basic long-term failure modes. The first is occlusion, which may be due to progression of the disease distally, resulting in the reduction of the blood flow below the thrombotic threshold velocity or due to some type of intimal hyperplasia. The second type of long-term failure mode is structural failure of the prosthesis itself or of the suture line. This chapter will concentrate on this second failure mode.

Processed Biological Prostheses

Biological prostheses can suffer from various forms of biological attack as well as mechanical damage.

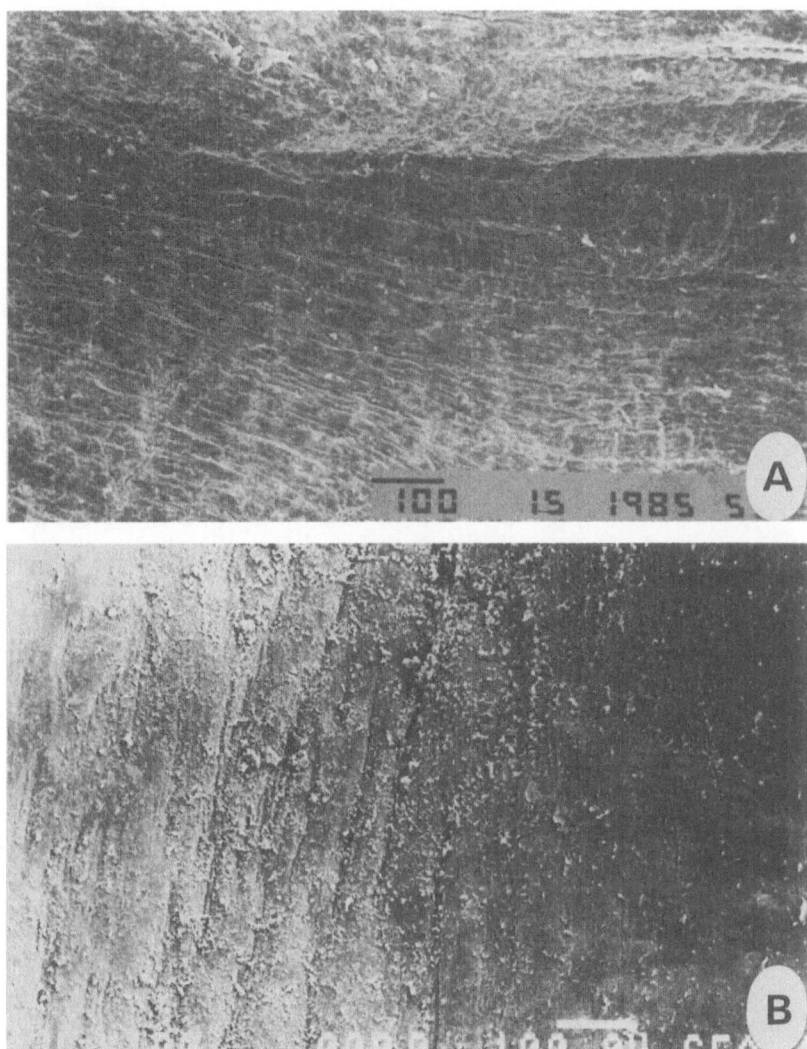

Fig. 4.9. a Reversed autologous saphenous vein after 21 days of implantation (× 100). **b** Meadox Dardik umbilical vein graft after 20 days of implantation (×100).

Mechanical Damage

Biological structures are sensitive to mechanical injury. Processed biological grafts have lost the capacity to repair themselves and this injury can lead to long-term failure. There are two major sources of mechanical injury to processed biological grafts.

Processing. Tissue is handled with forceps during harvesting. It is dissected free from surrounding tissue. For those arteries or veins with side branches (such as carotid arteries), these must be located and tied off. All of these operations are

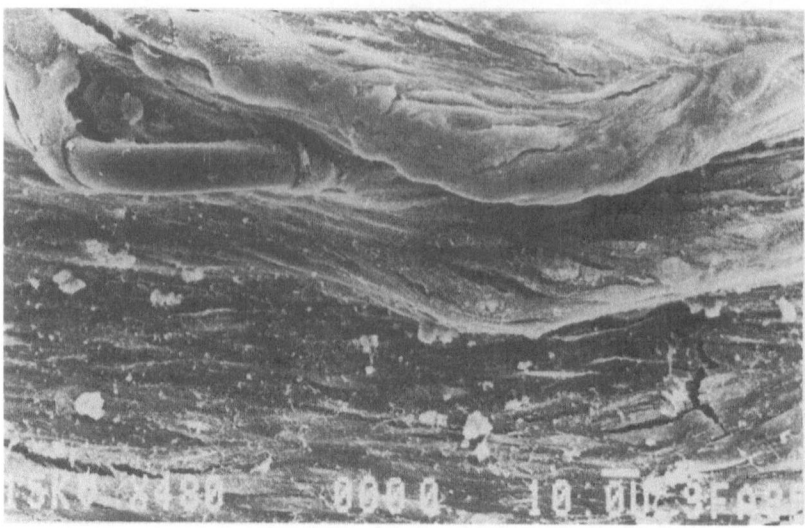

Fig. 4.10. Typical flow surface in a well-healed Bard Vasculour II graft after 6 months of implantation in a canine (×480).

potential sources of damage to the prostheses. However, the greatest potential for damage comes from the mandrels used to straighten and hold the vessel. Inserting and removing the mandrel can lead to damage of the intimal lining or other mechanical tears (Fig. 4.13).

Surgery. Biological grafts are susceptible to damage from improperly selected clamps. There is also the potential of damage from sutures. A delicate pre-

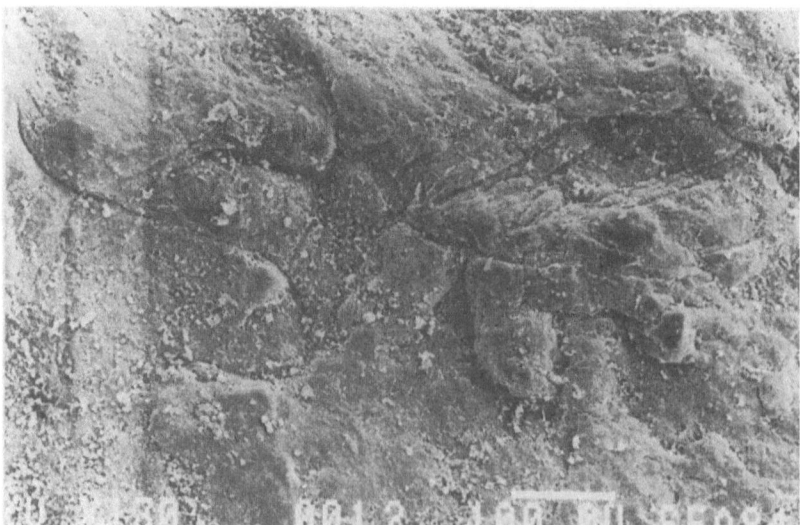

Fig. 4.11. Well-healed luminal surface in a Meadox Coopey Double Velour graft at 4 years in a human (× 130).

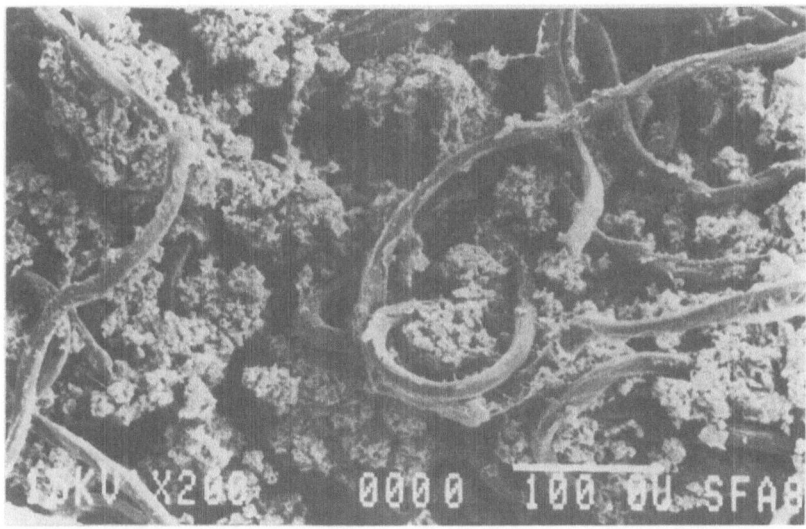

Fig. 4.12. Poorly healed Meadox Cooley Double Velour graft after 4 years of implantation in a human (×200).

caution must be taken to prevent suture pull-out. Suture holes will elongate under excessive tension.

Degradation

Autolysis starts as the vessel is removed from the donor. Processing must begin as soon as possible after 1emoval to stop the natural enzymatic degradation.

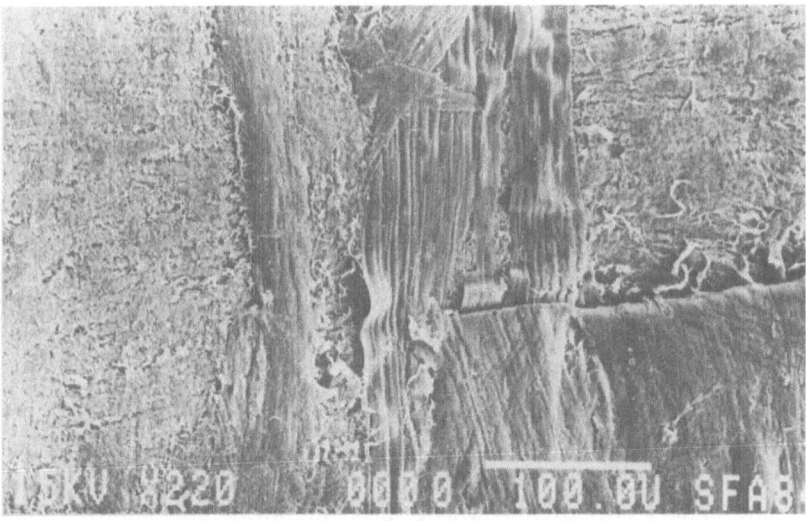

Fig. 4.13. Damaged luminal surface in umbilical vein graft (×220).

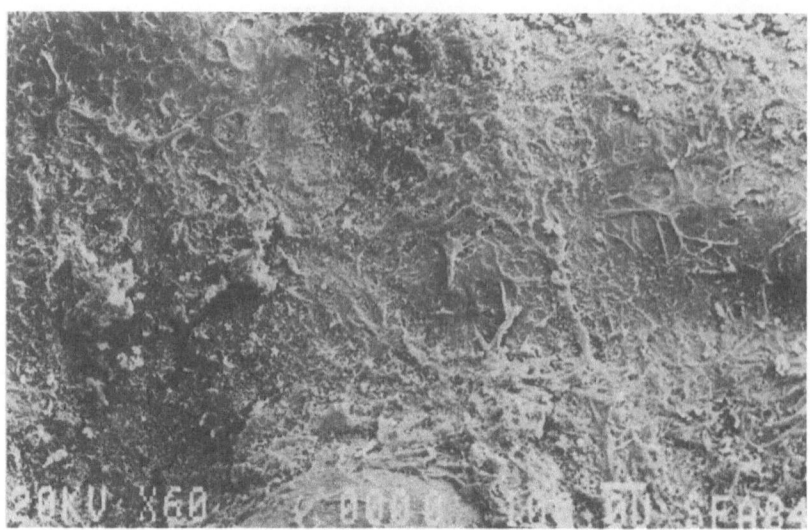

Fig. 4.14. Resorption of Biograft® after 5 years of implantation (×60).

Once the prosthesis is stabilized, either by crosslinking or by the complete removal of protein materials, the degradative process proceeds very slowly. Typical failures may occur several years after implantation, as shown in Fig. 4.14. There are two failure modes.

Calcification. Calcification can arise from host cell debris. However, this source is relatively rare as these prostheses cause little damage to cells. A more likely source is lipid absorption, which has been demonstrated early in implant history.

Mechanical Breakdown. Combining the effects of pulsating pressure, which causes the walls to thin, and enzymatic attack, either from the host or from bacteria, leads to aneurysms and genuine defects.

PTFE

PTFE, either in the form of textiles or as expanded PTFE, is a very inert material. No evidence of degradative changes in the material has been observed, even more than 20 years after implantation. However, it is susceptible to damage, particularly in the thin-walled expanded PTFE form.

Mechanical Damage

PTFE is a relatively soft or viscoelastic material. Thus, it can be deformed mechanically. The PTFE textile process used mandrels and held the material against the mandrel by winding yarn to form the crimps. This could deform

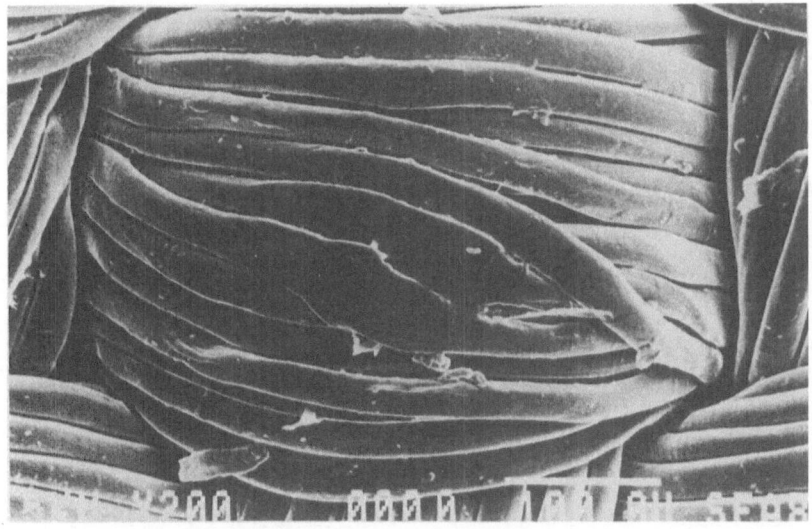

Fig. 4.15. A damaged woven PTFE graft which survived 19 years implantation (×200).

the yarn (Fig. 4.15). Similar damage to other PTFE prostheses is possible with mandrels, holding devices and pressure testing. The weakest direction in expanded PTFE is circumferential (see below). However, occasionally PTFE will split longitudinally, as shown in Fig. 4.16. The cause of this is unknown but may be affected by the rate tensile load is applied. For example, rapid stretching of an axillo-femoral graft when the arm is raised.

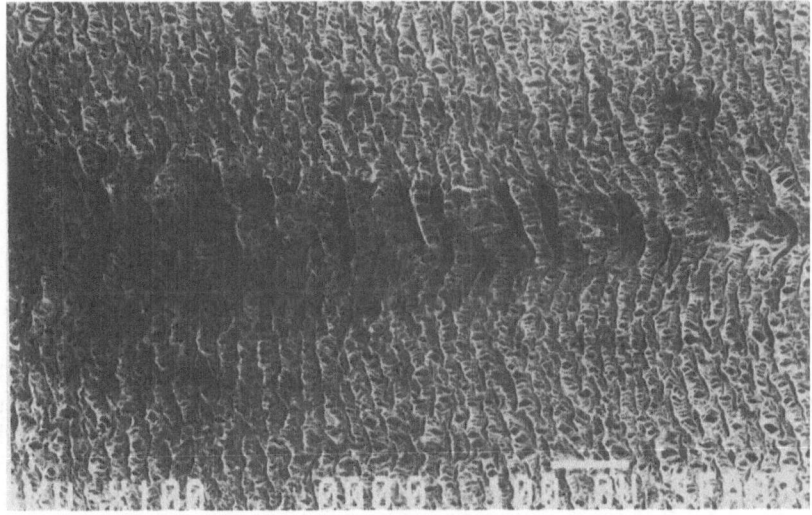

Fig. 4.16. Longitudinal tear in an expanded PTFE graft recovered after 14 months of implantation (×100).

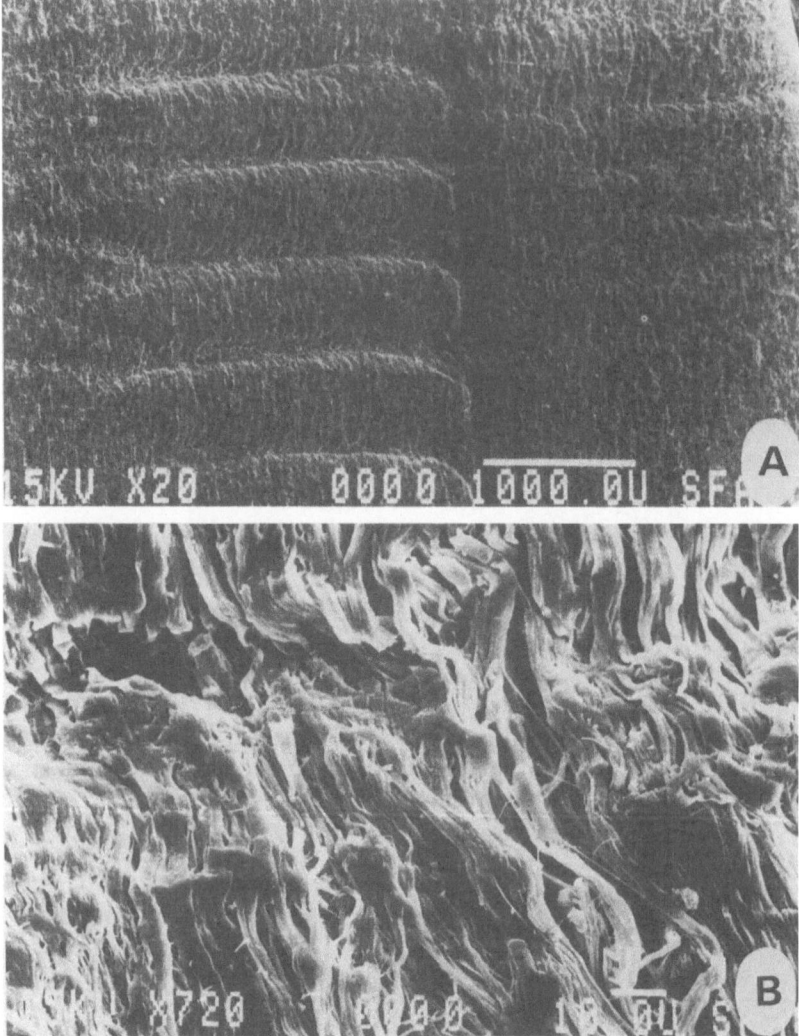

Fig. 4.17. Damage done to PTFE by vascular clamps (**a** ×20; **b** ×720).

Processing

Because of the inert nature and high melting point of PTFE, it is difficult to damage the material other than mechanically. However, expanded PTFE starts out as a resin. This resin, when formed into a tube, must be fused at high temperatures. Because PTFE is a good insulator (particularly in the porous form), sufficient time must be allowed for all parts of the PTFE to reach the proper temperature for sintering. If this does not occur, the material may split in the naturally weak longitudinal direction or may dilate.

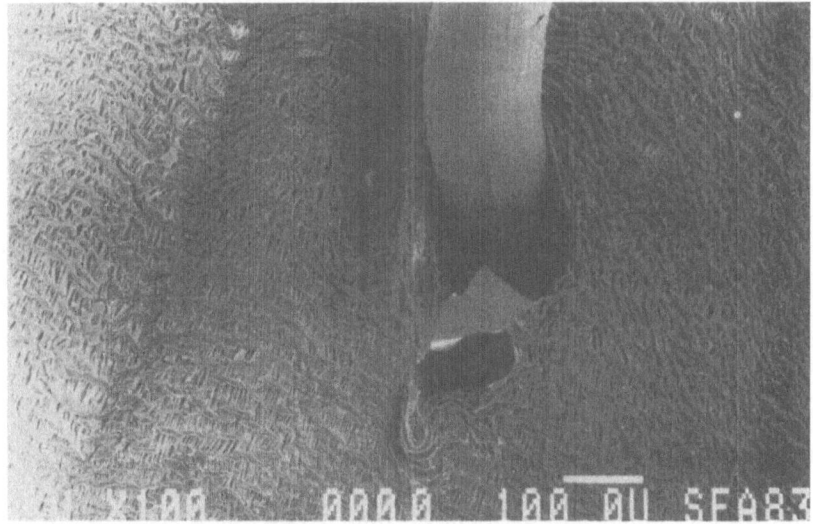

Fig. 4.18. Typical elongated suture hole in microporous PTFE (×100).

Surgical Damage

The same mechanism applies to surgical damage. Clamping will leave permanent deformation in an expanded PTFE graft (Fig. 4.17). Because of the non-elastic nature of the material, particular care must be taken with sutures. The oversized needles used with sutures and suture tension will result in elongated suture holes (Fig. 4.18). Care must also be taken to insert the

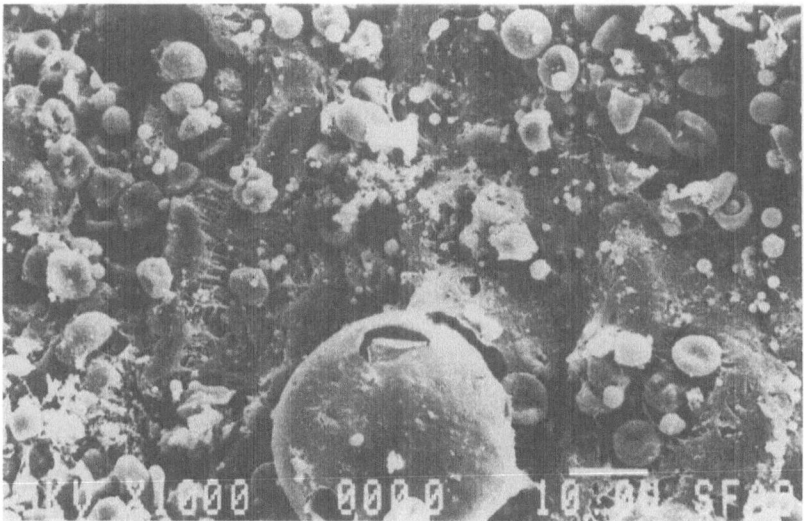

Fig. 4.19. Lipids, cholesterol and bacteremic colonization on an expanded PTFE after 18 months of implantation as a femoropopliteal bypass (× 1000).

sutures back from the anastomosis. One additional failure mode is calcification and infection. Figure 4.19 shows a PTFE graft with a lipid-bearing biofilm. This biofilm contains bacteria and may be due to improper sterilization or to a pre-existing infection in the host.

Fatigue

Any synthetic material is subject to fatigue failure, should the internal stresses exceed a threshold value. If the PTFE is sufficiently thin (or damaged), these stresses can cause long-term fatigue failures. The yarn filaments used in PTFE textile grafts were much larger than most yarn filaments, making this failure mode unlikely in textiles.

PET Vascular Prostheses

Although PET is much less viscoelastic than PTFE, as a synthetic it has the same basic failure modes. In addition, the polymer is not as inert as PTFE and can be susceptible to chemical attack and hydrolysis (at elevated temperatures) [78].

Surgical Damage

Although not as soft as PTFE, PET can still be damaged by clamping. Filaments can be flattened by improperly selected clamps. Filaments can also be broken or cut by severing tip needles (Fig. 4.20). The proper placement of

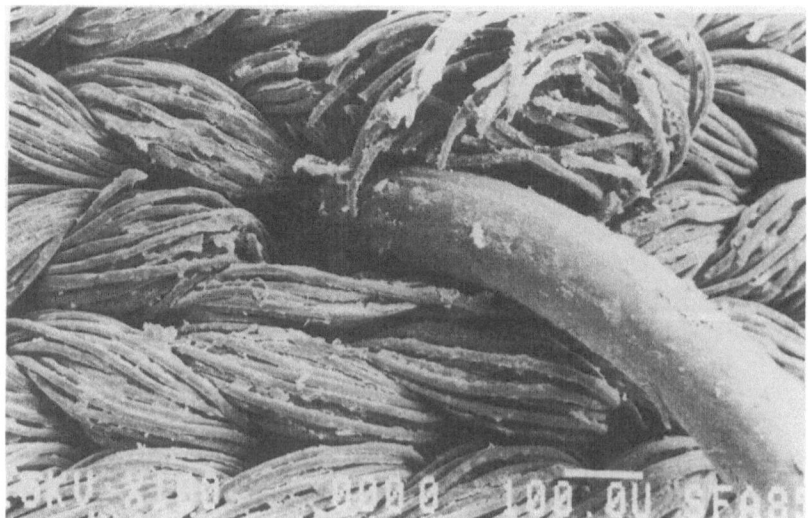

Fig. 4.20. Broken PET filaments caused by a suture and needle (×100).

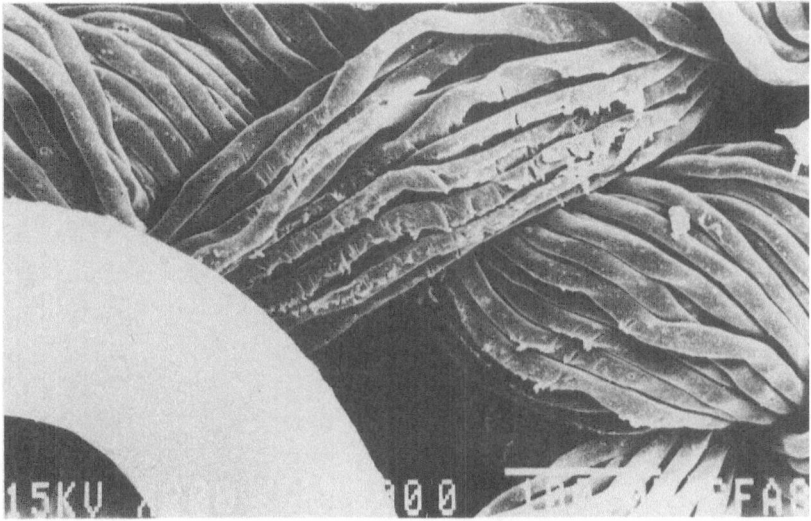

Fig. 4.21. Damaged caused by friction between suture and graft (graft implanted for 96 months) (×200).

sutures is dictated by the textile structure. Woven structures are much more susceptible to fraying and a bigger bite must be taken in these grafts. PET may also be damaged by excessive friction. Figure 4.21 shows such a damage caused by a suture.

Thermal Damage

PET has a much lower melting point than PTFE and care must be taken in the process not to exceed this point, particularly if the material is under pressure from clamps or yarn used to form crimps. Figure 4.22 shows the typical flattened filaments resulting from overheating. Because of the susceptibility of PET to hydrolysis, the atmosphere at higher temperature may also damage the grafts. For example, repeated autoclaving (particularly flash autoclaving) has been demonstrated to weaken PET.

Chemical Damage

PET is not as inert as PTFE. Some of the chemical cleaning processes proposed for PET can etch the polymer, leading to potential cracking under cyclic loading. In addition, some solvents can penetrate the filaments and be released over long periods of time with as yet unknown effects on the prostheses. Figure 4.23 demonstrates typical chemical damage to a graft which subsequently survived for 6 years after implantation.

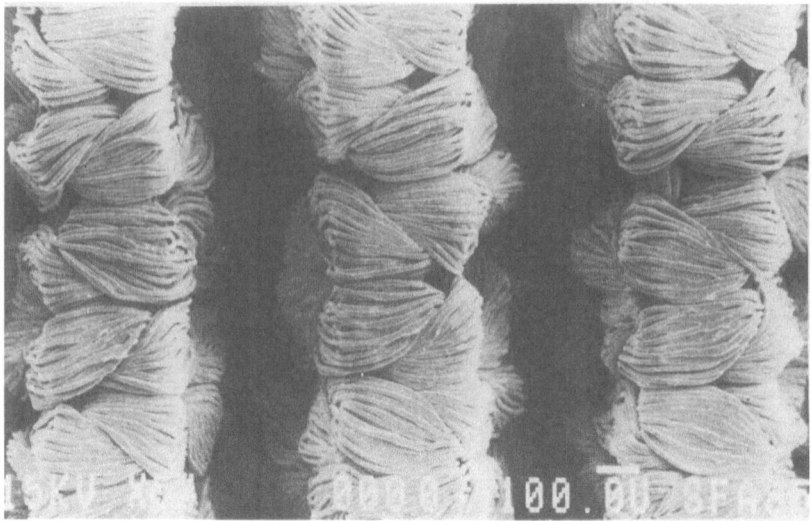

Fig. 4.22. Flattened filaments, probably caused by heated mandrel or excessive pressure from winding thread used to hold crimps to mandrel (×54).

Fatigue

There are two types of fatigue evidenced by PET textile prostheses: structural and polymer (or classical) fatigue.

Structural Fatigue. Structural fatigue occurs in textile structures that are loosely knit or woven. The bare structure is stabilized by the friction between yarns

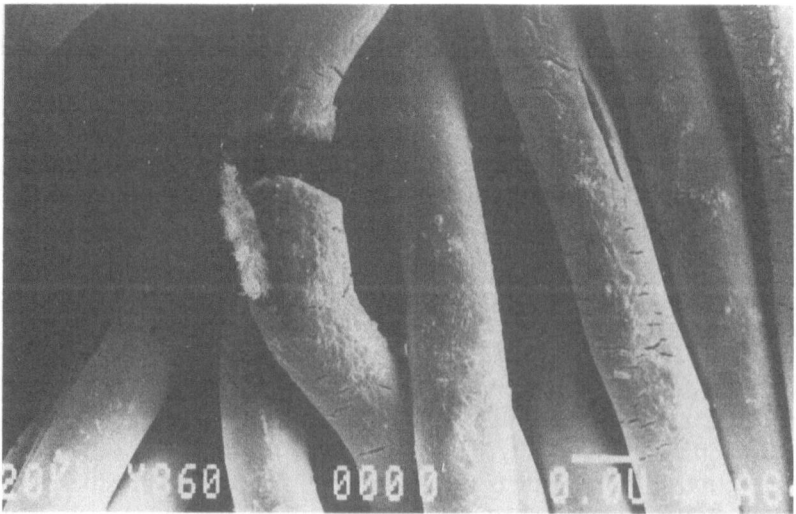

Fig. 4.23. Typical chemical damage to a PET graft explanted after 6 years (×860).

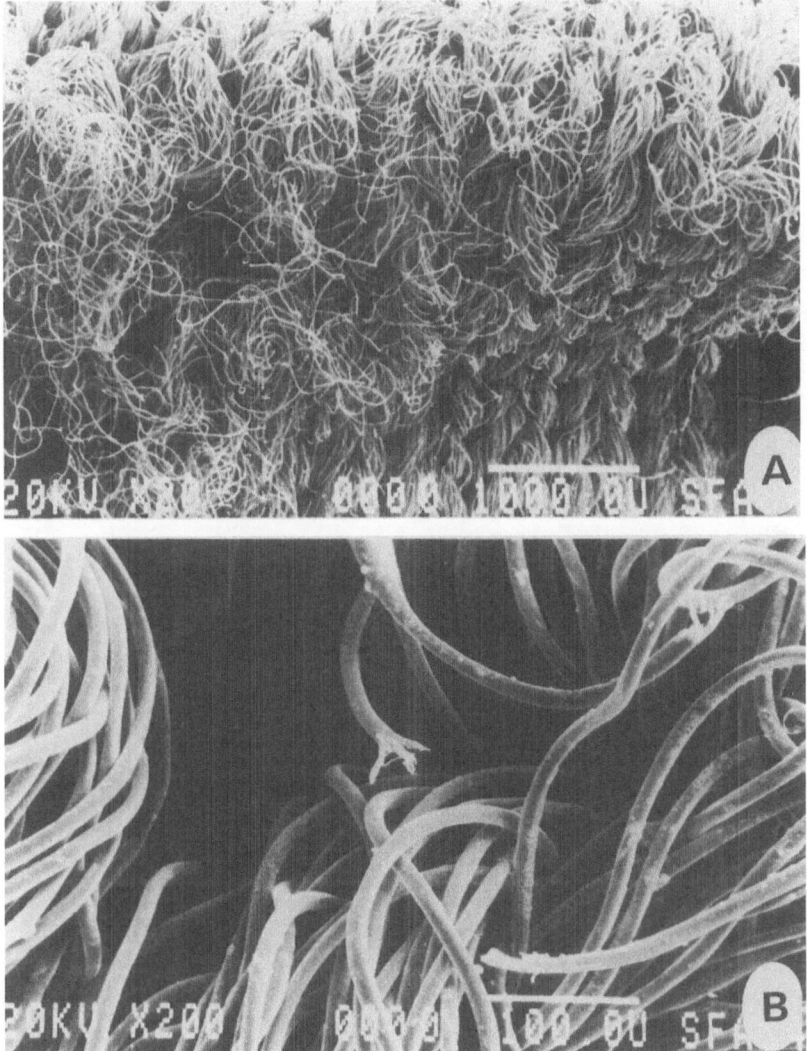

Fig. 4.24. Several holes appearing in a texturized weft-knit graft implanted for 2 years (**a** ×20); note splintered filament ends (**b** ×200).

and yarn tension. If this tension is too low and the friction is overcome, the structure shifts or stretches. This is partially reduced by any ingrowth in the implanted textile. However, if this ingrowth is insufficient or weak, the structure can shift. The graft then dilates and shortens.

Classical Fatigue. Classical fatigue occurs as the stresses in individual filaments exceed the endurance limit for PET. This can occur in damaged filaments or in thin-walled prostheses. Typical failures include splintered or fuzzy filament ends (Fig. 4.24), blunt ends (Fig. 4.25) and tapered ends (Fig. 4.26). The

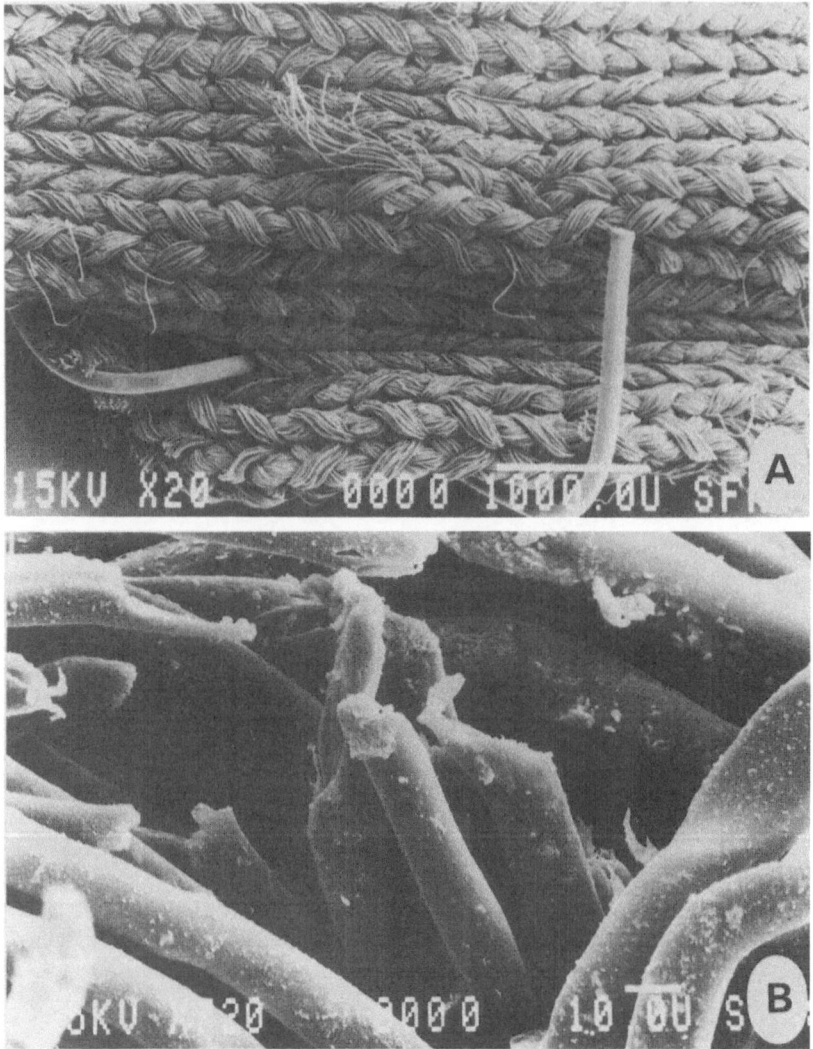

Fig. 4.25. Hole in a warp-knit graft implanted for 8 years (**a** ×20); note blunt ends of filaments (**b** ×720).

different configurations are caused by the different types of initial damage and/or different subsequent filaments loading patterns.

Degradation

To date, the only degradation that has been demonstrated in PET grafts has been in the coatings applied to hybrid grafts. If the coating is designed to degrade, this creates no problems. However, if (as in the case of the Sparks

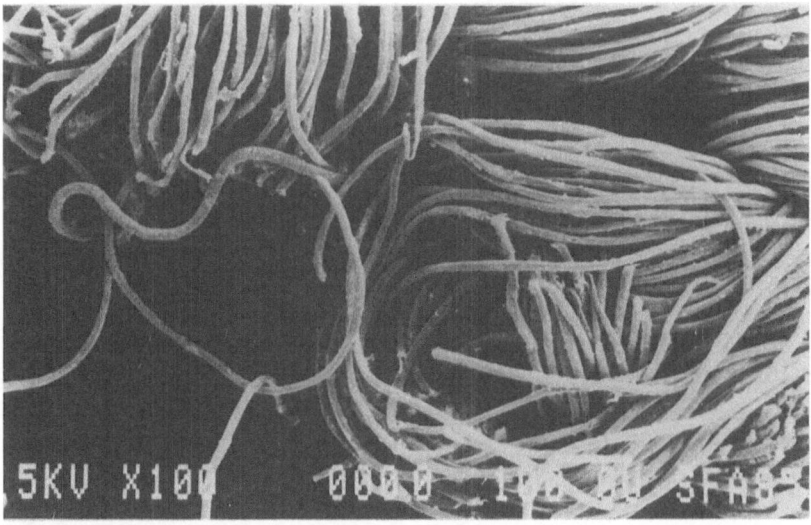

Fig. 4.26. Tear in a weft-knit graft after 6 years of implantation; note several tapered ends (×100).

mandrel shown in Fig. 4.27) the coating is necessary for graft function, this can be disastrous.

New Materials

Processed Biological Prostheses

Various new types of variants of processed human umbilical veins or bovine heterografts have been suggested. In most cases, they are either veins or arteries which have been treated chemically. A new version of the Sparks mandrel prepared from sheep and fixed in glutaraldehyde before implantation in humans has also been proposed [79]. All these models suffer from being resorbable and biodegradable and fail to stimulate angiogenesis. They should therefore be forgotten.

New Synthetic Grafts

Besides some of the unusual laboratory specimens being tried, polyurethane appears to stimulate a huge interest among investigators. These materials are easy to manipulate and further can be prepared to have a predetermined compliance. The most important models in this group are:

1. The laminated polyurethanes of Kardos [80].
2. The microporous replamineform structure obtained by incorporating the spicules of sea urchins to the polyurethane solution. After reticulation,

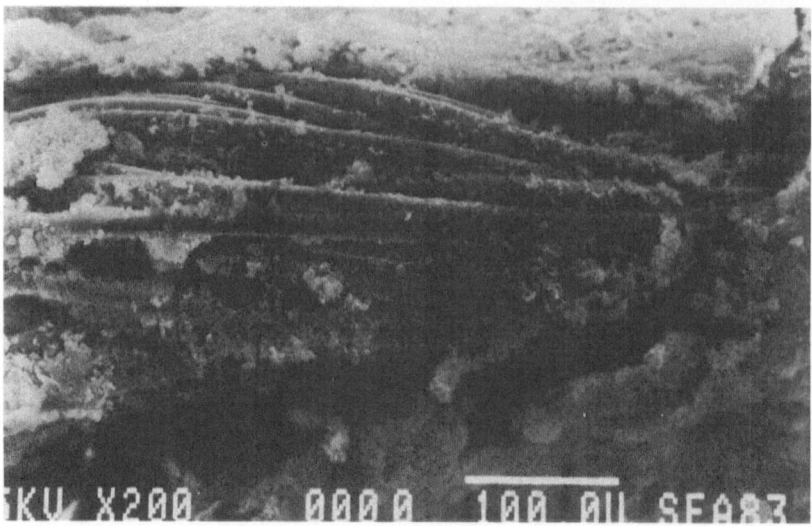

Fig. 4.27. Resorption of the Sparks mandrel after 10 years implantation (×200).

these spicules are dissolved in hydrochloric acid, thus leaving a microporous structure [81].

3. The Annis prostheses obtained by means of a process which electrostatically deposit polyurethane particles on a mandrel [82].

4. The Lyman graft obtained by successive immersion of a rod in a polyurethane solution [83].

5. The Ontario Research Foundation method, in which polyurethane filaments are extruded and wrapped on a rotating mandrel. Depending on the speed of rotation, grafts of various compliances are obtained [84].

6. The Mitrathane prosthesis, which is a closed cell, microporous, hydrophilic type of graft [85].

7. The composite and biodegradable Gogolewski graft of hydrophilic polyurethane [86].

Actually, all the polyurethanes are now the subject of intensive interest. However, as long as their stability has not been definitely established beyond any reasonable doubt, they should not be implanted in humans.

Conclusion

A review of current explant data indicates that current synthetic vascular grafts of PET and PTFE have enjoyed a good success in terms of biostability. PTFE grafts such as the one shown in Fig. 4.2 19 years after implantation or PET grafts such as the one shown in Fig. 4.28 after 10 years implantation prove their biostability. This is true for the vast majority of the synthetic grafts. The data

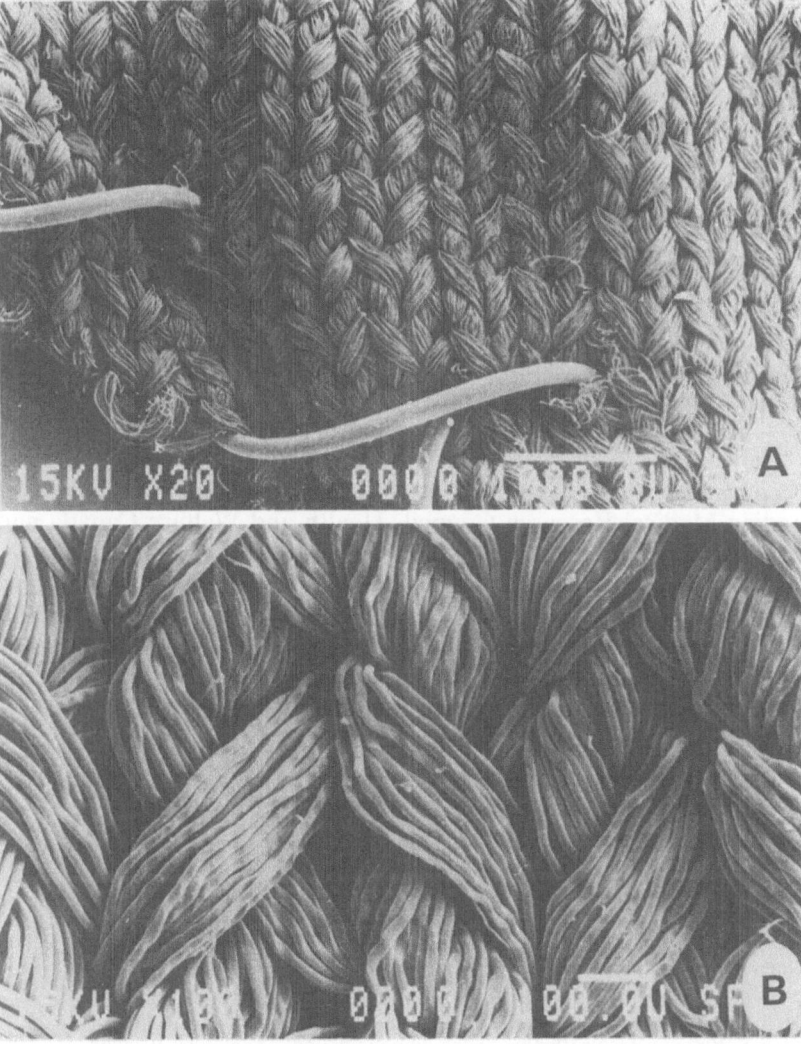

Fig. 4.28. Warp-knit Dacron graft after 10 years of implantation (**a** ×20; **b** ×100).

also demonstrate that these grafts must be treated with care, starting with carefully validated processes and easy handling at the time of surgery. Processed grafts of biological origin have not yet been able to match that success. New prostheses with improved flow surfaces must match the biostability of the existing grafts.

The great number of prosthetic models already marketed and the continuous emergence of new prototypes confirm the fact, if any confirmation was needed, that an ideal arterial prosthesis is not available. Would the quest for the perfect prosthesis finally end with some fortuitous discovery? Maybe. Meanwhile, we should not forget that these grafts are finally implanted in patients for the replacement of a segment of a diseased artery while the patient's vessels are the seat of arteriosclerotic lesions affecting numerous areas of their arterial system.

Experience has demonstrated three primary long-term failure modes which must be investigated: enzymatic degradation, hydrolysis and fatigue. Each of these must be tested prior to human implantation. Enzymatic degradation can be monitored by carefully controlling implant studies and storage in enzymatic solutions. Hydrolysis should be studied in two modes. The first mode is the potential damage done during autoclaving, should that be a possible mode of sterilization. The elevated temperature accelerates the effect. The second mode occurs over long periods of time (Nylon required 1–2 years) and should also be studied with simulators [87,88]. These simulators are designed to study the effect of pressure pulsation. Simulators can also be designed to study bending across a bony joint. Of course, these studies should take place in a buffered saline solution at or above body temperature.

Acknowledgements. Our research on arterial prostheses has been supported by the Canadian Medical Research Council, Health and Welfare Canada and the Quebec Heart Foundation. We would like also to give our thanks to the numerous colleagues and persons who have collaborated in our research work.

Disclaimer. The opinions expressed herein are solely those of the authors and do not necessarily reflect the views of the organization with which the authors are affiliated or those of the agencies which supported the work.

References

1. DeBakey M. The development of vascular surgery. Am J Surg 1979;137:697–738
2. Glickman MH, Hurwitz RL, Kimmins SA, Evans WE. Employment following peripheral vascular surgery: an increasingly critical issue. Surgery 1983;98:50–53
3. Hollier LH. Aortic and peripheral arterial disease. When is surgery warranted? Geriatrics 1982;37:85–94
4. Moore WS. Vascular reconstruction in the diabetic patient. Angiology 1978;29:741–748
5. Myers KA, King RB, Scott DF, Johnson M, Morris PG. The effect of smoking on the late patency of arterial reconstruction in the legs. Br J Surg 1978;65:267–271
6. Guidoin R, King M, Blais P, Marois M, Gosselin C, Roy P, Courbier R, David M, Noël HP. A biological and structural evaluation of retrieved Dacron arterial prostheses. In: Weinstein A, Gibbons D, Brown S, Ruff W (eds) Implant retrieval: material and biological analysis. SP 601, Washington DC, National Bureau of Standards, 1981, pp 29–129
7. Choux R, Payan MJ, Juhan-Vague I, Barrat E, Juhan C, Kadji H, Lebreuil G. Etude morphologique de différents types de greffons veineux. Essai de corrélation avec l'activité fibrinolytique pariétale. Ann Pathol 1982;2:293–300
8. Guidoin R, Roy PE, Bonnaud P, Marois M, King M, Beaudoin G, Hébert J, Gosselin C. Veines de stripping comme abord vasculaire secondaire pour l'hémodialyse: étude pathologique de greffons explantés. J Mal Vasc 1985;10:331–342
9. Hertzer NR, Beven EG. Venous access using the bovine carotid heterograft. Techniques, results and complications in 75 patients. Arch Surg 1978;113:696–700
10. Guidoin R, Gagnon Y, Roy PE, Marois M, Johnston KW, Batt M. The pathology of surgically excised human umbilical vein grafts. J Vasc Surg 1986;3:146–154

11. Maki Jr A, Hammerberg O. Clinical implications of bacterial glycocalyx. Can J Surg 1985;28:5-6
12. Cooke PA, Nobis PA, Stoney RJ. Dacron aortic graft failure. Arch Surg 1974;108:101-103
13. Reichle FA. Criteria for evaluation of new arterial prosthesis by comparing vein with Dacron femoro-popliteal bypass. Surg Gynecol Obstet 1978;146:714-720
14. Linton RR, Darling RC. Autogenous saphenous vein bypass grafts in femoro-popliteal obliterative arterial disease. Surgery 1962;51:62-73
15. Hall KV. The great saphenous vein used in situ as an arterial shunt after extirpation of the vein valves. Surgery 1962;51:492-495
16. Batson RC, Sottiurai VS. Non reversed and in situ vein grafts. Clinical and experimental observations. Ann Surg 1985;201:771-779
17. Bical O, Bachet J, Laurian C, Camilleri JP, Goudot B, Menu P, Guiomet D. Aorto-coronary bypass with homologous saphenous vein: long-term results. Ann Thorac Surg 1980;30:550-557
18. Ochsner JL, Lawson JD, Esking SJ, Mills NL, DeCamp PT. Homologous veins as an arterial substitute: long-term results. J Vasc Surg 1984;1:306-313
19. Piccone Jr NA, Sika J, Ahmed N, LeVeen HM, Discala V. Preserved saphenous vein allografts for vascular access. Surg Gynecol Obstet 1978;147:385-390
20. Bocking JK, Roach MR. The elastic properties of the human great saphenous vein in relation to primary varicose veins. Can J Phys Pharmacol 1974;52:153-157
21. Lachance S, Guidoin R, Cardou A. Contrôle de qualité des prothèses artérielles d'origine biologique: nécessité de disposer d'un banc d'essais in vitro. Rev Europ Tech Biomed 1984;6:341-345
22. Beaudoin G, Guidoin R, Gosselin C, Marois M, Roy PE, Gagnon D. Caractéristiques physiques des veines de stripping conservées à 4°C et susceptibles d'être utilisées comme substituts artériels. J Mal Vasc 1985;10:147-151
23. Axthelm SC, Quarter JM, Strickland SFL. Antigenicity of venous allografts. Ann Surg 1979;189:290-293
24. Balderman SC, Montes M, Schwartz K, Hart T, Bhayana JN, Gage AA. Preparation of venous allografts. A comparison of techniques. Ann Surg 1984;200:117-130
25. Sheiner N. Peripheral vascular surgery: alternate anatomical pathways and the use of allograft vein as arterial substitute. In: Current problems in surgery. Year Book Medical Publishers Inc, Chicago, 1978, vol 5
26. Domergue J, Bouhaddioui N, Barnéon G, Marchal G. Survie indéfinie d'allogreffes pancréatiques sous cyclosporine A chez le rat. J Chir 1984;121:195-201
27. Rosenberg DML, Glass BA, Rosenberg N, Lewis MR, Dale WA. Experience with modified bovine carotid arteries in arterial surgery. Surgery 1970;68:1064-1072
28. Rosenberg N. The bovine arterial graft and its several applications. Surg Gynecol Obstet 1976;142:104-108
29. Rausis C, Erasmi H, Gremion G, Horsch S. Vascular replacement in small-calibre arteries. Helv Chir Acta 1983;50:407-412
30. Guidoin R, Marois D, Zeltzer J, Bonnaud P, Marois M, Leblond P, Sheiner N, Gosselin C, Roy P. Complications évolutives associées à l'utilisation d'une hétérogreffe bovine comme abord vasculaire. Can J Surg 1984;27:72-77
31. Guidoin R, Domurado D, Couture J, Dubé S, Marois M, Sigot MF, Martin L, BenSlimane S. Chemically processed bovine heterografts of the second generation as arterial substitutes: a comparative evaluation of three commercial prostheses. J Cardiovasc Surg 1989;30:202-209
32. Dardik H, Ibrahim IM, Jarrah M, Sussman BC, Dardik II. Three year experience with glutaraldehyde stabilized umbilical vein for limb salvage. Br J Surg 1980;67:229-232
33. Mindich B, Silverman M, Elguezabel A, Flores L, Sheka RP, Levowitz BS. Human umbilical cord vein for vascular replacement: preliminary report and observation. Surgery 1977;81:152-160
34. Guidoin R, Noël HP, Dubé S, DeEstable-Puig RF, Marois M, King M. Long-term follow-up of the processed human umbilical cord vein as an infra-renal aortic substitute in non human primates. J Vasc Surg 1985;2:715-723
35. Esquivel CO, Bjorck CG, Bergqvist D, Bergentz SE. Heparinized human umbilical vein grafts. Delayed heparin desorption after alcohol treatment. Eur Surg Res 1983;15:289-296
36. Boontje ABH. Aneurysm formation in human umbilical vein grafts used as arterial substitutes. J Vasc Surg 1985;2:524-529

37. Edwards WS. Arterial grafts of Teflon. In: Sawyer PN, Kaplitt MJ (eds) Vascular grafts. Appleton-Century-Crofts, New York, 1978, pp 173–176
38. Harrison JH. Synthetic materials as vascular prostheses. I. Comparative study in small vessels of nylon, dacron, orlon, ivalon sponge and teflon. Am J Surg 1958;95:3–15
39. Harrison JH. Synthetic materials as vascular prostheses. II. A comparative study of nylon, dacron, orlon, ivalon sponge and teflon in large blood vessels with tensile strength studies. Am J Surg 1958;95:16–24
40. Edwards WS. Clinical experience with Teflon grafts. In: Wesolowski SA, Dennis C (eds) Fundamentals of vascular grafting. McGraw-Hill, New York, 1963
41. Boyd DP, Midell AI. Woven teflon aortic grafts. An unsatisfactory prosthesis. Vasc Surg 1971;5:148–153
42. Couture J, Guidoin R, King M, Marois M. Textile Teflon arterial prostheses: how successful are they? Can J Surg 1984;27:575–582
43. Soyer T, Lemphinen M, Cooper P, Norton L, Eiseman B. A new venous prosthesis. Surgery 1972;72:864–872
44. Matsumoto H, Hasegawa T, Fuse K, Yamamoto M, Saigusa M. A new vascular prosthesis for a small caliber artery. Surgery 1973;74:519–523
45. Campbell CD, Goldfarb D, Rodney R. A small arterial substitute: expanded microporous polytetrafluoroethylene, patency vs porosity. Ann Surg 1975;182:138–143
46. Haimov M, Giron F, Jacobson II JH. The expanded polytetrafluoroethylene graft. Three years experience with 362 grafts. Arch Surg 1979;114:673–677
47. Bergan JJ, Veith FJ, Bernard VM, Yaor JST, Flinn WR, Gupta SK, Scher LA, Samson RH, Towne JB. Randomization of autogenous vein and PTFE grafts in femoro-distal reconstruction. Surgery 1982;92:921–930
48. Weisel RD, Johnston KW, Baird RJ, Drezner AD, Oates TK, Lipton IH. Comparison of conduits for leg revascularization. Surgery 1981;89:8–15
49. Chignier E, Guidollet J, Heynen Y, Serres M, Clendinnen G, Louisot P, Eloy R. Macromolecular histological, ultrastructural and immunocytochemical characteristics of the neointima developed within PTFE vascular grafts. Experimental study in dogs. J Biomed Mater Res 1983;17:623–636
50. Formichi M, Jausseran JM, Guidoin R, Marois M, Bergeron P, Gosselin C, Corubier R. Analyse de prothèses artérielles en téflon microporeux après exérèse chirurgicale. J Mal Vasc 1986;11:248–255
51. Guidoin R, Doyon B, Blais P, Domurado D, Boyce B, Marois M, Martin L, Roy J, Gosselin C. Effects of traumatic manipulations on grafts, sutures and host arteries during vascular surgery procedures. Experiments on dogs. Res Exp Med 1981;179:1–21
52. King M, Blais P, Guidoin R, Prowse E, Marois M, Gosselin C, Noël HP. Polyethylene terephthalate (Dacron) vascular prostheses: material and fabric construction aspects. In: Williams DF (ed) Biocompatibility of clinical implants materials. CRC Press, Boca Raton, 1981, vol II, pp 177–207
53. Reichle FA, Stewart GJ, Essa N. A transmission and scanning electron microscopic study of luminal surfaces in Dacron and autogenous vein bypasses in man and dog. Surgery 1973;74:945–960
54. Wesolowski SA, Fries CC, Karlson KE, DeBakey ME, Sawyer PN. Porosity: primary determinant of ultimate fate of synthetic vascular grafts. Surgery 1961;50:91–96
55. Wesolowski SA, Fries CC, Hennigar G, Fox LM, Sawyer PN, Sauvage LR. Factors contributing to long-term failures in human vascular prosthetic grafts. J Cardiovasc Surg 1964;5:544–567
56. Wesolowski SA, Fries CC, Martinez A, McMahon JD. Arterial prosthetic materials. Ann NY Acad Sc 1968;146:325–344
57. Hussey HH. Arterial replacement: failure of synthetic prostheses. JAMA 1976;235:848
58. Noon GP, DeBakey ME. DeBakey Dacron prosthesis and filamentous velour graft. In: Sawyer PN, Kaplitt MJ (eds) Vascular grafts. Appleton-Century-Crofts, New York, 1978, pp 177–184
59. Sauvage LR, Berger K, Nakagawa Y, Wood SJ, Mansfield PB. An external velour surface for porous arterial prostheses. Surgery 1971;70:940–953
60. Turner RJ, Hoffman HL, Weinberg SL. Knitted Dacron double velour grafts. In: Stanley JC (ed) Biologic and synthetic vascular prostheses. Grune and Stratton, New York, 1982, pp 509–522

61. Knox WG. Aneurysm occuring in a femoral artery Dacron prosthesis five and one-half years after insertion. Ann Surg 1962;156:827–830

62. Koopmann MDE, Brands LC. Degenerative changes in Dacron external velour vascular prostheses. J Cardiovasc Surg 1980;21:159–162

63. Lynn RB. Knitted Dacron ultralightweight grafts: a warning. Can J Surg 1979;22:593

64. Guidoin R, King M, Hood R, Marois M, Martin L, Maini R. New polyester arterial prostheses from Great Britain: an in vitro and in vivo evaluation. Ann Biomed Eng 1986;14:351–367

65. Herring MB, Gardner A, Glover J. A single-staged technique for seeding vascular grafts with autogenous endothelium. Surgery 1978;84:498–504

66. Graham LM, Vinter DV, Ford JW, Khan RH, Burkel WE, Stanley JC. Endothelial seeding of prosthetic vascular grafts. Arch Surg 1980;115:929–933

67. Clarke JMF, Pittilo RM, Nicholson LJ, Woolf N, Marston A. Seeding Dacron arterial prostheses with peritoneal mesothelial cells: a preliminary morphological study. Br J Surg 1984;71:492–494

68. Herring MB, Gardner AL, Glover JL. Seeding of human arterial prostheses with mechanically derived endothelium: the detrimental effect of smoking. J Vasc Surg 1984;1:279–289

69. Chvapil M, Krajicek M. Use of collagen in the construction of an arterial prosthesis. Med Trends Vasc Surg 1970;1:120–140

70. Domurado D, Guidoin R, Marois M, Martin L, Gosselin C, Awad J. Albuminated Dacron prostheses as improved blood vessel substitutes. J Bioeng 1978;2:79–91

71. Moore WS, Chvapil M, Leiffert G, Keown K. Development of an infection-resistant vascular prosthesis. Arch Surg 1981;116:1403–1407

72. Grinnell F, Feld M, Minter D. Cell adhesion to fibrinogen and fibrin substrate: role of cold insoluble globulin (plasma fibronectin). Cell 1980;19:517–525

73. Sparks CH. Autogenous grafts made to order. Ann Thorac Surg 1969;8:104–113

74. Guidoin R, Thevenet A. Noël HP, Mary H, Marois M, Gosselin C, King M. Le Sparks-mandril comme prothèse artérielle. Un concept ingénieux, un échec complet. Que faut-il en retenir. J Mal Vasc 1984;9:277–283

75. Eldor A, Hoover EL, Pett Jr SB, Gay Jr WA, Alonso DR, Weksler BB. Prostacyclin production by arterialized autogenous venous grafts in dogs. Prostaglandins 1981;22:485–498

76. Guidoin R, Marois M, Martin L, Noël HP, Laroche F, Gosselin C, Côté R, Bénichoux R, Blais P. Processed human umbilical veins as arterial substitutes: evaluation in canine models. Biomaterials 1980;1:82–88

77. Guidoin R, Gosselin C, Martin L, Marois M, Laroche F, King M, Gunasekera K, Domurado D, Sigot-Luizard MF, Blais P. Polyester prostheses as substitutes in the thoracic aorta of dogs. I. Evaluation of commercial prostheses. J Biomed Mater Res 1983;17:1049–1077

78. King M, Guidoin R, Blais P, Garton A, Gunasekera K. Degradation of polyester arterial prostheses: a physical or chemical mechanism? In: Fraker AC, Griffin CD (eds) Corrosion and degradation of implant materials: second symposium. ASTM Special Technical Publication 859, 1985, pp 294–307

79. Ketharanathan V, Christie BA. Glutaraldehyde-tanned ovine collagen conduits as vascular xenografts in dogs. A preliminary report. Arch Surg 1980;114:967–969

80. Kardos JL, Mehta PS, Apostolou SF, Thies C, Clark RE. Design, fabrication and testing of prosthetic blood vessels. Biomater Med Devices Artif Organs 1974;2:387–396

81. Hiratzka LF, Gocken JA, White RA, Wright CB. In vivo comparison of replamineform silastic and bioelectric polyurethane arterial grafts. Arch Surg 1979;114:698–702

82. Annis D, Bornat A, Edwards RO, Higham A, Loveday B, Wilson J. An elastomeric vascular prosthesis. Trans Am Soc Artif Intern Organs 1978;24:209–213

83. Lyman DJ, Albo Jr D, Jackson R, Knutson K. Development of small diameter vascular prostheses. Trans Am Soc Artif Intern Organs 1977;23:253–261

84. Leidner J, Wong EWC, MacGregor DC, Wilson CJ. A novel process for the manufacturing of porous grafts: process description and product evaluation. J Biomed Mater Res 1983;17: 229–247

85. Gilding DK, Reed AM, Askill IN, Briana S. Mitrathane^R: a new polyether urethane urea for critical medical applications. Trans Am Soc Art Intern Organs 1984;30:571–576

86. Gogolewski S, Pennings AJ, Lommen E, Wildevuur CRH, Nieuwenhuis P. Growth of a neo-artery induced by a biodegradable polymeric vascular prosthesis. Makromol Chem Rapid Comm 1983;4:213–219

87. Botzko K, Snyder R, Larkin J, Edwards WS. In vivo/in vitro life testing of vascular prostheses. In: Syrett BC, Acharya A (eds) Corrosion and degradation of implant materials. ASTM STP 684, 1979, pp 76–88
88. Marceau D, Cardou A, Guidoin R, King M, Gosselin C. Développement d'un système d'essai pour l'étude du comportement dynamique des prothèses artérielles alloplastiques: le vivocycleur. Rev Europ Tech Biomed 1984;6:31–38

Chapter 5

Heart Valve Replacements: Problems and Developments

A.P. Yoganathan, H. Reul and M.M. Black

Introduction

Heart valve prostheses have been used successfully since 1960. As stated by Roberts [1] the 1960s will probably be remembered most in the annals of cardiology as the decade during which cardiac valve replacement became a successful reality. Of the more than 50 different cardiac valves introduced over the past 25 years, many have been discarded due to their lack of success, and of those remaining several modifications have been made or are being made at the time of this writing. The five most commonly used basic types of prosthetic valves at present are: caged ball, caged disc, tilting disc, bi-leaflet and bio-prostheses. At present over 75 000 prosthetic valves of different designs are used annually throughout the world. Even after 25 years of experience the problems associated with heart valve prostheses have not been totally eliminated. The most serious problems and complications associated with heart valve prostheses are: thromboembolism, tissue overgrowth, infection, tearing of sewing sutures, red cell destruction (haemolysis), valve failure due to material fatigue or chemical change, damage to the endothelial tissue lining of the vessel wall adjacent to the valve and leaks caused by failure of the valve to close properly. Thromboembolism, tissue overgrowth, red cell destruction and endothelial damage are directly related to the fluid dynamics associated with the various prosthetic heart valves and need to be addressed in more detail by investigators studying biofluid mechanics. The other problems are indirectly related to fluid mechanics. Problems relating to valve failure due to material fatigue or chemical change also need to be studied, especially in relation to bioprostheses.

Tissue bioprostheses gained widespread use during the mid-1970s. The major advantage of tissue bioprostheses compared to their mechanical counterparts is that they have a lower incidence of thromboembolic complications. There-fore, tissue valves for a large part can be used without anticoagulants. Unfortunately, the tissue bioprostheses clinically used at present also have major disadvantages such as relatively large pressure drops compared to some of the mechanical valves (especially in the smaller sizes), jet-like flow through the valve leaflets, material fatigue and/or wear of valve leaflets, and calcifi-cation of valve leaflets, especially in children and young adults. Because of these drawbacks, valve manufacturers are now developing newer designs of bioprostheses and trileaflet valves made from polymeric materials.

The ideal heart valve prosthesis has not yet been designed and probably will never exist. An ideal valve should:

1. Be fully sterile at the time of implantation and be non-toxic.
2. Be surgically convenient to insert at or near the normal location in the heart.
3. Conform to the heart structure rather than the heart structure conforming to the valve (i.e. the size and shape of the prosthesis should not interfere with cardiac function).
4. Show a minimum resistance to flow so as to prevent a significant pressure drop across the valve.
5. Have minimal reverse flow necessary for valve closure, so as to keep the incompetence of the valve at a low level.
6. Show long resistance to mechanical and structural wear.
7. Be long-lasting (25 years) and maintain its normal functional performance (i.e. must not deteriorate with time).
8. Cause minimum trauma to blood elements and the endothelial tissue of the cardiovascular structure surrounding the valve.
9. Show a low probability for thromboembolic complications without the use of anticoagulants.
10. Be sufficiently quiet so as to not disturb the patient.
11. Be radiographically visible.
12. Have an acceptable cost.

Mechanical Valves

The use of a caged-ball valve in the descending aorta became obsolete with the development of what today is still referred to as the Starr-Edwards ball-and-cage valve in 1960, as illustrated in Fig. 5.1. In concept it was similar to the original Hufnagel valve but was designed to be inserted in place of the excised diseased natural valve. This form of intracardiac valve replacement in the mitral position was reported by Starr [2] and for aortic and multiple valve replacements by Cartwright et al. [3]. Since 1962, the Starr-Edwards valve has undergone many modifications in order to improve its performance in terms of reduced haemolysis and thromboembolic complications. However, the changes have involved materials and techniques of construction and have not altered the overall concept of the valve design in any way.

Other manufacturers have produced variations of the ball and cage valve, notably the Smeloff-Cutter valve and the Magovern prosthesis. In the case of the former, the ball is slightly smaller than the orifice. A subcage on the proximal side of the valve retains the ball in the closed position with its equator in the plane of the sewing ring. A small clearance around the ball ensures easy

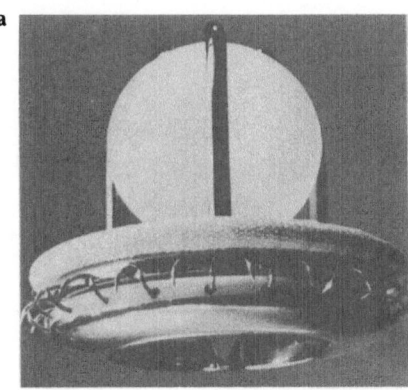 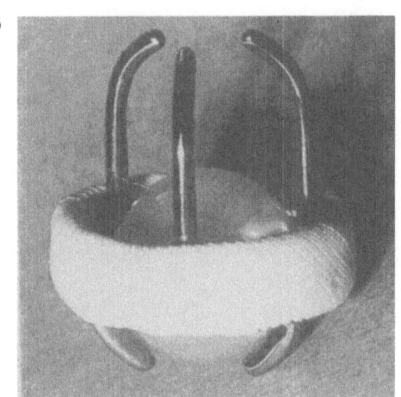

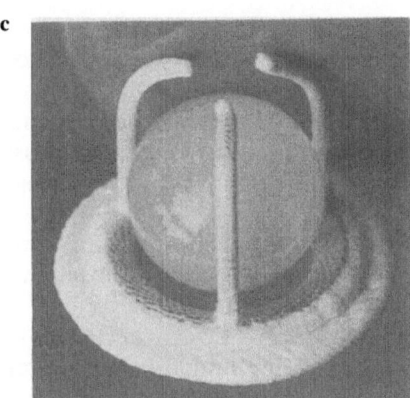 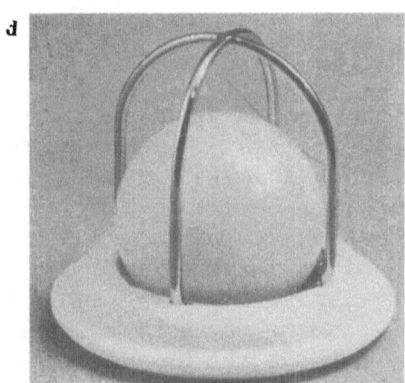

Fig. 5.1. Ball valves: **a** Starr-Edwards; **b** Smeloff-Cutter; **c** Braunwald-Cutter; **d** Magovern-Cromie.

passage of the ball into the orifice. This clearance also gives rise to a mild regurgitation which was felt, though not proven, to be beneficial in preventing thrombus formation. The Magovern valve is a standard ball-and-cage format which incorporates two rows of interlocking mechanical teeth around the orifice ring. These teeth are used for inserting the valve and are activated by removing a special valve holder once the valve has been correctly located in the prepared tissue annulus. The potential hazard from dislocation from calcific annulus due to imperfect placement was soon observed. This valve is no longer in use.

Due to the high profile design characteristics of the ball valves, especially in the mitral position, low profile caged disc valves were developed in the mid-1960s. Examples of the caged disc designs are the Kay-Shiley and Beall prostheses which were first introduced in 1965 and 1967 respectively (Fig. 5.2). These valve designs were used exclusively in the atrioventricular position.

a
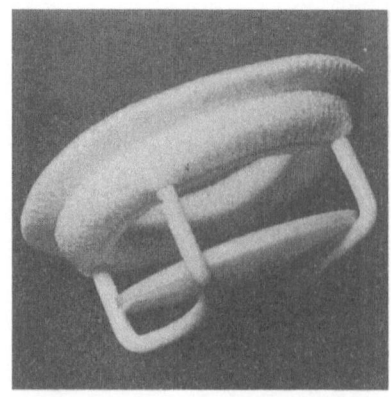

b
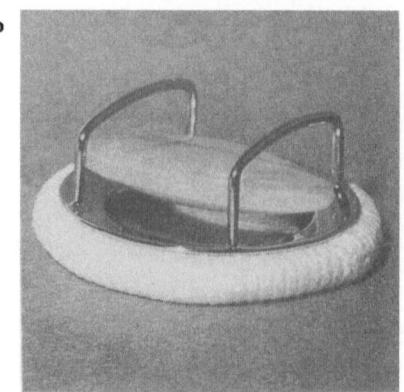

Fig. 5.2. Disc valves. **a** Beall. **b** Kay-Shiley.

However, due to their inferior haemodynamic characteristics caged disc valves are rarely used today.

Even after 25 years of valve development, the ball-and-cage format remains the valve of choice amongst some surgeons. However, it is no longer the most popular mechanical valve, having been superseded, to a large extent, by tilting-disc or hinged-leaflet valves.

This latter group of valves, some which are shown in Fig. 5.3, overcomes two major drawbacks of the ball valve, namely, large profile height and excessive occluder-induced turbulence in the flow through and distal to the valve.

The most significant developments in mechanical valve design occurred in 1969 and 1970 with the introduction of the Björk-Shiley and Lillehei-Kaster tilting-disc valves. Both prostheses involve the concept of a "free" floating disc which, in the open position, tilts to an angle depending on the design of the disc-retaining struts. In the original Björk-Shiley valve, the angle of tilt was 60° for the aortic, and 50° for the mitral model. The Lillehei-Kaster valve has a greater angle of tilt of 80°, but in the closed position is preinclined to the valve orifice plane by an angle of 18°. In both cases the closed valve configuration permits the occluder to fit into the circumference of the inflow ring with virtually no overlap, thus reducing mechanical damage to erythrocytes. A small amount of regurgitation backflow induces a "washing out" effect of "debris" and platelets and theoretically reduces the incidence of thromboemboli.

The obvious advantage of the tilting-disc valve is that in the open position it acts like an aerofoil in the blood flowing through the valve, and induced flow disturbance is substantially less than that obtained with a ball occluder. Although the original Björk-Shiley valve employed a "Delrin" occluder, all present-day tilting-disc valves use pyrolitic carbon for this component. It should also be noted that the "free" floating disc can rotate during normal function, thus preventing excessive contact wear from the retaining components on one particular part of the disc.

Tilting-disc valves remain popular although central-orifice tissue valves, as discussed below, are gaining in usage. Various improvements to this form of

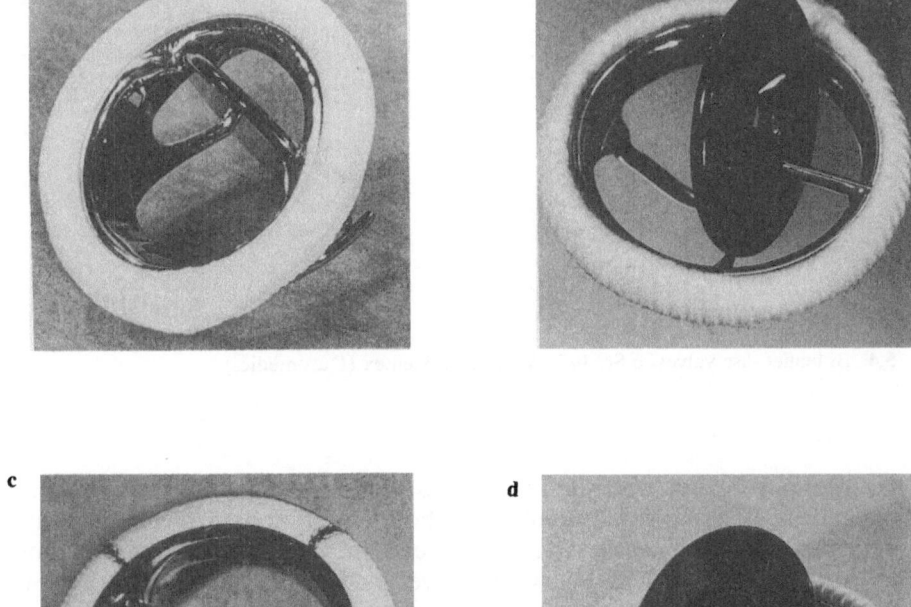

Fig. 5.3. Tilting or pivoting disc valves. **a** Björk-Shiley. **b** Medtronic-Hall. **c** Omni-Science. **d** Lillehei-Kaster.

mechanical valve have been developed but have tended to concentrate on alterations either to the disc geometry as in the Björk-Shiley concavo-convex design, or to the disc retaining system as with the Medtronic-Hall and Omni-Science valve designs.

Perhaps the most interesting development has been that of the bileaflet all-pyrolitic carbon valve produced by St. Jude Medical Inc. and introduced in 1978. This design incorporates two semicircular hinged pyrolitic carbon occluders which in the open position provide minimal disturbance to flow. The leaflets pivot within grooves made in the valve orifice hanging. In the fully open position the leaflets are designed to open to an angle of 85°. Early clinical results with this valve design are encouraging and it is very popular in the small sizes due to its superior haemodynamic characteristics. The newly introduced (1983) Hemex valve is similar in concept to the St. Jude, except that it incorporates curved leaflets (Fig. 5.4).

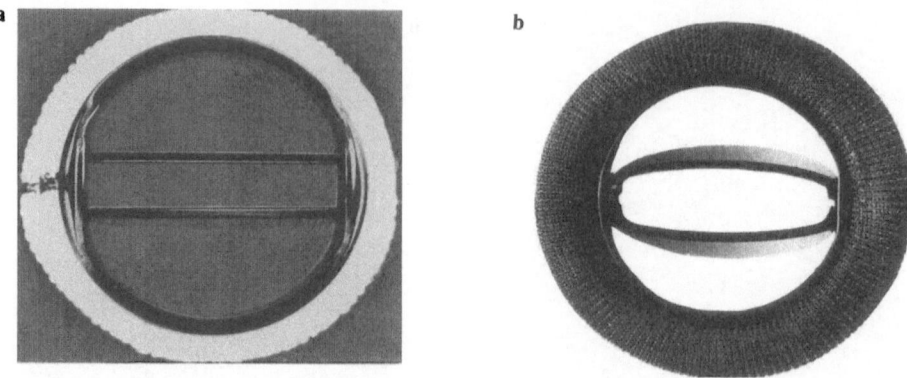

Fig. 5.4. Bi-leaflet disc valves. **a** St. Jude Medical. **b** Hemex (Duromedics).

The informed reader will realize that this section on mechanical valves has highlighted a relatively small number of the many various forms which have been made. However, those that have been included are either the most commonly used, or are those which have made notable contributions to mechanical valve design.

The majority of mechanical valves in current clinical use do offer patients reasonable hope for several years of event-free survival, even though they bear no morphological comparison to natural valves.

Tissue Valves

One major disadvantage with the use of mechanical valves is the need for continuous anticoagulation therapy to minimize the risk of thrombosis and thromboembolic complications. Furthermore, the haemodynamic function of even the best types of mechanical valves differs significantly from that of normal heart valves. An obvious step, therefore, in the development of heart valve substitutes was the application of naturally-occurring heart valves. This was the basis of the approach to the use of treated human aortic valves removed from cadavers for implantation in place of their diseased counterparts.

The first of these procedures was carried out by Ross [4] in 1962 and the overall results so far have been satisfactory [5]. This is, perhaps, not surprising since the replacement valve is optimum both from the point of view of structure and function. In the open position these valves provide unobstructed central orifice flow and also have the ability to respond to deformations induced by the surrounding anatomical structure. As a result, such substitutes are less damaging to the blood when compared with the rigid mechanical valve. The main problem with these cadaveric allografts, as far as may be ascertained, is that they are no longer living tissue and therefore lack that unique quality of cellular regeneration typical of normal living systems. This makes them more vulnerable to long-term damage.

An alternative approach is to transplant the patient's own pulmonary valve into the aortic position. This operation was also first carried out by Ross [6] in 1967, and his study of 176 patients followed up over 13 years showed that such transplants continued to be viable in their new position with no apparent degeneration [5]. This transplantation technique is, however, limited in that it can only be applied to one site.

The next stage in the development of tissue valve substitutes was the use of autologous fascia lata either as free or frame-mounted leaflets. The former approach for aortic valve replacement was reported by Senning [7] in 1966, and details of a frame-mounted technique were published by Ionescu and Ross in 1966 [8]. The approach combined the more natural leaflet format with a readily available living autologous tissue. Although early results seemed encouraging, Senning [9] expressed his own doubt on the value of this approach in 1971, and by 1978 fascia lata was no longer used in either of the above, or any other, form of valve replacement. The failure of this technique was due to the inadequate strength of this tissue when subjected to long-term cyclic stressing in the heart. This situation might have been avoided if adequate analysis of the mechanical behaviour of fascia lata had been undertaken.

In parallel with the work on fascia lata valves, alternative forms of tissue leaflet valves were being developed. In these designs, however, more emphasis was placed on optimum performance characteristics than on the use of living tissue. In all cases the configuration involved a three-leaflet format which was maintained by the use of a suitably designed mounting frame. It was realized that naturally-occurring animal tissues, if used in an untreated form, would be rejected by the host. Consequently, a method of chemical treatment had to be found which obviated this antigenic response but did not degrade the mechanical strength of the tissue.

Formaldehyde has been used by histologists for many years to arrest autolysis and "fix" tissue in the state in which it is removed. It had been used to preserve biological tissues in cardiac surgery but, unfortunately, was found to produce shrinkage and also increase the "stiffness" of the resulting material. For these reasons, formaldehyde was not considered ideal as a method of tissue treatment.

Glutaraldehyde is another histological fixative which has been used especially for preserving fine detail for electron microscopy. It is also used as a tanning agent by the leather industry. In addition to arresting autolysis, glutaraldehyde produces a more flexible material than does formaldehyde, with improved strength characteristics due to increased collagen crosslinking. Glutaraldehyde has the additional ability of reducing the antigenicity of xenograft tissue to a level at which it can be implanted into the heart without significant immunological reaction.

In 1969, Kaiser et al. [10] described a valve substitute using an explanted glutaraldehyde-treated porcine aortic valve which was mounted on to a rigid support frame. Following a modification described by Reis et al. [11], in which the rigid frame was replaced by a frame having a rigid base ring with flexible posts, this valve became commercially available as the Hancock Porcine

Xenograft in 1970. It remains one of the two most popular valve substitutes of this type, the other being the Carpentier-Edwards Bioprosthesis introduced commercially by Edwards Laboratories in 1976. This latter valve uses a totally flexible support frame.

In this type of prosthesis, the use of the intact biologically formed valve obviates the need to manufacture individual valve cusps. Whilst this has the obvious advantage of reduced complexity of construction, it does require a facility for harvesting an adequate quantity of valves so that an appropriate range of valve sizes of suitable quality can be made available. This latter problem did not occur in the production of the three-leaflet calf pericardium valve developed by Ionescu et al. The construction of this valve involves the moulding of fresh tissue to a tricuspid configuration around a support frame and, whilst held in this position, the tissue is treated with glutaraldehyde solution. The valve, marketed in 1976 as the Ionescu-Shiley Pericardial Xenograft, is currently the most popular valve of its type. Examples of mounted porcine valves and bovine pericardium valves are shown in Fig. 5.5. Clinical results so far obtained with tissue valves indicate their superiority to mechanical valves with respect to a lower incidence of thromboembolic complications. For these reasons the use of tissue valves increased significantly during the mid and late 1970s.

It is interesting to note that, as is the case with mechanical valves, all the popular tissue prostheses are manufactured in the United States of America and, until recently, there was no competition from other countries in this field. However, the first commercially-available British tissue valve, the Wessex Porcine Bioprosthesis manufactured by Wessex Medical Laboratories Limited, has recently begun a series of clinical trials having successfully completed both laboratory evaluation and animal trials. Other examples are the Swiss-made Xenomedica and the Canadian Bioimplant valves.

Despite the generally satisfactory haemodynamic performance of tissue valves, recent reports on clinical experience with these valves increasingly indicate time-dependent structural changes such as calcification and leaflet wear, leading to valve failure and subsequent replacement [13–16]. The problem of valve leaflet calcification is more prevalent in children and young adults. Therefore, tissue valves are rarely used in children and young adults at the present time. Such problems have not been eliminated by the glutaraldehyde tanning methods so far employed, and it is not easy to see how these drawbacks are to be overcome, unless either living autologous tissue is used or the original structure of the collagen and elastin are chemically enhanced. On the latter point there is, as yet, much room for further work. For instance, the fixing of calf pericardium under tension during the moulding of the valve cusps will inevitably produce "locked-in" stresses during fixation, thus changing the mechanical properties of the tissue [17]. A valve configuration which does not involve fixation moulding of the cusps would be advantageous.

The design of a new pericardium valve, presently being developed by Black et al. [18] in Sheffield, allows the valve cusps to be formed using fully fixed, unstressed pericardium. Furthermore, this valve is specifically designed for the mitral position and is consequently of a bicuspid form. The design also incorporates a differentially flexible frame. This allows the base ring to deform from

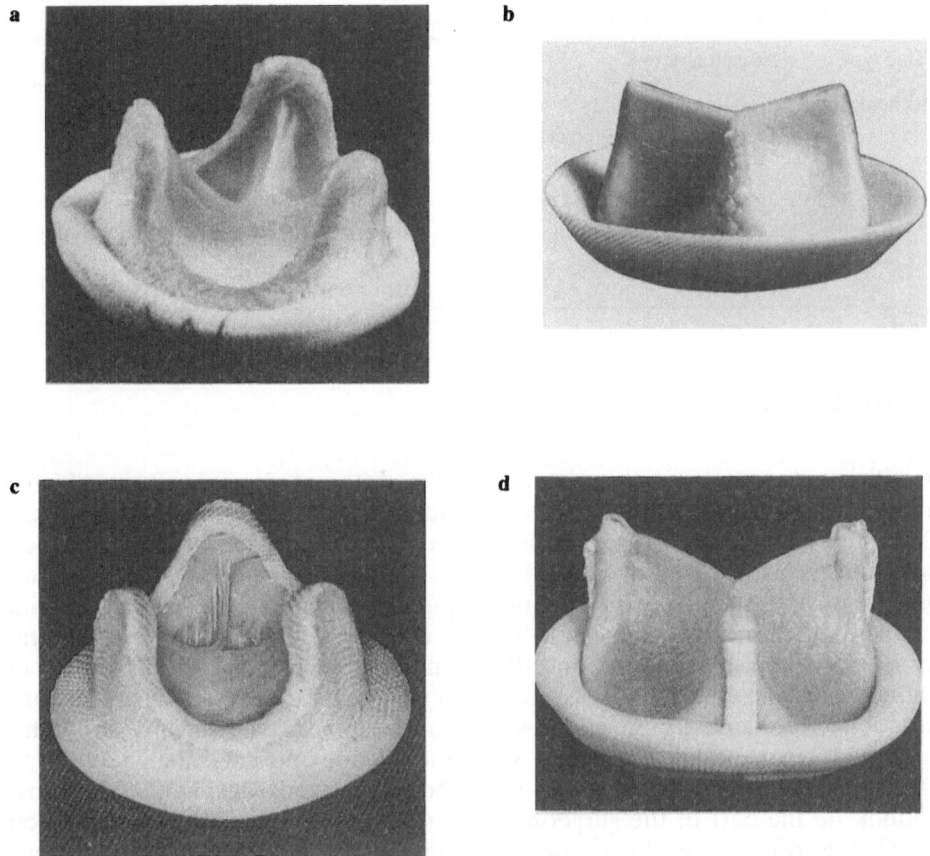

Fig. 5.5. Bioprostheses. **a** Ionescu-Shiley pericardial. **b** Mitroflow pericardial. **c** Hancock porcine. **d** Wessex porcine.

circular in diastole to an approximate D-shape in systole, thus reproducing the physiological behaviour of the normal mitral valve annulus during the cardiac cycle.

There are also attempts to develop leaflet valves from man-made materials such as block-copolymers or modified polyurethanes [19,20]. The major advantages of such a valve type would be better reproducibility and cost. The currently tested valve exhibits sufficient fatigue life of more than 400 million cycles and good haemodynamics but, on the other hand, also shows severe leaflet calcification after implantation times of more than 100 days in calves. It is expected that these problems will be reduced by further modifications of the material and/or by using new materials.

Table 5.1. Advantages and disadvantages of mechanical and tissue valves

Valve type	Advantages	Disadvantages
Mechanical	Long-term durability	Unnatural form
	Consistency of manufacture	Patient usually requires long-term anticoagulant therapy
Tissue	More natural form and function	Unproven long-term durability
	Less need for long-term anticoagulant therapy	Consistency of manufacture is more difficult
		In vivo calcification

Conclusions

It will be obvious from the above that the different designs of heart valve substitutes currently available have individual advantages and disadvantages. Certainly, none of the present prostheses could be regarded as ideal, or even optimum, replacements for natural valves. To identify in detail the good and bad points of each valve would require a publication in its own right and would not add significantly to the value of this chapter. However, in very general terms, valve type advantages and disadvantages can be classified as shown in Table 5.1. From this table it is clear that surgeons are faced with a difficult situation when deciding on the most appropriate valve type for any particular patient. In many cases a surgeon will tend to use one particular valve type almost to the total exclusion of any other. This does not imply a narrow outlook on the part of the surgeon, but rather a natural scepticism in relation to what is often clinically unsubstantiated information provided by various manufacturers regarding new valve products.

For the present, the surgeon has to make his own assessment of the potential advantages and disadvantages of any particular design. Whilst the apparent long-term durability of mechanical valves is immediately attractive, problems of maintaining large and increasing numbers of patients on optimum anti-coagulation therapy can lead to logistic difficulties. Incidence of significant levels of haemolysis due to mechanical damage can also militate against their extensive use by many surgeons.

References

1. Roberts WC. Am J Cardiol 1976;38:633
2. Starr A. Surg Forum 1960;11:258–260
3. Cartwright RS, Palick WE, Ford WB, Giacobine JW, Zubritsky SA, Ratan RS. JAMA 1962;180:6–12
4. Ross DN. Lancet 1962;ii:487
5. Wain EH, Greco R, Ignegeri A, Bodnar E, Ross DN. Int J Artif Organs 1980;3:169–172
6. Ross DN. Lancet 1967;ii:956
7. Senning A. Acta Chir Scand [Suppl] 1966;356B:17–20

8. Ionescu MI, Ross DN. Lancet 1969;ii:335–338
9. Senning A. Thoraxchirurgie, 1971;19:304–308
10. Kaiser GA, Hancock WD, Lukban SB, Litwak RS. Surg Forum 1969;20:137–138
11. Reis RL, Hancock WD, Yarborough JW, Glancy DL, Morrow AG. J Thorac Cardiovasc Surg 1971;62:683–689
12. Ionescu MI, Mary DAS, Abid A. In: Stalpaert G et al. (eds) Late results of valvular replacements and coronary surgery. European Press, Ghent, p 56
13. Ferrans VJ, Spray TL, Billingham ME, Roberts WC. Am J Cardiol 1978;41:1159
14. Ferrans VJ, Boyce SW, Billingham ME, Jones M, Ishihara R, Roberts WC. Am J Cardiol 1980;46:721
15. Oyer PE, Stinson EB, Reitz BA, Miller DC, Rossiter SJ, Shumway NE. J Thorac Cardiovasc Surg 1979;78:343
16. Yoganathan AP. Prosthetic heart valves: a study of in vitro performance. Phase I final report, FDA Contract no. 223-81-5000, April 1982 (NTI S no. PB 83-134478)
17. Reece IJ, Van Noort R, Martin TRP, Black MM. Ann Thorac Surg 1982;33:480–485
18. Black MM, Drury PJ, Tindale WB. Proceedings of the European Society for Artificial Organs 1982;9:116–119
19. Ghista DN, Reul H. J Biomech 1977;10(56):313
20. Reul H. In: Planck H et al. (eds) Polyurethanes in biomedical engineering. Elsevier Science Publishers, Amsterdam, 1984, pp 257–277

Chapter 6

Cardiac Assist Devices

D.F. Gibbons

Introduction

The ultimate objective of any program developing a ventricle pump is to join two artificial ventricles together to form a total artificial heart. However, an initial objective has been to develop an assist pump, or ventricular assist device, for weaning a patient whose heart will not spontaneously beat after open heart surgery, by artificially assuming some fraction of the right and/or left ventricle pumping load until the heart can overcome the trauma and assume the total load [1,2].

Effectively, the problem resolves itself into two separable but related tasks, the development of a fatigue-resistant pumping diaphragm and one which does not induce thrombus formation. The former is controlled by the development of a material, specifically an elastomer, together with a mechanical design which minimizes the elastic strain of the diaphragm during pumping; the second is controlled by another material parameter, thrombus resistance, coupled with mechanical design which optimizes the development of non-turbulent fluid dynamics during the pumping cycle. Another factor, which affects the choice of material for the outside housing of the ventricles, is whether the ventricle is extrathoracic as compared with para- or intrathoracic. When designed for use in the latter two positions the housing material must also be tolerated by the biological system. Most of the physiological factors which are important to the operation of the pump, such as pumping rate and synchronous or non-synchronous pumping mode, introduce no significant material restrictions. Table 6.1 gives some typical physiological specifications for an artificial ventricle.

Figure 6.1 schematically illustrates the components from which a single pumping chamber (ventricle) is constructed. The blood enters the pumping chamber (diastole) through the inflow conduit C_i, and inflow valve V_i as the diaphragm moves from position D_s to position D_d. The diaphragm then expels the blood (systole) through the outflow valve V_o and conduit C_o as the diaphragm moves back to position D_s.

The housing, H, provides the rigid structure needed to hold the valves, support the diaphragm, and through which a connector penetrates which carries the leads necessary for the activation of the diaphragm, either pneumatically or electrically, and a connection to the compliance chamber,

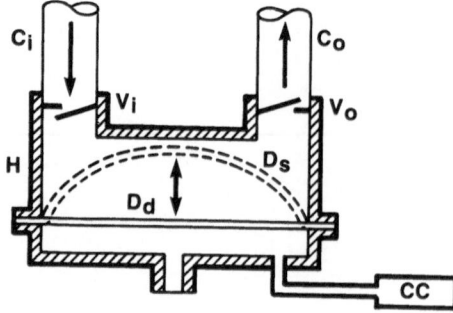

Fig. 6.1. Schematic illustration of the components from which a single pumping chamber (ventricle) is constructed. For explanation of abbreviations see text.

CC, which is necessary when the ventricle is para- or intrathoracic and not vented.

The requirement for the material from which each of these components is made is to allow that component to perform its function without compromise to the host tissue, that is blood or connective tissue, over the designed lifetime of the ventricle, e.g. 2 weeks, 2 years or longer. Before discussing the different materials which may be used to fabricate each component, the basic ventricle designs which are currently being used clinically or in clinical trials, will be briefly described. Conceptually, the "axio-symmetric" design (Fig. 6.2a) is the simplest and, as its name suggests, is a cylindrical chamber with a valve at each end [3]. A cylindrical elastomer bladder (ventricle) is placed inside the housing between the inlet and outflow valves. Pneumatic constriction of this bladder pushes blood out through the outflow valve (systole) and relaxation of the bladder allows blood to enter through the inlet valve (diastole). The major disadvantage of this design is that it is not anatomical, i.e. the inflow and outflow valves are at opposite ends of the pumping chamber, whereas they are at the same end in the natural ventricle. This non-anatomic geometry can be tolerated in an acute (weaning) ventricular assist device, but is not acceptable for consideration as half of a total artificial heart.

Figure 6.2b shows schematically the hemispherical diaphragm or bladder pump [4]. A pressure increase behind the diaphragm causes a movement of the diaphragm from the base and initiates systole, which expels blood through the outflow valve. Returning the pressure to atmospheric or providing a slight vacuum initiates diastole and causes the diaphragm to return and blood to enter through the inflow valve. A variation of this design which eliminates the seam between the housing and diaphragm has been developed [5]. This is achieved by using a sac (bladder) as the ventricle which is attached to the housing at the

Table 6.1. Typical physiological specifications for an artificial ventricle

Pumping rate 80–120 beats per minute
Stroke volume 60–100 ml
Pumping capacity, up to 10–12 l/min
Optional R wave, synchronization
Ability to decrease pumping capacity to ~5 l/min

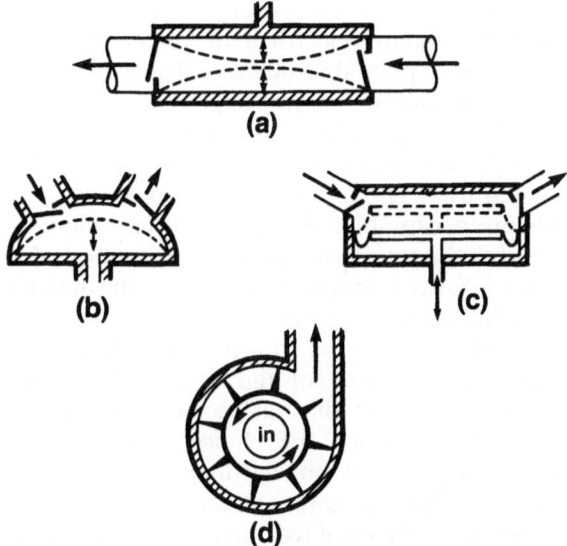

Fig. 6.2a–d. The basic ventricle designs currently being used clinically or in clinical trials. **a** The "axio-symmetric" design. **b** The hemispherical diaphragm or bladder pump. **c** The pusher plate design. **d** A turbine.

inflow and outflow valves, positions at which seams already exist. This is important in that elimination of the seam removes an additional site at which blood stasis, and thus thrombus, may be initiated. Application of a pneumatic pressure between the housing and the sac causes the sac to collapse, thus expelling blood through the outflow valve in a manner similar to the diaphragm design.

Figure 6.2c schematically illustrates the pusher plate design [6], in which motion of the plate, either by pneumatic pressure or a mechanical linkage, initiates the systolic and diastolic phases of pumping. Sealing the blood chamber is accomplished by an elastomeric rolling seal at the circumference which is bonded to the pusher plate and clamped at the housing junction.

Figure 6.2d schematically illustrates an entirely different pump concept, namely a turbine [7]. Rotation of the rotor causes blood to be drawn in through the inlet conduit and expelled through the outlet conduit; no valves are required. This is a non-pulsatile pump, although a pressure wave simulating the pulsatile nature of the other pumps may be superposed by rhythmically varying the speed of the rotor.

Housing

As already stated, the purpose of the housing is to provide a rigid structure in which to locate the valves and pumping chamber-ventricle, and on which to attach the inflow and outflow conduits. If self-powered, the housing will support the power source (electrical motor). The housing must provide connectors for the driving system (electrical or pneumatic leads) as well as a compliance chamber for implantable devices. Table 6.2 lists materials which have been used for fabrication of the housing.

All of the materials are well tolerated by tissue. The metal alloys have the disadvantage of weight and radio-opacity (X-rays are useful in determining valve status) but when used acutely to wean patients after open heart surgery, all of the materials are acceptable. However, for chronic applications, including paired ventricles for the total artificial heart, reduction of the mass together with the advantage of X-ray transparency favours the polymers. Each of the polymers has acceptable tissue tolerance.

In the design of ventricle such as shown in Fig. 6.2b (except the bladder design) or 6.2c, the inner surface of the housing forms part of the blood contacting surface. Treatment of this surface in order to make it acceptably non-thromobogenic may influence the choice of material for the housing. Porous metal surfaces prepared by powder metallurgical techniques have been shown to develop a stable, thin, adherent thrombus covering (pseudoneointima) in animal investigation [8]. Chemical treatment of the metal surface will allow a polyurethane, such as Biomer, to be cast on the surface [9], thus making the surface acceptable for short-term (weaning) applications. In the future, devices for chronic application may use chemical treatments utilizing radiation or chemically-induced free radical polymerization [10] to produce acceptable non-thrombogenic surfaces; such considerations will play an important role in determining the material of choice for the housing.

Diaphragm

The choice of an acceptable biomedical material represents one of the more difficult issues in the development of an artificial ventricle. The material must be first and foremost an elastomer, in order that it may reproducibly be moved back and forth during the pump cycle. Second, the elastomer must not exhibit fatigue failure over the designated lifetime for the device. Third, the material surface must have an acceptably low propensity for thrombus initiation. Finally, the elastomer must be capable of being formed into the shape dictated by the

Table 6.2. Ventricle housing materials

Epoxy Resin (Hysol)[a]
Epoxy (Hysol)/fibreglass composite
316 LVM stainless steel
Titanium or titanium 6Al-4V alloy
Polysulphone[b] (machined or moulded)
Polycarbonate[c] (machined or moulded)

---

[a] Hysol Division, Dexter Corp., Olean, New York.
[b] Union Carbide, e.g. P-1700, Union Carbide, Danbury, CT.
[c] For example, Lexan 144, General Electric, Pittsfield, MA.

pump design in such a way that its mechanical and surface properties meet the design specifications and at the same time do not introduce any processing contaminants.

The criteria of fatigue resistance represents one which is particularly restricting because an average heart rate of 70 beats per minute amounts to approximately 40 million beats (cycles) per year. A fatigue life of 10^7 cycles is normally considered to represent the ultimate in design criteria! Everything must be done in the design to reduce the maximum strain to which the diaphragm is subjected since fatigue life is controlled by maximum strain per cycle as well as the individual material characteristics. There is no absolute method available to evaluate the fatigue life of elastomers. Most commercial applications use data from various types of reversed bending cycle instruments [11] and many different methods have been used in polymer research, especially to accelerate the test in order to obtain hopefully useful data within a reasonable time period [12]. Table 6.3 lists diaphragm materials. There is no question, however, that the development of elastomeric materials with improved fatigue resistance will play a significant part in realizing the objective of a long-lived artificial ventricle.

Design of the ventricle also plays an important factor in defining the "degree" to which the material from which the diaphragm is made should be able to eliminate or retard the induction of thrombus. A critical factor is the residence time of blood at the diaphragm surface, the ideal being that all blood which enters during diastole shall be expelled at the next systolic episode. Unsteady state flow conditions meet this ideal most closely if the blood "front" were analogous to "plug" flow, i.e. each blood element having the same

Table 6.3. Diaphragm materials

Silicone-polyurethane elastomers
Cardiothane[a]

Polyurethane elastomers
Biomer[b] (urea-urethane) MDI-PTMG
Hemothane[c] (urea-urethane) MDI-PTMG
Mitrathane[d] (urea-urethane) MDI-PTMG
TLC-15 series[e] (urea-urethane) MDI-PTMG with additives
Pellethane[f] 2363-80A (urethane) MDI-PTMG
Tecoflex[g] hylene W-PTMG

Polyolefin elastomers
Hexsyn[h] (polyhexene)
Bion[i] (polyhexene)

[a] Kontron Instruments, Everett, MA.
[b] Ethicon Corp., Sommerville, NJ.
[c] 3M Corp., St. Paul, MN.
[d] Mitral Medical Ltd., Wheat Ridge, CO.
[e] Thoratec, Berkeley, CA.
[f] Dow Chemical Co., Midland, MI.
[g] Thermedics Inc., Woburn, MA.
[h] Goodyear Tire and Rubber Co., Akron, OH.
[i] Lord Corp., Erie, PA.

velocity. This flow mode, however, maximizes blood/interface shear stresses, which lead to haemolysis, etc. (the centrifugal turbine pump approximates such a flow pattern). The other extreme flow pattern would be streamlined (lamellar) flow which minimizes interface shear stresses and therefore haemolysis, but increases residence time since each blood volume element has, in principle, a different velocity through the device. As the regions of turbulence have been removed and residence times much greater than a cycle have been eliminated, thrombus formation and subsequent embolization have been decreased. An early philosophy was to coat the surface of the diaphragm with fibrils [13], similar to the velour concept in vascular grafts, in order to stabilize and anchor any thrombus which formed. Fibril-coated surfaces, however, have been demonstrated to be inferior to smooth surfaces on many counts [14] and smooth surfaces are now uniformly used by the main design groups.

Under the flow and surface shear conditions present in a pump no thrombus should be developed. It is not possible to predict such conditions from in vitro assays. Long-term behaviour will in all probability be dictated by very slow surface chemistry changes produced by hydrolysis and/or enzyme-related degradation [15]. Platelet and/or leukocyte attachment at the blood-contacting surface may influence subsequent thrombus growth but also provides a nidus for local calcification to occur [16]. Of more serious concern, however, is influence of the calcium mineral (either phosphate or apatite) on the mechanical properties of the diaphragm. In the presence of the flexing diaphragm the mineral may abrade the diaphragm surface [17] and so initiate a fatigue crack which would eventually cause failure and rupture of the pump diaphragm.

Valves

A wide variety of valve types, most of which are regularly used in clinical practice, are used as the inflow and outflow valves for artificial ventricles. Table 6.4 lists a number of the valves used in the various pump designs which have been developed. In most cases choice of valve is dictated by ventricle

Table 6.4. Valves used in the artificial ventricle

Type	Materials
Björk-Shiley (hinged)	Pyrolytic carbon, Delrin 150; 316 LVM alloy base ring/pivot
Medtronic (hinged)	Delrin 150; Ti6-4 alloy Base ring/pivot
Tissue valves (tricuspid)	Glutaraldehyde treated; porcine[a] Dura mater – hand fabricated[b]

[a] Hancock Laboratories, Anaheim, CA.
[b] Cleveland Clinic Foundation, Div. Artificial Organs, Cleveland, OH.

design. The occluder seat diameter, pressure drop and dynamic opening/ closing time all affect the ventricle flow and emptying characteristics.

The synthetic materials from which the valves are constructed are principally pyrolytic carbon [18] or delrin occluders and the natural tissue valves. The cage, hinge and seat are usually fabricated from 316 LVM stainless steel, Ti or Ti-6Al-4V alloy or cobalt case alloys (all alloys with extensive histories of clinical use in orthopaedics) [19]. Under the conditions used, namely high flow rate, all of the materials are reasonably non-thrombogenic. The major problems are in minimizing gaps between the valve seat and the bladder and conduit. Very small "cracks" at these interfaces have been demonstrated to initiate thrombus formation, presumably due to a small volume of stagnant flow. In order to overcome this problem the tendency is to use valves where the ring extends past the occluder and pivot in both directions, so that these surfaces can be machined flat and parallel; in valves used for clinical valvular replacement, i.e. where a sewing ring is used, these surfaces are highly polished but not necessarily flat.

The second most important factor is wear resistance in the hinge or restraining strut region. Wear in these regions is usually the cause of valve malfunction. It should be appreciated that wear is influenced by both design and the materials at the "bearing" surfaces. In caged valves any rubbing between the cage struts and occluder will lead to wear. The early valve occluders were fabricated from polymers and wear was a problem particularly with polytetrafluoroethylene (PTFE, i.e. Teflon) [20]. For hinged valves, e.g. Lilliehei/ Kastner, Björk-Shiley and St. Jude, the wear is associated with the hingebearing surfaces. Failure of polymeric occluders as a result of "grooving" where they impacted against the struts was a major factor leading to the development of the pyrolytic carbon components. The pyrolytic carbon occluders, hinge and struts are particularly wear resistant. The formulation containing approximately 10% silicon in the form of silicon carbide in the pyrolytic carbon is responsible for the superior wear resistance. The only major cause of failure is mistreatment during assembly of the valve itself or insertion of the valve in the housing: ceramic materials (pyrolytic carbon) are inherently brittle and cracks or high stress concentrations may lead to a delayed fracture failure mode. Because the output characterisitics of any ventricle are under external control, it is also possible to "over drive" the pump and cause excessive impact stress between occluder and seat or hinge at the extremes of opening and closing, which may cause impact failure in pyrolytic carbon (ceramic) occluders and hinge assemblies [21]. This is rare, however, and is a consequence of the valve being retained in a rigid housing, as opposed to soft tissue surrounding the sewing ring in clinical valve prosthesis replacements. Nevertheless, the trend is to use polymeric materials for the occluder.

Natural tissue valves will essentially deteriorate, usually as the result of calcification [22]. However, this will only be a problem for truly long-term chronic usage in total artificial heart applications, similar to those seen in prosthetic valve applications.

Conduits

The conduits which join the pump to the arterial system (left atria to ascending aorta) are usually fabricated from standard polyethylene terepthalate (PET, i.e. Dacron) vascular graft material [23]. The graft used is usually a low porosity, tightly woven, crimped PET prosthesis (not a velour). The graft is usually moulded into a thermoplastic polyurethane to ensure precise fitting and streamline flow conditions at the outflow and inflow connectors. It is essential that no or minimal blood turbulence and/or stasis occur in this connector. In many cases the moulded connector region and PET graft are then uniformly coated with a segmented polyurethane, such as Biomer or Hemothane [24]. If in the surgical procedure and pump placement, the conduit routing requires bends which may cause kinking and collapse of the graft, the graft is usually reinforced on the outside by a helical stainless steel or polymeric coil. When it is anticipated that pumps are to be used for longer term support than weaning there is need to ensure as best possible that no thrombus is developed in the support circuit. To this end active non-thrombogenic treatments of the blood contacting surfaces are being actively explored. The process which has been most thoroughly evaluated both experimentally and clinically is the end attachment of low molecular weight heparin [25] which has demonstrated improvement in performance.

Compliance Chamber

If the ventricular assist device is totally implanted, it is necessary to compensate for the volume of gas which is moved out of and back into the space between the back of the diaphragm and the housing at diastole and systole respectively. This is not a problem when the pump is extrathoracic, but is a problem if the pump is intra- or parathoracic and not vented. The problem is solved by connecting the space behind the diaphragm to a compliant space (chamber) which is also implanted either intrathoracically or subcutaneously. The requirements for such a chamber are that:

1. Its walls shall remain compliant so that impedance to diaphragm motion is not materially altered with time.
2. The mechanical interaction between the chamber walls and the surrounding tissue shall remain consistent, or approximately so.
3. The chamber shall be impermeable to fluids or gases which may condense in the chamber when the dew point reaches 37 °C.
4. The external surface of the compliance chamber shall not cause an inflammatory response, i.e. is "biocompatible".

At the present time, only a few experiments to provide a totally implantable system without an air vent have been carried out. A typical system consists of a flat "hot water bottle" shape a chamber fabricated from an elastomer and covered with a PET velour to allow tissue adhesion [26]. The fibrous tissue

Table 6.5. Permeability of elastomeric polymers to moisture

	Transmission rate (average) (g/cm/day)[a]
Biomer	0.020
Tecoflex	0.022
Silicone rubber	0.021
Butyl rubber (isobutylene-isoprene)	Not detectable

[a] Using ASTM D-814 procedure; data from [27].

anchoring the outside of the chamber does not tend to lower the compliance when situated in the thoracic space of a calf for up to 6 months. However, earlier experiments with similar configurations placed subcutaneously did cause extensive fibroplasia which caused a considerable decrease in chamber compliance [27]. The PET velour can be considered an inert stable material for this application.

A major problem with a non-vented system is that of the water permeability of the elastomeric component. Most current elastomers used in ventricular assist devices are permeable to water (Table 6.5); however, the butyl rubbers have a considerably lower permeability for water. At the time of writing, laminates of butyl rubber with a polyurethane such as Biomer are capable of considerably reducing the moisture condensation problem [28].

References

1. Gaines WE, et al, Studies Leading to an Artificial Heart for Clinical Application, Contemp Surg 1986;24(5):41
2. Pierce WS, Circulation, Artificial Hearts and Blood Pumps in the Treatment of Profound Heart Failure 1983;68:883
3. Bernhard WF, LaFarge CG, Robinson TC, et al, An Improved Blood–Pump Interface for Left-Ventricular Bypass, Ann. Surg. 1968;168:750
4. Nose Y, Topaz S, Sen Gupta A, et al, Artificial Hearts Inside the Pericardial Sac in Calves, Trans. Am. Soc. Artif Intern Organs 1965;11:225
5. Pierce WS, Meyers JL, Donachy JG, et al, "Approaches to the Artifical Heart", Surgery 1981;90:137
6. Harasaki H, Kambic H, Whalen R, et al, "Comparative Study of Flocked vs. Biolized Surface for Long-Term Assist Pumps", Trans. Am. Soc. Artif Intern Organs 1980;26:470
7. Golding LR in "Assisted Circulation" 3rd Ed., Edited Unger F, Academic Press, N.Y. (1984).
8. MacGregor DC, Pilliar MR, Wilson GJ, et al, "Porous Metal Surfaces: A Radical New Concept in Prosthetic Heart Valve Design". Trans, Am. Soc. Artif Intern Organs 1976;22:646
9. Blubaugh A, et al, e.g., Progress Report, NIH Contract NO1-HV.02911–2, May, 1981, Div. Art. Organs, Cleveland Clinic.
10. "Hydrogels for Medical and Related Applications", Edited Andrade JD, ACS Symposium Series 31, American Chemical Society, Wash. D.C., 1978, p. 1.
11. ASTM Annual Book of Standards. Philadelphia, PA., USA. Vol. 901. D813–87, "Standard Test Method for Rubber Deterioration - Crack Growth" and D1052–85, "Standard Method for Measuring Rubber Deterioration - Cut Growith Using Ross Flexing Apparatus".

12. "Biocompatible Polymers, Metals and Composites", Ed. Szycher M, Society of Plastics Engineering, Inc., 1983, Chap. 21.
13. LaFarge CG, et al, "Hemodynamic Studies During Prolonged Mechanical Circulatory Support", Trans. Am. Soc. Artif Intern Organs 1972;18:186
14. Olsen OB, et al, "The Haemocompatibility of Fibril-Coated and Smooth Elastic Materials Compared with Polyurethanes in Total Heart Replacement". Chap. 58, "Evaluation of Materials", Edited Winter GD, et al, J Wiley and Sons, NY. 1980.
15. "Polyurethanes in Biomedical Engineering", Progress in Biomedical Engineering, 1, Ed. Planck H, Egbers E. and Syre I, Elsevier, Amsterdam, 1984, p. 93.
16. Murray JD, "Dystrophic Calcification in Blood Pumps", M.S. Thesis, Case Western Reserve University, 1982.
17. Whalen RL, Snow JL. Harasaki H and Nose Y, "Mechanical Strain and Calcification in Blood Pumps", Trans. Am. Soc. Artif Intern Organs 1980;26:487
18. Bokros JC, LaGrange LD and Schoen FJ, "Chemistry and Physics of Carbon", Ed. Walker P, Marcel Dekker, N.Y. 1972;9:103
19. "Biocompatibility of Orthopedic Implants", Vol. 1, CRC Press, Ine., Boca Raton, Florida (1982).
20. Clark RE, Pavloric TA, Knight BE, et al, "Quantification of Wear, Hernolysis and Coagulation Deficits in Patients with Beall Mitral Valves", Circulation 1977;56:139
21. Joyce LD, et al, "Response of the Human Body to the First Permanent Implant of the Jarvik-7 Total Artificial Heart", Trans. Am. Soc., Artif Intern Organs 1983;29:81
22. Levy RJ, et al, "Vitamin K-dependent Calcium Binding Proteins in Aortic Valve Calcification", J. Clin, Invest 1980;65:563
23. Snyder RW and Botzko KM, "Woven, Knitted, and Extermally Supported Dacron Vascular Prostheses", Chapter 28, "Biologic and Synthetic Vasculat Prostheses", Ed. Stanley JC, et al. Grune and Stratton, N.Y., 1982.
24. Murabayashi S, et al, "A Flexible, Noncollapsible and Impermeable Inflow Graft for Long-Term Implantable Left Ventricular Assist System (LVAS)", Trans. Am. Soc. Artif Intern Organs 1984;30:526
25. Pasche B, et al. Thrombin inhibition on surfaces with covalently bonded heparin. Thromb Res 1986;44:739
26. Snyder A, Rosenberg G, Weiss W, et al, "Chronic Animal studies in a Motor-Driven LVAD and an Implanted Compliance Chamber", Trans. Art. Soc. Artif Intern Organs 1984;30:92
27. Sato N, et al, "Compliance Chamber - System Integration Studies", Trans. Art. Soc. Artif Intern Organs 30:545
28. McGec MG, et al, "Use of a Composite Biomer/Butyl Rubber/Biomer Material to Prevent Transdiaphragmatic Water Permeation During Long-Term, Electrically Actuated Left Ventricular Assist Device (LVAD) Pumping", Trans. Am. Soc. Artif Intern Organs 1980; 26:299

Subject Index